INNOVATIONS IN PAIN MANAGEMENT

A Practical Guide for Clinicians

Volume 1

INNOVATIONS IN PAIN MANAGEMENT

A Practical Guide for Clinicians

Volume 1

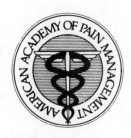

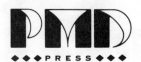

Edited by
RICHARD S. WEINER, PhD
Executive Director
American Academy of
Pain Management

Published by
PAUL M. DEUTSCH PRESS

Editorial Staff:
Production Editor and Book Designer: Ann Groom
Managing Editor: Myrene O'Connor
Production Assistant: Stephanie Murphy
Publication Specialist: Debra Kramer

Copyright © 1990
Paul M. Deutsch Press, Inc.
A Paul M. Deutsch Company
2208 Hillcrest Street
Orlando, FL 32803

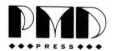

ISBN: 1-878205-13-7
Library of Congress Card Catalog Number: 90-84153

Cover design by Groom Design, Inc.
Printed in the United States of America

DEDICATION

In order to treat something, we must first learn to recognize it.

—Sir William Ostler

This book is dedicated to the multitude of individuals and families who live each day coping with pain and to the new breed of health care professionals dedicated to the multidisciplinary team approach to pain management.

Richard S. Weiner, Ph.D.
Executive Director
American Academy of Pain Management

INTRODUCTION

by Arnold Fox, M. D.

I began seeing patients as a second year medical student, well over 30 years ago. As a medical student, an Intern, a Resident, and finally, a full-fledged Internist and Cardiologist, I got to know pain as well as any physician can. Of course, my knowledge was always one step removed. No one can possibly "know" pain as well as the patient does.

When I was a young medical student, patients were treated as passive receptacles for the medicines and surgeries we were so eager to use. We doctors made the diagnosis, we prodded and poked the patient, we called for X-rays and neurologic studies. During Grand Rounds at the giant Los Angeles County Hospital, pain patients would be brought in on their wheel chairs and crutches. The great doctor with his white hair and long white coat, stethoscope dangling from his neck, would make his pronouncements. Then the nurses and orderlies would wheel the patient away to begin treatment. As I look back through the years I see that doctors, my teachers, were brilliant indeed. Unfortunately, they worked with a philosophy inherited from the 18th century, that of the omnipotent, omnipresent physician who "waves his hand" over the silent, awe-struck patient.

The 30-some years that have passed have seen great advances in medical technology. More importantly, the same years have seen a revolutionary upheaval in medical philosophy. We physicians now realize that chronic pain can be a very complex problem that refuses to yield to an injection or two, or a quick surgery. The "grand old doctor" working by him or herself is often not enough.

All across the country, physicians have wisely discarded that outdated and so often ineffectual approach. Instead, we're asking allied health professionals to join with us, to share their knowledge and experience as we work, together with the patient, to control chronic pain.

I remember so many patients with chronic pain who were in and out of the hospitals during the 1950s and 1960s, patients whom we frankly did not help. We went it alone, without the help of a psychologist to handle emotional upsets, without the assistance of a skilled social worker to identify and rectify certain home problems, without dentists, chiropractors, physical therapists, and others at our side.

Toward the end of the 1960s, this began to change. I watched the new approaches evolving. I remember how our allied health professional struggled for recognition, fought to have their voices heard. By the 1970s, many new modalities were used for chronic pain: biofeedback, meditation, acupuncture, nutrition, hypnosis, electrotherapy, group therapy, and more. I believe that the 1970s saw the power shift from the physician back to the patient, where it belongs. Very wise people pointed out that the patient does not live in a vacuum. Like everyone else, pain patients are part of a family, a circle of friends, they have an occupation, they belong to various social, cultural, and religious groups. We've learned that all these have to be taken into consideration, for pain is a multi-faceted experience strongly influenced by all the things which make us who we are.

Improvements in diagnostic procedures paralleled, and to some extent spurred the philosophical development. We went from X-rays to CAT scans to MRI's and PETs. In the mid-70s the first of the endorphins were discovered, those marvelous hormone substances secreted by various cells which modulate our perception of pain.

Finding the endorphins was perhaps the most exciting discovery of all, for it gave us even more reason to make the patient the senior partner on the team. After all, we know that our attitude influences our endorphin levels, as well as the levels of other substances in our bodies. The patient controls his or her outlook on life, and their outlook influences their endorphins.[1] If we give control back to the patient, if we treat the patient as a person rather than a passive receptacle, if we include their family; if we do these things, and more, we can help better the patient's outlook. If we do that, we help influence their very biochemistry, for the better.

As a physician who learned the old way of treating pain, yet who sees the tremendous advances of the new way, I am excited about playing a small role in helping the launch the American Academy of Pain Management. It's exciting to work with other health professionals, to learn their techniques and philosophies. I've learned a great deal from the psychologists, dentists, chiropractors, podiatrists, registered nurses, medical social workers, and others who make up the Academy, who help the patient along in this great experiment called life. I've been so glad to learn that when I can't help a patient, there are others who can.

The American Academy of Pain Management is to the commended for bringing together the various professions and disciplines dedicated to healing. *Innovations in Pain Management* provides a useful and practical guide for all the pain professionals.

---

[1]See Fox, A. and Fox, B., *DLPA To End Chronic Pain and Depression,* Pocket Books, 1985.

PREFACE

by Pierre L. LeRoy, M.D., F.A.C.S., C.C.E.

Pain is virtually a universal experience. Mankind is born in a painful process, and while certain pains have beneficial end results, we still must seek to alleviate this pernicious disorder. The purpose of this book is to provide a broad understanding of both pain medicine and pain management which is rapidly becoming a field of specialization. Individual chapters will deal with the rapidly changing scientific and theoretical concepts applicable to the everyday problems of diagnostic and treatment programs that face the many different health professionals who have a special interest in pain management and who wish to improve their professional development.

There are many descriptors of pain, from the ancient Book of Job to contemporary literature and medical books. Edmund Burke's "pain and pleasure are simple ideas incapable of definition" succinctly expresses the pain rubic. However, Cervante's "Other men's pains are easily borne" states precisely the dilemma health professionals face daily. We intend to examine these issues in depth and offer solutions in the text.

Pain is a subjective sensory experience that produces unpleasant sensations first associated with psychological and behavioral changes followed later by structural differences. Thus, it can serve as a warning sign of conditions within the human body mechanism. In this sense, pain can be considered beneficial. However, when pain becomes intractable and chronic, serving no useful purpose, it can be as destructive and pernicious to the life process as any disease entity. Because of the organized efforts of our world health resources, it now appears that pain syndromes may well be manageable within our lifetimes.

We have come a long way in working towards our pain management needs. Primitive man managed pain by both plants and herbs and by praying to the deities in search of a remedy for pain. Medications for pain management have significantly improved—from using the poppy plant or chewing on willow bark 2000 years ago, to the turn of the 19th century when morphine and acetylsalicylic acid were isolated. Much more has transpired since then. This book will review the current and continuing complex changes in pharmacology.

The book's format is designed to facilitate the health professional's need to keep pace with the avalanche of new information which is published almost daily on the subject of pain management. Each chapter covers specific subjects designed toward an integrated whole with specific supplements made available as priorities of interest and technological breakthroughs develop.

This book will explore the dynamics of pain pathophysiology determined through current basic research, clinical experience, and outcome studies. It will consider the possible role of culture and genetics within the pain syndromes since we are still not certain if there is a hereditary, as well as a familial factor.

The pathophsiology of pain is an unique, personal, individualized, subjective, and objective, response pattern. Do the quality and quantity of immune and neurotransmittal substances play a vital role in pain's acute and chronic manifestations? The study of chronic pain raises many questions. Is chronic pain then a "deficiency syndrome"? If so, how do we inhibit facilitation? How do we facilitate the inhibition? What is the role of cytochrome C? Why reactive depression? Why premature aging? How do we rehabilitate patients with complex chronic pain syndrome? What are the ethical and cost considerations? These remain provocative problems that will be discussed in this book.

Advances have been made in pain management since the middle of this century due to the efforts of many, but one individual, Dr. John. H. Bonica, stands out above all others in his accomplishments; working toward the goal of the increased awareness and need for a new discipline in pain medicine. Through his continued personal efforts and with his unique ability to stimulate others, there is now a better grasp of the complex pain mechanisms based on the anatomic, physiologic, pharmacologic, and neuropsychologic principles of algology. This is exciting because as late as the 1950s a relative medical inertia prevailed.

The enlightenment continues to gain momentum in greater depth. Since the 1950s, Dr. Bonica has been joined by many persons who have each made significant contributions in this new field. As a result, pain management is no longer a seemingly inexorable task, but fits into scientifically definable, subjective, and objective responses that are often intermixed. The reader is referred to Dr. Bonica's latest outstanding text *Pain Management* second edition, which reviews a milestone of significant progress.

At the direction of Dr. Bonica and others who founded the International Association of Study of Pain (I. A. S. P.) and later through its Taxomony Committee, chaired by Professor Mersky of Canada, this dedicated group of people labored for years and finally developed a concensus that universally suits the many faces of pain. They concluded that "Pain is an unpleasant experience that we primarily associate with tissue damage or disease, or describe in terms of tissue damage, or both."

The complex psycho-biological integrating systems responses to pain perception were wonderfully simplified by Dr. J. Loeser who states, "Pain is perceived nociception" thereby clarifying our basic understanding but, at the same time, raising many unanswered questions. How is nociception perceived? These questions will be addressed in this book.

The scope of pain as a medical problem is staggering. Statistics vary even from the World Health, National Institute of Health (NIH) and other sources depending on the methodology employed. Pain causes a considerable burden on private and public concerns, lost work days, insurance costs, etc. There are an estimated 20 million people who suffer from migraine headaches; 70 million with various types of back pain; millions of others who are racked annually with medical disease and injuries resulting in chronic pain syndrome that remain underdiagnosed or under-treated. Most feared of all is the pain associated with cancer, afflicting an estimated 800,000 Americans and perhaps 18,000,000 people worldwide.

A growing understanding of more specific pain syndromes are now better understood, too. For example, the Reflex Sympathetic Dystrophy Syndrome (RSDS), first classically described by Weir Mitchell in 1864 and through the continuing efforts of Drs. Bonica, Le Riche, Ochoa, Schwartzman, and others, helped in its awareness. Specifically, RSDS can be diagnosed earlier, but still remains a baffling, disabling disorder in its pathophysiology as well as its treatment. It is considered a C-fiber disorder.

Now is the time "to speak of many things" as Alice in Wonderland noted. Theories trying to explain pain have been evolving for several centuries and have varied widely since Descartes' 17th century simplistic view of a straight line theory from reception to perception followed by variable physical and emotional responses. A classic advance was reached with Melzak and Wall's gate theory in 1965, proposing complex integrated gating mechanisms operating at first at spinal and later at different levels, eventually influencing other ascending and descending neural pathways in afferent-efferent integrating systems.

World class contributors attempting to explain complex interactions of pain from Pavlov to Abel-Fessard, Arnoff, Bonica, Crue, Finnision, Iaggo, Leibskind, Mersky, Ochao, Sears, Sternback, Tollison, and so many others are already standing of the shoulders of anatomic, physiological, and clinical giants as will be seen in the succeeding chapters, which review historical changes in medical thoughts of the physician scientist.

Peripheral and central integration of pain perception is still relatively poorly understood because central and other biasing mechanisms involve complex neuropsychological and cognitive processes. We are retrospectively reminded of the eloquent 19th century Sherringtonian concept of the "enchanted loom of the brain" that still challenges all health professionals to undertake the research to not only understand but diagnose and treat this universal distress that afflicts so many. We are also mindful, too, of the many important contributions that come from non-experts who, at times must compete with the Ivory Tower of established medical hierarchy, for they, too, have their theories and practical suggestions. We should continue to encourage this dialogue and to take counsel from these contributors.

History reminds us that medicine of the 20th century has profited from the contributions of 17th, 18th, and 19th century philosophers and scientists. Now we move into the new age of neuropsychopharmacology started by chemist Thudicum's neuro-chemical concepts at the turn of the century to more specific understanding of the neurotransmitter substances whose concentrations and fleeting existence have eluded investigators of the centuries, awaiting new instrumentation, which resulted in a change in our theories. Scientific discussions are now possible about qualitative and quantitative decisions made at the microsynaptic junction of 70 microns. This achievement had to wait for the development of advanced techniques employing electron microscopy and specially trained staffs available only at major University Centers, the National Institute of Health, and other laboratories supported by basic science funding.

We should recall that in the first half of the 20th century, two basic substances were thought to be the principal ingredients of the physiologic function of neural transmission ... adrenalin and acetylcholine. Since then, with additional advances now include 16 neurotransmitters, including endorphins and the elusive presynaptic substance P, which have recently been identified as part of the chemical messenger family by Drs. Kostertiz, Pert, Sweet, Snyder, and efforts of many others. These have greatly advanced our present knowledge of pain transmission and modulation. Doctor Snyder has postulated that there must be at least 200 chemical messengers needed at the synapse to explain everything. What challenge!

There have been studies in the anatomical aspects of pain. New philosophies behind patient care of those suffering from chronic pain are emerging. Grouping patients into well-organized programs should be both humanitarian and cost-effective. Such programs have been developed by Drs. Aire, Addison, Hendler, Rosemoff, Seres, Shealy, and others to name a few and could serve as ongoing basic clinical training programs. University-based pain centers are developing within hospital settings at Johns Hopkins, Jefferson, UCLA, and other prestigious institutions as well as other clinics, each contributing in their respective ways towards one goal—the humanitarian aspect of cost-effective patient care.

In addition to the theoretical and clinical progress in diagnosis and treatment, important new laboratory contributions now allow us to understand things we cannot see, for pain still cannot be imaged. Imaging studies have made great advances.

X-ray technology, demonstrating both structural and physiologic changes through the years, has greatly improved but still has significant limitations as will be seen in subsequent chapters.

Our ability to see structured abnormalities is improved by third-generation computerized axial tomography (CT), advances in Magnetic Resonance Imaging (MRI) combining electromagnetic and computer principles, for which Drs. Purcell and Block received the Nobel Prize. These will be addressed in later chapters of this book.

New tests, for example, the single proton emission computerized tomography (S.P.E.C.T.) and proton emission tomography (P.E.T.) are becoming important. Progress in medical thermography is taking its place in medical testing armanentarium, helping to assess and differentiate neuropathic, vascular, skeletal, and myofascial pain syndromes that frequently co-exist with each other and must be differentiated for treatment as well as reimbursement purposes. These tests demonstrate functional or patho-physiologic changes before structural changes, which is the real goal as we move into the 21st century.

Advances in non-imaging tests, such as electromyography (E.M.G.), compliment our understanding of nerve action potential, depolarization, ionic shift, and repolarization all brought to scientific respectability in the crucible of many scientific debacles. Early physiologists, such as Galvaini, Duchenne, Beevor, and others made basic contributions to the understanding of today's peripheral electrophysiology. Recent contributions of Drs. Aminoff, Brazier, Basmajian, De Luca, Moore, and others continued to produce more accuracy of diagnosis.

Progress in spinal, auditory, and visual evoke potentials test hold promise for new applications in pain medicine for better interpretations of changes in latency and abnormal wave forms. These help clinically interpret complex peripheral pain mechanisms as the rapid signal passes from peripheral receptor to lower and upper neuron integrated systems producing effective responses needed for clinical correlation. These will be subjects of later chapters.

The electroencephalograph (EEG) has enriched the overall concept of evaluating headache syndromes associated with chronic pain. The contributions of Berger, Gastaut, Gibbs, Gloor, Goldenman, Kellway, Kooi, and Walter are being helped by today's deep brain stereotaxic recordings pioneered by Spiegal, Wycis, Cooper, Gildenburg, and others.

Once diagnosis is made, what about treatment? As we progress in our fundamental understanding of medications we are reminded of the contributions of the Shamans, who still practice their art of healing, searching for the principles based on their empirical observations while imploring the spirits. They helped lay the groundwork for the development of the modern principles of current opiate and non-opiate analgesic pharmacology. Classic contributions of the 18th century understanding of the complex arachniconic cascade, which is now helping in the design of better and more specific idealized analgesics.

Today, there are basically three groups of analgesics for pain treatment: the opiates, non-narcotics, and adjuvants. These have special indications pertaining to relative and absolute contradictions that will modulate peripheral receptors, afferent, ascending, and central as well as descending pathways. The search continues for the principal agent that is receptor specific and yet lacks significant undesirable side-effects that can affect sleep, mental capability, gastric, renal, hepatic physiology, and cause habituation. Chapters in the book will deal in depth with this part of pain management.

The surgery of pain is based on interruption of anatomic pathways which included peripheral nerves, spinal cord, and brain de-afferent procedures. For the past 50 years, neurosurgical techniques have continued to improve in their techniques based on the contributions of Drs. German, Groff, Peet,

Ray, Matson, Scott, and others. However, long-term follow-up studies demonstrate that pain pathways exist and recurrence occurs following surgery on primary, sensory pain pathways. This has lead to many new surgery techniques that will be discussed, including neural augmentation and modulation procedures employing implantation systems. Contributions from Drs. Black, Burton, Campbell, Long, Nashold, North, Ray, and other experts in de-afferentation surgery are providing a great deal of data. The question is exemplified by Dr. German's observation, "They do so much with so little" can not we do more!

Research in pain management at the basic experimental, investigatory, and clinical levels must continue since each contributes to each other in important breakthroughs but not always in the same sequence or time frame. We are reminded of the important observation of industrial chemist and intellectual giant, Dr. Sinnes, who has always insisted at the national level that funding must continue for basic science research. Education in science, too, must be a national priority going to the level of the elementary school child hoping to spark genius and enthusiasm early.

Lack of the perfect analgesic, and because of the relatively unsatisfactory results of surgical operations designed to disconnect or de-afferent anatomic pain pathways, eventually lead to the alternative use of electrotherapy. There is now a better understanding of transducing electrical impulses into the body without invasion since the 1900s by Duchenne and others, contributing to early treatment. This was eventually followed by today's topical pain modulation technique.

Breakthroughs in advanced transcutaneous stimulation techniques through the initial efforts of bioengineers, Avery and Mauer and later by Drs. Burton, Ray, Shealy, Sweet, and others, produced a consortium of effort in the 1970s to devise specific pain modulation implantation systems that had to pass the pre-market clearance test regulations imposed by the strict 1986 Device Act. Chapters on electro-mechanical devices will offer more detail.

Associations, such as the American Association of Medical Instrumentation (A.A.M.I.) and the Biomedical Association are basically providing strong interface for pain patients by linking together physician, patient, hospital, and biomedical engineers cooperating in developing and designing pain-related devices and publishing important breakthroughs as the reader will see in later chapters.

Investigators seem to be adhering to the eloquent observation in William Shakespeare's *Hamlet*:

Disease desperate grown
by desperate appliance are relieved,
Or not at all.

Pain due to cancer in the future will perhaps have more alternatives for its treatment thanks to the research done today in areas unthought of years ago. Scientists are aware that cancer pain is based on different mechanisms. Cancer pain has its special problems with the oncologist making significant clinical progress in managing their problem from non-cancer pain with new cancercidal drugs and adjurvants to help modulate pain, especially in the terminally ill. The efforts of Drs. Foley, Houde (at the Sloane Kettering Institute), and many others are to be lauded in this difficult task that afflicts such a large patient population. Chapters will review current therapy in oncology.

The scientific and medical communities have formed organizations to try to improve the insights of our present understanding. These have improved a Tower of Babel situation only made possible through Dr. Bonica's concept of developing a global perspective for communication, it became known as the International Association for the Study of Pain. The fundamental goal of this prestigious organization is to bring together scientists and medical specialists to communicate with each other informally and promote an ongoing data base. The I.A.S.P. founded a periodical journal call *Pain* with an Editorial Board that is composed of experienced senior scientists, who voluntarily contribute their time to study on-going problems through standing committee systems. The prestigious Board currently consists of J. J. Bonica, Seattle, WA; A. Iggo, Edinburgh; J. D. Loeser, Seattle, WA; and W. Noordenbos, Amsterdam, forming a global communication network for the study of pain.

At the national level, the American Pain Society was founded and has brought together basic scientists, clinicians, psychiatrists, and psychologists to stimulate scientific advancement and sponsor national and regional meetings with other associations. Where else could a clinician meet and have dialogue with a rat physiologist? Other major publications and journals discussing pain management, diagnosis, and treatment such as the *Clinical Journal of Pain*, founded by Dr. Arnoff, provide the reader with an important, continuing data base.

Other groups and associations have also made important contributions, such as the American Chronic Pain Association, an all-volunteer organization based on prinicples of learned skills in nursing, communicate promptly important new skills.

The Reflex Sympathetic Association, founded in 1984 by devoted Audrey Thomas, R. N. and Roselyn and Francis Davis, whose own children are RSDS patients, has made tremendous strides in pioneering changes that bring a prestigious advisory board to help patients personally understand Dr. Tollison's belief, "No pain is hopeless." The reader is referred to Dr. Tollison's informative publication *Pain Management* which offers a broad scale of current clinical subjects providing the reader with a very special and experienced data base.

Through continuing efforts at decentralization, the development of regional associations, such as the Eastern, Midwestern, and Western Pain Societies with their various affiliates, continue to aid research in a spirit of academic competition. Each group contributes in its own way to the total body of knowledge. The development of more regionally oriented societies, such as the Delaware Valley Pain Association, sponsored through the efforts of Thomas Jefferson Medical University serves as a model to bring together the doctor, the nurse, and other clinicians to discuss, expand, and debate the various subjects of pain medicine.

Local community conferences, primarily designed for participating patients, such as Pain Update series held at the historic Delaware Academy of Medicine, has provided for the past five years topics of interest to patients and professionals concerning chronic pain syndromes as a community service.

In 1988, the American Academy of Pain Management (A. A. Pain Management) was formed. The Academy was founded on the concepts of Drs. Weiner, Shealy, Travell, and others who perceive important new trends. The Academy is a forum for clinicians across disciplines. The Academy strives to raise standards of professionalism through education and training. Certification by the Academy signals to one's peers a commitment as well as a minimum of training and experience related to the field of pain management. This book is a symbol of that commitment.

Jonathan Swift's "vision is the ability to see things invisible" aptly summarizes the important medical insights in this compendium of experts who will clarify much of the misinformation that has crept into the health care delivery system. It will also provided consensus leadership in pain management with better cost-effective humanitarian patient care as the ultimate goal.

SUGGESTED READINGS FROM THE PREFACE

1. *Celebrations of Life,* Rene DuBos
2. *The Lives of a Cell, Notes of a Biology Watcher,* Lewis Thomas
3. *Cellular Pathology,* as based upon *Physiological and Pathology Histology*
4. *Medical Engineering,* Editor-in-Chief, Charles Dean Ray, M.S., M.D., F.A.C.S., F.R.S.H. (London)
5. *Hans Berger on the Electroencephalogram of Man,* translated from the original German version and edited by Pierre Gloor
6. *Magnetism and Its Effects on the Living System,* Albert Roy Davis and Walter C. Rawls., Jr.
7. *Invention, Discovery, and Creativity,* A.D. Moore
8. *What Mad Pursuit: A Personal View of Scientific Discovery,* Francis Crick
9. *Current Therapy of Pain,* edited by Kathleen M. Foley, M.D. and Richard M. Payne, M.D.
10. *Dictionary of Rheumatic Diseases,* prepared by the Glossary Committee, American College of Rheumatology
11. *Text of Pain,* Robert D. Wall and Ronald Melzack

SUGGESTED PUBLICATIONS RELATED TO PAIN MANAGEMENT

1. *The Pain Practitioner,* a quarterly newsletter published by the American Academy of Pain Management.
2. *Pain,* this is the official journal of the International Association of the Study of Pain. It is published monthly, providing a forum for the dissemination of research in the basic and clinical sciences of multidisciplinary interest.
3. *The Clinical Journal of Pain,* the official journal of the American Academy of Pain Medicine, published quarterly, presenting results of original clinical research.
4. *The Journal of Pain and Symptom Management,* published quarterly and provides professionals with research and clinical information on pain and other symptoms. Many articles concern cancer pain.
5. *Pain Management,* a bimonthly journal intended as a practical guide for primary care physicians on the subject of clinical pain management.

EDITOR'S NOTE

by Richard S. Weiner, Ph.D.

HISTORICAL TREATMENT OF PAIN

Throughout millennia, problems associated with pain and attempts to control pain have historically been one of the principle reasons that individuals have sought health care. Alleviating pain is not a recent concern. Relief of suffering has been the helping professions primary objective throughout time. However, the way we view pain and the treatments available have altered considerably.

Individuals in pre-scientific cultures felt less control over their environment than is common in contemporary society. Consequently, people sought explanations and meaning for their lives in mystical, supernatural, or God-like concepts. The common thread was a feeling of very limited control over events. Attribution theory has been offered by social psychologists to explain coping mechanisms by which people ascribe a cause to an unpleasant event in the hope of establishing a difference between themselves and the "inflicted one." Such a process could comfort one into a belief of invulnerability. Thus, early men and women attributed pain to evil, at times vengeful spirits, who invaded the body of an unworthy host. However, these spirits were amenable to negotiation. Culturally differentiated rituals were used to exorcise the pain. That ancient communities paid great attention to the treatment of pain is suggested by one of the earliest vocational specialties developed by humanity: the medicine man or witch doctor. Throughout recorded history, the healer or reliever of pain was given a special status in his or her community.

Ancient healers or shamans practiced a sacred art and were viewed as catalysts who could negotiate with an angry God or who could, by ritual, restore balance with nature. In this orientation, intervention was possible but the final outcome was not within the control of mortals. The context of the illness and pain represented more of a wholeness than presently exists in disease of the body, disease of the mind, or disease of the spirit. An illness affected the total person, who consisted of an integration of these components.

Philosophically, this concept changed when Descarte conceptually separated the body from the soul and described pain as a signal of mechanical dysfunctioning. As a result, narrow specialties, often fragmented and with little common language, developed. While such an epistemological approach has resulted in great scientific breakthroughs in many areas of acute health care, it has often created a barrier in our understanding of intractable pain.

THE PROFESSIONAL ENVIRONMENT OF PAIN MANAGEMENT

In recent years, great strides have been made in our ability to help individuals who suffer from pain. We have gone beyond the historical method of providing treatment in which a sole practitioner works with a chronic pain patient. Interdisciplinary and multidisciplinary pain clinic facilities have demonstrated a new service delivery approach to pain management. There has been a phenomenal growth in the number and variety of inpatient and outpatient clinics. Professionals from several disciplines who work together have re-introduced an awareness that pain patients experience physical, emotional, interpersonal, financial, and spiritual problems. This reintegrated blend of art and science within the team concept help establish the pain practitioner as a renaissance healer.

In 1988, the American Academy of Pain Management was incorporated in order that clinical pain practitioners from all disciplines could work together for the purpose of developing standards for practice, codes of ethical conduct, and for the purpose of establishing a certification process for clinical pain practitioners.

CONTINUING EDUCATION

The present work represents a continuing commitment by the American Academy of Pain Management in assisting pain practitioners to more fully understand the art and science of pain management. The authors whose work is presented in this text are among the leaders in pain management. They write with a vision based on experience. The collection of their wisdom, represented here, is relevant for pain management clinicians and professionals from all disciplines who wish a consultative state-of-the-art resource for their practice. *Innovations in Pain Management,* is intended to be an updatable resource. Additional chapters will be written and as new insights are gleaned from the real world of pain management, revisions will allow expansion; both increasing the value of this project and creating a living resource which shall not soon become outdated.

Each chapter has been written to allow the reader to independently read topics of interest and thus may be viewed as a self-contained study. The collection of chapters allows an authoritative self-study on many of the pressing issues faced by pain practitioners. The writing style of each author has been left intact, further highlighting the unique contributions of each chapter to the total project.

Although we have come a long way in our understanding of the impact of pain and in our ability to help reduce the toll of pain on the lives of our patients/clients, we have not yet eliminated the scourge of pain. It is my hope that *Innovations in Pain Management* will help illuminate our present ability and encourage future analysis.

ACKNOWLEDGEMENTS

Many people helped bring this project to fruition. I am indebted to Junis Merchant for typing and to Rose Steele whose humor helped us complete these tasks. I must recognize Kathryn Weiner for her valuable insights and I am beholden to my children, Rebecca and Jason Weiner, for reminding me of both the beauty of life and the fragility of life. I also wish to acknowledge and recognize the assistance of the publisher, Paul M. Deutsch Press, without whose commitment to this project the first steps could never have been taken.

CONTRIBUTING AUTHORS

Editor
Richard S. Weiner, Ph.D.
Executive Director, American Academy of Pain Management
National Board of Certified Counselors
International Academy of Professional Counseling and
   Behavioral Medicine
American Board of Medical Psychotherapists
American Association of Family Counselors and Mediators
International Association for the Study of Pain
American Pain Society

Preface
Pierre L. LeRoy, M.D.
American Board of Neurological Surgery
Founding Director, American Pain Society
American College of Surgeons
Board of Examiners for Clinical Engineering
Congress of Neurological Surgeons
International College of Thermology
International Association for the Study of Pain

Introduction
Arnold Fox, M.D.
Commissioner, California Board of Medical Quality Assurance
American College of Cardiology
Fellow, American College of Angiology
Fellow, International College of Applied Nutrition
International Academy of Preventive Medicine

Chapter 1
C. David Tollison, Ph.D.
Editor, *Journal of Pain Management*
Director, Pain Therapy Center of Greenville
Greenville Hospital System
Senior Vice President, Pain Therapy Centers
   Greenville Health Corporation
   Greenville, South Carolina

Chapters 2 and 4
C. Norman Shealy, M.D., Ph.D., D.Dc.
American Board of Neurological Surgery
American Board of American Psychotherapists
Fellow, American College of Surgeons
Founding President, American Holistic Medical Association
Fellow, American College of Preventative Medicine

Biofeedback Certification Institute of America
International Association for the Study of Pain
Director, Shealy Institute for Comprehensive Health Care
Clinical and Research Professor
   Forest Institute of Professional Psychology

Roger K. Cady, M.D.
   Medical Director, Shealy Institute for Comprehensive
      Health Care

Chapters 3 and 13
B. Eliot Cole, M.D.
   American Board of Psychiatry and Neurology
   American Society of Neuroimaging
   American Academy of Neurology
   American College of Emergency Medicine
   International Association for the Study of Pain
   Clinical Assistant Professor
      Department of Psychiatry and Behavioral Sciences
      University of Nevada School of Medicine
   Medical Director
      Hospice of Northern Nevada
      Saint Mary's Regional Medical Center

Chapter 5
Richard Materson, M.D.
   Past President, Fellow, American Academy of Physical Medicine
      and Rehabilitation
   American Association for Electromyography and
      Electrodiagnosis
   Diplomate, American Board of Physical Medicine and
      Rehabilitation
   American Academy for Cerebral Palsy and Development
      Medicine
   National Rehabilitation Association
   Vice-President for Medical Affairs and Medical Director,
      National Rehabilitation Hospital and Washington Pain and
      Rehabilitation Center, Inc.

Chapter 6
Nelson Hendler, M.D., M.S.
   Clinical Director, Mensana Clinic
   Assistant Professor of Neurosurgery, Johns Hopkins University
      School of Medicine
   Psychiatric Consultant

Chapter 7

Margaret S. Texidor, Ph.D.
Assistant Professor, Tulane Medical School
National Board of Certified Counselors
National Academy of Certified Clinical Mental Health Counselors
American Board of Medical Psychotherapists
Past President, Louisiana Mental Health Counselors Association

Chapter 8

Robert B. Supernaw, Pharm. D.
Associate Dean and Professor, University of the Pacific School of
    Pharmacy
Fellow, American College of Clinical Pharmacy
American Pharmaceutical Association
American Society of Hospital Pharmacists

Arthur Harralson, Pharm. D.
Vice Chairman, Department of Pharmacy Practice
Associate Professor of Clinical Pharmacy
    School of Pharmacy
    University of the Pacific

Chapter 9

William N. Harsha, M.S., M.D., J.D.
American Board of Orthopedic Surgery
American Academy of Neurological and Orthopedic Surgeons
American College of Legal Medicine
American Academy of Pain Medicine
International College of Surgeons
International Association for the Study of Pain

Chapter 10

Steven D. Waldman, M.D.
Director, Pain Consortium of Greater Kansas City

Chapter 11

Michael Gallagher, D.O.
Assistant Dean for Clinical Affairs
Director, University Headache Center
    University of Medicine and Dentistry of New Jersey
    School of Osteopathic Medicine

Chapter 12

Charles McNeill, D.D.S.
Director, Craniofacial Pain, TMJ Clinic
University of California
    School of Dentistry
    San Francisco

Consultant, Thorndike Memorial Library
Harvard University, School of Medicine
Diplomate, American Board of Pain Management
Fellow, Royal Society of Health
Fellow, American Society of Podiatric Medicine
Fellow, American Association of Hospital Podiatrists
Fellow, American Academy of Podiatry Administration
Fellow, American Society of Podiatric Dermatology
Trustee, California College of Podiatric Medicine

Chapter 18
Joseph A. Kwentus, M.D.
American Board of Psychiatry and Neurology
Certified in Psychiatry and Neurology
Association of Sleep Disorder Centers
Certification in Polysomnography

Chapter 19   *Volume 2*
Joseph V. Uricchio, Jr., M.D.
Diplomate and Fellow, American Academy of Orthopaedic
Surgeons
Past President, Academy of Neuromuscular Thermography
American College of Legal Medicine
American Pain Society
Eastern Orthopaedic Society
Southern Pain Society
Southern Orthopaedic Association
Board of Directors, State of Florida Reflex Sympathetic
Dystrophy Association

Chapter 20
Scott Havsy, D.O., FAANaOS
Orthopedic and Industrial Medicine
Diplomate, American Academy of Pain Management
Member, The American College of Sports Medicine
Member, The American Osteopathic College of Sports Medicine

Chapter 21
Donald B. Taylor, Jr., D.C.
Commmissioner, California State Board of Chiropractic
Examiners
California Chiropractic Association
Past Vice President, San Joaquin-Stanislaus Chiropractic
Society
Certified Independent Medical Examiner in Worker's
Compensation

Chapter 22
C. K. Fernando, M.A., L.P.T.
Past Fulbright Scholar
Past Associate Clinical Professor
 University of Illinois, Department of Physical Therapy
Director, Forest Hills Therapy Center

Chapter 23
Daniel L. Kirsch, Ph.D.
Former Clinical Director, The Center for Stress and Pain-Related
 Disorders, Columbia-Presbyterian Medical Center, New York
Designer, Alpha-Stim Technology
Editor, *American Journal of Electromedicine*

Fred N. Lerner, Ph.D., D.C.
Director of Continuing Education, National Institute of Elec-
 tromedical Information, New York
Clinical Director, Medical Dental Evaluations, Beverly Hills,
 California
Former Associate Dean, Graduate School of Electromedical
 Sciences, City University Los Angeles

Chapter 24
Stephen A. Lawson, M.S., C.R.C., C.I.R.S.
National Rehabilitation Association
National Rehabilitation Counseling Association

Chapter 25
William N. Harsha, M.S., M.D., J.D.
American Board of Orthopedic Surgery
American Academy of Neurological and Orthopedic Surgeons
American College of Legal Medicine
American Academy of Pain Medicine
International College of Surgeons
International Association for the Study of Pain

CHAPTER CONSULTANTS

Jerry M. Fabrikant, D.P.M.
Diplomate, American Board of Podiatric Surgery
Diplomate, American Board of Podiatric Orthopedics
Fellow, American College of Foot Orthopedists
Fellow, American College of Foot Surgeons

Bob Gant, Ph.D.
Past President Division 12, American Psychological Association
Diplomate, American Board of Professional Neuropsychology
Diplomate, Academy of Behavioral Medicine
American Board of Clinical Hypnosis
Fellow, Academy for Psychosomatic Medicine
National Academy of Neuropsychology

Mary M. Garcia, Pharm. D.
American Society of Hospital Pharmacists
American Pharmaceutical Association
California Society of Hospital Pharmacists

Joseph Lee, M.D.
American Board of Anesthesiology
American College of Anesthesiology
American Academy of Pain Medicine
International Association for the Study of Pain
American Pain Society

Carl H. McNeely, R.N., B.S.N., M.Ed.
American Nurses Association
Clinical Nurse Dual Diagnosis, Substance Dependence Unit
Previous Staff Experience: Surgical, Oncology Unit, Burn Intensive
Care Unit, Medical Psychiatric Unit

Ward B. Studt, M.D.
Fellow, American Academy of Orthopedic Surgeons
Fellow, American College of Surgeons
American Board of Orthopedic Surgeons

Jerry W. Taylor, D.M.D.
Fellow, Academy of General Dentistry
American Dental Association
International Academy of Gnathology
Craniomandibular Institute

Contents

SECTION 1

The History of Pain Management

SECTION 2

The Elements of Multidisciplinary Pain Management Including Classification and Assessment

SECTION 3 ▮▮▮▮▮▮▮▮▮▮

The Treatment of Commonly Occuring Pain Syndromes

SECTION 4 ███████████████

Manual and Electromedicine

SECTION 5 ███████████████

Work Disability and Litigation

LIST OF ILLUSTRATIONS

Section 1
THE HISTORY OF PAIN MANAGEMENT

Chapter 1

THE MAGNITUDE OF THE PAIN PROBLEM:

The Problem in Perspective
C. David Tollison, Ph.D.

Dr. Tollison describes the magnitude of pain as an epidemic touching the lives of pain sufferers, family members, and society in general. Dr. Tollison is to be admired in his ability to clearly describe the impact of pain in terms both of suffering and dollar expenditures. The examples that he uses illustrate how the experience of pain affects all of us and sets the tone for the chapters that follow.

Chapter 1

THE MAGNITUDE OF THE PAIN PROBLEM:

The Problem in Perspective

C. David Tollison, Ph.D.

The magnitude of human pain and suffering is both profound and escalating. Few medical problems are more complex and perplexing. Statistics are staggering, but statistics alone do not paint the entire picture. While statistics give us a data base from which to address the problem of pain, statistics do not offer us an appreciation for the impact of pain upon the individual patient, family friends, and community.

More than 75 million Americans suffer chronic, handicapping pain (Tollison, 1987). These individuals have typically suffered through several years of agony, undergone two or more failed surgeries for pain relief, are restricted in their jobs if not totally unable to work, take various and multiple medications for pain, experience chronic sleep disturbance and marital and family dysfunction, suffer depression and emotional distress, and are physically and psychologically depleted (Tollison, 1982).

Surprised? Many people are surprised since chronic pain seems such an innocuous problem to those fortunate individuals who do not know the daily agony of unremitting discomfort. In this era of rampant heart disease, coronary surgery, organ transplantation, cancer, leukemia, and other dreaded diseases and life-saving interventions, the problem and treatment of benign pain too often fails to impress. As a population, we have been conditioned to fear only the worst, the lifethreatening, and the dramatic. Consequently, we jog, exercise, quit smoking, maintain healthy diets, attend stress inoculation workshops, and make every effort to avoid those diseases that endanger our lives.

And chronic pain? It goes without saying that intractable benign pain generally poses no major direct threat to our longevity, nor does it draw enough national attention to warrant even a storyline in an episode of one of the many television medical shows. But while we are fast gaining a healthy respect for and knowledge of those issues and problems that affect the quantity of life, what steps are we taking to ensure the quality of our existence?

We as a nation are particularly illiterate in the management of one of the most costly, frequent, and painful disorders plaguing the quality of life. It is true that no one dies from benign pain, but many victims suffer a disabled and pleasureless existence. In addition, an alarming percentage of severely afflicted chronic pain patients have no interest in longevity, but await death and its end to suffering with anticipation.

Perhaps a truly meaningful and enjoyable life cannot be measured only in terms of longevity. We have only to consider the chronic pain victim whose every movement produces disabling pain to know that life must be a careful balance between quantity and quality. While heart disease, hypertension, cancer, leukemia, and other well-known problems certainly interrupt the quantity of life, chronic pain is gaining recognition as a major social, personal, industrial, and economic disruption in the quality of life.

It is unfortunate that if the average person on the street were to be asked about chronic pain, it is likely that he or she would have little or nothing to say. Ask the same person about alcoholism, however, and you will probably hear about the very serious ramifications of this disease. Yet the annual expenditure on chronic pain is estimated at over $65 billion whereas the expenditure on alcoholism, a far more publicized disease, is estimated at approximately $30 billion (Tollison & Kriegel, 1989). Despite ranking behind only heart disease and cancer as our nation's third greatest health care problem (Tollison, 1987), chronic pain remains a national mystery. Many of us who work in the field of chronic pain share with our patients a mounting frustration over the national inattention and ignorance of one of our most costly, disrupting, and distressing health problems—chronic pain.

In order to examine the magnitude of the phenomenon we term chronic pain, we will briefly address three different aspects: prevalence, economic impact, and the psychosocial impact of pain. Our objective is not to compile a statistical volume, but rather to present an overview of the magnitude of pain and a data base from which practitioners may clinically approach the problem.

PREVALENCE

Seventy-five to 80 million people in the United States are estimated to suffer chronic pain, and this is generally considered a conservative estimate (Kotarba, 1983). Millions of these individuals are either partially or totally disabled from social and vocational pursuits. Chronic low back pain, for example, affects almost 31 million Americans and represents the most common cause of disability in persons less than 45 years of age (White & Gordon, 1982). Striking victims during their most productive years, low back pain accounts for more than 8 million physician office visits annually and some 89 million workdays lost each year (Taylor & Curran, 1985). Twenty percent of all occupational injuries involve the back and research suggests that six percent of Americans will suffer a back injury during their lives that will disable them for six months or longer (Nordby, 1981). Finally, it is interesting that the incidence of low back pain is reportedly increasing at a rate 14 times faster than the growth of the population (Taylor & Curran, 1985).

The alarming incidence of chronic pain is not restricted to the lumbar spine. Twenty to 50 million Americans suffer arthritis pain, and 600,000 new cases of arthritis are diagnosed each year (Arthritis Foundation, 1976). Workers lose almost 108 million workdays annually because of multiple joint pain, including arthritis.

The most prevalent of all painful disorders is, however, headaches. Headaches strike 70 to 80 percent of the American population at least once per month (Tollison & Tollison, 1982). Of those suffering more frequent headaches, over 15 million Americans are believed to suffer from migraine, while another 25 million are affected by muscle contraction headaches (Tollison & Tollison, 1982). American workers lose close to 157 million workdays each year due to headache pain, an affliction that also represents the most frequent cause of school absenteeism (Taylor & Curran, 1985).

ECONOMIC IMPACT

There is also a second element of pain that can be objectively measured. The economic impact of pain, particularly chronic pain, is impressive and growing.

The annual cost of chronic pain includes the expense of medical diagnostics and treatment, compensation for lost wages, lost productivity, personnel replacement costs, and others (Snook, 1987). Medical costs and lost wages are frequently covered by various types of insurance. In the United States there are three major types of disability insurance: Social Security disability insurance (a federal program), workers' compensation insurance (usually a state regulated program), and private health insurance. Most of our information on the economic impact of pain comes from insurance statistics.

Chronic low back pain is not only one of the most frequently occurring pain disorders, it is also one of the most expensive. Chronic back pain is estimated to cost $16 billion annually in the United States, and a large percentage of back injuries fall within the domain of workers' compensation. Back injuries, for example, represent 20 percent of all reported occupational injuries, yet account for over 32 percent of workers' compensation expenditures (Snook, 1987). Additional occupational research suggests that back injuries and pain cost an average of $15,000 per incident, and that 10 percent of the reported cases represent 79 percent of the total costs (Snook, 1987).

The most comprehensive estimate of annual back pain costs was published in 1984 by Holbrook and his colleagues for the American Academy of Orthopaedic Surgeons (Holbrook, et al., 1984). The primary data sources were three surveys conducted by the National Center of Health Statistics: (1) the 1977 National Health Interview Survey, (2) the 1977 National Hospital Discharge Survey, and (3) the 1977 National Ambulatory Medical Care Survey. All costs were adjusted to 1984 dollars and represented an estimated total cost of back pain of $16 billion. Inpatient services represented the largest portion of direct costs. The authors reported that physician fees and drug costs were relatively high when compared with other musculoskeletal conditions, indicating greater dependence on surgical specialists and widespread use of prescription medicines.

An interesting study of compensable back pain costs was published in 1981 by Liberty Mutual Insurance Company (Antonakes, 1981). The author reported that Liberty Mutual paid over $217 million for workers' compensation back injuries in 1980, or almost one million dollars for every working day. At that time, Liberty Mutual represented approximately nine percent of the insured workers' compensation market, while the entire insurance industry represented approximately 52 percent of the total market. The remainder of the market was represented by state and federal funds (35 percent) and selfinsurers (13 percent). Assuming that other insurance carriers had similar experiences as Liberty Mutual, and the total workers' compensation cost of back pain in the United States can be estimated at $46 billion.

Given the incidence and costs associated with chronic pain, most American employers have considered workers' compensation insurance to be a necessary cost of conducting business. Research would substantiate this opinion, particularly with regard to back pain. It has been calculated, for example, that in order to offset a minor $500 compensation loss if paid directly out of company profits rather than insurance (Anonymous, 1984):

- A restaurant must serve 1,940 lunches at $3.00 each
- A supermarket must ring up 1,540 sales of $25.00 each
- An electronics factory must build 20 color television sets at $400 each
- A bakery must sell 47,620 loaves of bread at 75 cents a loaf

- A garment manufacturer must sell 640 men's shirts at $15.00 each
- A publisher must sell 25,315 newspapers at 25 cents each
- A furniture manufacturer must make 120 chairs at $50.00 each
- A tool maker must manufacture 910 hammers at $10.00 each
- A department store must sell 12,500 pairs of boys socks at $1.25
- An appliance factory must make 1,350 electric irons at $10.00 each

The economic impact of chronic pain can also be measured by investigating the cost of analgesic medication. Analgesic medicines represent the largest volume sales category of all prescription and over-the-counter drug sales alike. Research suggests that over $900 million is spent each year in our country on nonprescription pain-reducing drugs, and over $100 million is spent on aspirin alone (Tollison, 1987). To put the figures for aspirin alone in perspective, consider that Americans swallow 20,000 tons of aspirin a year, or 225 tablets for every man, woman, and child. The total cost of chronic pain in America is estimated at between $65$70 billion a year (Tollison, 1987). Consider that this estimate equates to over $330 per year for every man, woman, and child in the United States.

PSYCHOSOCIAL IMPACT

Chronic pain is not a terminal condition but rather an illness that extends over time and one that has substantial impact on all aspects of human functioning—psychological, social, vocational, and behavioral— as well as physical. The extent of objectively measured physical impairment experienced by victims of chronic pain may vary with the nature of the pain syndrome and the extent of pathology. The extent of disability (or the human response to impairment) is, however, not always directly proportional to the extent of tissue or structural damage. Moreover, chronic pain patients have typically been subjected to numerous medical and surgical interventions, largely without success. The "average" chronic pain patient treated at one interdisciplinary pain treatment center, for example, is described as a 42-year-old male with complaints of lower back pain lasting over three years who is vocationally disabled, has failed to respond to an average of 1.86 surgeries, is taking 1.92 analgesic medications (including narcotics), has consulted an average of 6.8 health care providers, and who is clinically depressed (Tollison et al., 1989).

On the basis of such extensive adjustive demands and the failures of the health care system to alleviate the complaints of pain, it is hardly surprising that most chronic pain victims suffer significant emotional difficulties, impairment of integrated functioning, demoralization, depression, and global psychosocial impact.

It is generally accepted that the majority of chronic pain victims suffer depression and, in fact, considerable research exists in support of that assumption. While the prevalence of depression in the general population has been estimated to range from nine to 14 percent (Comstock & Helsing, 1976), the typical rates of depression in chronic pain patients has been estimated to range from 30 to 100 percent (Turk et al., 1987).

Blumer and Heilbronn (1982), in an extension of Engel's model (Engel, 1959), attempt to explain the relationship between chronic pain and depression by hypothesizing that chronic pain represents a muted depressive state in a painprone individual. According to this model, pain and depression are viewed as manifestations of a single, common disease process. Specifically, the painprone disorder is considered as a masked "depressive equivalent . . . the prime expression of a muted depressive state" (p. 381). According to Blumer and Heilbronn, there are four core clinical features of the painprone personality: (2) somatic complaints (continuous complaints of obscure origin, hypochondriacal preoccupation, desire for surgery); (2) "solid citizen" mentality (denial of conflicts, idealization of self and family relations, ergomania, prepain workaholism, and relentless activity); (3) depression (post-pain anergia, lack of initiative, inactivity, fatigue, anhedonia, inability to enjoy social life and sex, insomnia, depressed mood, and despair; and (4) history (family or personal history of depression and alcoholism, past abuse of spouse, crippled relative, relative of chronic pain).

A variety of other hypothetical models exist that attempt to explain the relationship between pain and depression, but it is the existence of the relationship and not the theoretical explanation that directly impacts the patient. While psychological factors are known to influence pain expression, the burden of pain itself can produce profound emotional distress. Recognition that the psyche and soma are interrelated in complex ways is the basis for much painrelated research and promise for more effective future clinical practice.

SUMMARY

Chronic pain remains one of the most prevalent, challenging, and influential problems facing our society. Its impact is widespread, from the individual pain victim, family, friends, and community, to an economic influence on business, industry, and even our national health care system. While both prevalence and cost of pain continue to escalate, so too does the personal devastation of pain upon the victim.

There is, however, hope and promise for the future. With increasing public and scientific attention being directed to pain — its victims and its impact — is the expectation of more effective clinical management of one of mankind's oldest maladies. In the subsequent chapters of this text, the interdisciplinary diagnosis and treatment of pain will be carefully explored and outlined. As health care providers with an interest in pain, our responsibilities have been poignantly summarized by Albert

Schweizer: "We must all die. But that I can save (a person) from days of torture, that is what I feel as my great and even new privilege. Pain is a more terrible lord of mankind than even death itself."

REFERENCES

Anonymous (1984). What does a work injury really cost. *Journal of American Insurance, 2*, 6.

Antonakes, J. A. (1981). Claims costs of back pain. *Best's Review, 9*, 36.

Arthritis Foundation. (1976). *Arthritis.* Atlanta: American Arthritis Foundation.

Blumer, D., & Heilbronn, M. (1982). Chronic pain as a variant of depressive illness. The painprone disorder. *Journal of the Nervous and Mental Disease, 170*, 381-406.

Comstock, G. W. & Helsing, K. J. (1976). Symptoms of depression in two communities. *Psychological Medicine, 6*, 551-563.

Engel, G. L. (1959). Psychogenic pain and the pain prone patient. *American Journal of Medicine, 26*, 899-918.

Holbrook, T. L., Grazier, K., Kelsey, J. L., & Stauffer, R. N. (1984). *The frequency of occurrence, impact, and cost of selected musculoskeletal conditions in the United States.* Park Ridge, Illinois: American Academy of Orthopaedic Surgeons.

Kortaba, J. R. (1983). *Chronic pain: It's social dimensions.* Beverly Hills, California: Sage.

Nordby, E. J. (1981). Epidemiology and diagnosis in low back injury. *Occupational Health and Safety, 50*, 38-42.

Snook, Stover H. (1987). The costs of back pain in industry. In R. A. Deyo (Ed.), *Occupational Back Pain* (p.1). Philadelphia: Hanley and Belfus.

Taylor, H. & Curran, N. M. (1985). *The nuprin pain report.* New York: Louis Harris.

Tollison, C. D. (1982). Chronic benign pain: An innovative program for South Carolina. *Journal of The South Carolina Medical Association*, 379-383.

Tollison, C. D. (1987). *Managing chronic pain.* New York: Gardner Press.

Tollison, C. D. & Kriegel, M. L. (1989). *Interdisciplinary rehabilitation of low back pain.* Baltimore: Williams and Wilkins.

Tollison, C. D. & Tollison, J. W. (1982). *Headache: A multimodal program for relief.* New York: Sterling Publishing.

Tollison, C. D., Kriegel, M. L., Satterthwaite, J. R., Hinnant, D. W., & Turner, K. P. (1989). Comprehensive pain center treatment of low back workers compensation injuries. *Orthopaedic Review, 10*, 1115-1126.

Turk, D. C., Rudy, T. E., & Stieg, R. L. (1987). Chronic pain and depression. *Pain Management, 1*, 17-25.

White, A. A. & Gordon, S. L. (1982). Synopsis: Workshop on idiopathic low back pain. *Spine, 7*, 141-149.

Chapter 2

THE HISTORY OF PAIN MANAGEMENT

C. Norman Shealy, M. D., Ph. D., D. Sc.
Roger K. Cady, M. D.

Doctors Shealy and Cady trace the early references of pain control attempted by the Chinese, Egyptians, and Arabians. Treatment included: exercise, heat, massage, opium, natural herbs, and electrical stimulation. The first major innovation in pain treatment, nitrous oxide, is attributed to the work of Joseph Priestley. Advances in neurophysiology during the 19th century included discoveries of codeine, aspirin, ether, needles and syringes, hypnosis, and neurosurgical ablative techniques.

The reader will better understand the theory of specific nerve energy, pattern theory, psychological theory, and the gate theory in their historical contribution to our understanding of pain transmission. A detailed listing of developments in the pain field are chronologically presented in chart form.

A deposition on this topic is included in the Appendix section entitled, "Depositions."

Chapter 2
THE HISTORY OF PAIN MANAGEMENT

C. Norman Shealy, M. D., Ph. D., D. Sc.
Roger K. Cady, M. D.

Most people fear death less than they fear continuing pain. Indeed, many individuals who commit suicide during terminal or potentially fatal illnesses do so to avoid pain to themselves, and philosophically to spare their families psychological suffering. Bonica (1990) has estimated that 15-20% of the population have acute pain and 25-30% have some form of chronic pain. The Nuprin Pain Report (1986) suggests that pain affects a huge majority of Americans each year. Obviously any consideration of pain has to begin with an understanding that pain is a natural part of life, and has been a major factor in human development throughout time. Prehistorical evidence through archaeological findings suggests that the most primitive of populations suffered from diseases which would be expected to involve pain, and in every civilization in the history of the world there are numerous references to the plague of pain. The concept of counter-stimulation through rubbing, massaging, or pressure on painful points or around painful areas probably had been used throughout history. Theory and management have indeed evolved together.

At least 4,500 years ago the Chinese already had a well-developed system of pain management—acupuncture. Competent pain medicine clinicians today recognize that acupuncture remains one of the most powerful treatments for both acute and chronic pain. Although we are not as certain of the details involved, it is equally certain that the Chinese used herbs, and very early in their history, opioids or narcotics.

In recorded history the ancient Egyptians chronologically stand next in line. The Egyptians appear to have believed that pain was inflicted by either God or a disincarnate spirit, and as in India, the Egyptians considered the heart to be the center of sensation. The ancient Indians attached much more significance to the emotional roots for pain. Looking forward in history, the ancient Greeks introduced the concept that the brain was the organ in which sensation became conscious, although that concept, introduced by Alcmaeon, was vigorously fought by Aristotle who considered the heart the center of sensation. Hippocrates, the "father of medicine", had a concept that was very similar to the Chinese five element theory, except that the Chinese included only four humors: blood, phlegm, yellow bile, and black bile. An excess or deficiency in one of the humors was supposed to lead to pain. Eventually the reality of the brain as the seat of sensation did succeed, and it was the ancient Greeks who demonstrated that the brain and the peripheral nerves were intimately connected, and that there were two types of nerves, those for muscle control and those for sensation. Ancient Rome added relatively little to the concept of pain, but Galen demonstrated the central and peripheral nervous system as well as cranial and spinal nerves and sympathetic trunks. Even then Galen continued to follow Aristotle's concept of pain being "a passion of the soul".

The center of civilization moved to Arabia approximately 1,000 years ago where Avicenna described 15 different types of pain and treatment, including exercise, heat, massage, opium, and other natural herbal remedies. Paracelsus, who died only 450 years ago, advocated the use of opium and natural herbs, but added various electrical stimulation techniques, massage, and exercise.

Remarkably, even William Harvey, who described the circulation of the blood, considered the heart to be the site where pain was felt. Descartes, who is often attacked by holistic philosophers as the individual who tore the body and mind apart, nevertheless made great contributions to the concept of pain. Unfortunately, as with much early philosophy, he was rather inaccurate. He considered that pain was a direct transfer through a tubular structure, and that strong impulses were transferred directly from the periphery to the brain. He is credited as essentially having created the first "specificity" therapy for pain transmission.

Although opium and undoubtedly alcohol were used as analgesics from very early times, in many cultures exorcism and various religious ceremonies were also an integral aspect of pain control. Nevertheless, many early cultures used surgical trephination of the skull for headache; and acupuncture, moxibustion, massage, physical exercise, and diet have all been used for pain control in a variety of cultures. In ancient Egypt, Greece, and Rome, electric shock was used for the treatment of gout, headache, and neuralgia, through the use of the electric fish.

The first major innovation in pain treatment in almost 2,000 years occurred in the late 18th century when Joseph Priestley introduced nitrous oxide, and it was later found to be a significant analgetic. Throughout the 19th century great progress was made in neurophysiology in general, and pain physiology in particular. Johannes Muller introduced "The Doctrine of Specific Nerve Energies" in 1840.

Other important 19th century innovations were the isolation of morphine from crude opium, and discoveries of codeine, aspirin, ether, needles and syringes, cocaine (especially as a local anesthetic), hypnosis, the first neurosurgical procedures for ablation of peripheral nerves of the spinal cord in the management of pain, electrotherapy, hydrotherapy, diathermy, and the introduction of x-ray, both for diagnostic and therapeutic purposes.

During the mid to latter portion of the 19th century the specificity theory became the dominant concept of most scientists. Just as Galen, Avicenna, Descartes and Muller had theorized, specificity seemed to consolidate the idea of specific pathways and specific receptors for pain. It is interesting that as early as 1858, Schiff had demonstrated analgesia by sectioning of the anterior quadrants of the spinal cord of an animal, and it was over 50 years later that a clinician in Philadelphia introduced the concept of spinal cordotomy in the human being. Von Frey (1894) discovered specific end organ receptors for pain and touch and expanded Muller's concept to include warmth and cold.

The origin of the pattern theory, another dominant pain theory, was introduced by Goldscheider (1894) who believed that certain patterns of nerve activation were produced by summation of sensory input from the skin in the dorsal horn. This theory was more formalized when Nafe (1934) introduced the concept that all sensation is the result of the patterns spatially and temporally of nerve impulses rather than being the result of specific receptors or pathways. Building upon this, Sinclair (1955) and Weddell (1955) emphasized that all fiber endings, except those innervating hair follicles, are similar and that it is only the pattern that is important in sensory discrimination. Unfortunately, both the specificity and the pattern theories were incomplete.

Hardy, Wolff, and Goodell (1952) objected to the pattern and specificity theories and insisted that there was a difference between reception of pain and reaction to pain, and they perhaps more than any authors of their time, introduced the concept of major cognitive psychological, emotional factors important in chronic pain management. There are numerous other minor theories related to pain, but the next major innovation and that which sparked the most intense change in management of pain in the past 5,000 years was that of gate control.

Melzack and Wall (1965) introduced the theory that the information coming in over C-fibers is modulated through presynaptic inhibition from incoming Beta fibers in the substantia gelantinosa. This "gating" mechanism depends upon the relative quantity of information coming in over the larger fibers versus the smaller fibers. Thus, there are two major ways in which pain "gets through" the gate: either through damage to the Beta fibers which allows spontaneous pain or sensory deprivation pain, or there is activation of the C-fibers by excess stimulation through inflammation or pressure upon the C-fibers (Fig. 1).

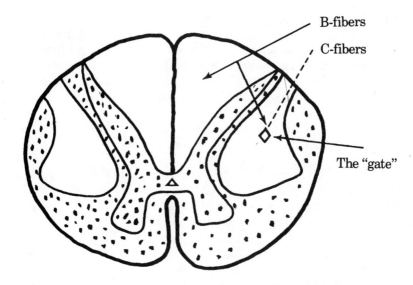

Fig. 1. The dorsal columns are "pure" projections of Beta fibers. The gate is closed by increased input of Beta fibers and opened by excessive "C" fiber activity.

Later work by Shealy (1966) demonstrated physiologically that approximately 60% of C-fiber activity is crossed to the opposite side (Fig. 1) of the spinal cord and distributed fairly diffusely in all parts of the spinal cord except the dorsal columns. That is, 60% of the total volume of central distribution of C-fiber activation goes contralaterally, not into the spinothalamic tracts, but throughout the entire gray and white matter of the cord other than the dorsal columns; and 40% is similarly distributed ipsilaterally. Strong stimulation of Beta fibers is capable of inhibiting at this initial spinal gate the activity from the dorsal columns (Shealy, 1966, 1967).

It appears that the major contribution to the spinothalamic tracts is the input from the gamma-delta fibers which primarily bring in acute or sharp brief pain as well as touch, vibratory sensation, etc. The dominant role of the dorsal columns seems to be something like an FM radio station, modulating input from the other sensory fibers.

Shealy (1966, 1967), after discussing the gate control theory with Wall and Melzack, reasoned that stimulation of the dorsal columns would conceivably antidromically inhibit the gate; and he demonstrated this initially in animals and later in human beings. Both Melzack and Wall, in their original theory, emphasized that there were descending controls of the gates coming from the cortex and other central brain locations as well as the peripheral control through the Beta fibers. Shealy (1967) had demonstrated adequate safety of long-term stimulation of the dorsal columns, in cats and monkeys, to insert the first dorsal column stimulator in a human being suffering from terminal metastatic cancer.

In 1967, Shealy resurrected an old external electrical stimulator, the Electreat (R), and began encouraging the engineers at Medtronic, Inc., to make a modern solid state electrical stimulator. Shealy, working in collaboration with Long, and each working independently, prompted Norman Hagfers who left Medtronic to form StimTec, Inc., and Donald Maurer, at that time still with Medtronic, to produce the first two solid state transcutaneous electrical nerve stimulators. Shealy had already demonstrated the two most useful types of electric current for pain relief were either the spike or the square wave. Various TENS devices began to be introduced in the early in 1970s, and have used both square waves and spikes, although most current ones use some form of modified square wave. The largest known collection of material related to the use of electrical stimulation for various purposes is the Bakken Library of Electricity and Light, 5337 Zenith Avenue, South Minneapolis, MN 55416. Earl Bakken is one of the co-founders and is the Chief Executive of Medtronic, Inc.

In 1969, following Shealy's presentation of the results in his first eight cases of dorsal column stimulation, a national Dorsal Column Study Group was formed, the purpose being to have a number of neurosurgeons doing the procedure and monitoring results over a five-year period. Sweet declined joining the Dorsal Column Study Group and, as a result of that, two companies began manufacturing dorsal column stimulators, Medtronic and Avery. During the next few years the Dorsal Column Study Group inserted approximately 480 dorsal column stimulators. In the fall of 1972, Avery began advertising dorsal column stimulators as a therapeutic technique for all neurosurgeons, and in the spring of 1973, Medtronic followed suit.

Unfortunately, in going from a research project to a clinical application, the design of the electrodes was changed from a solid platinum plate to a tinsel wire electrode. The solid platinum plate electrodes had proven remarkably sturdy and efficacious. Numerous problems developed with the tinsel wire electrodes which seemed to polarize and develop increased impedance or break fairly easily. The thickness of the machine-made electrodes was also greater than that of the solid platinum plate which led to increased technical difficulties. As a result, Shealy permanently stopped doing dorsal column stimulation in 1974 because he reasoned that the technology had not been adequately researched to make it a widely clinically useful procedure. Shealy, in his first paper on dorsal column stimulation, had emphasized the possibility of inserting dorsal column stimulators percutaneously, and it is worth noting that today a variety of percutaneous dorsal column stimulators are available with less risk than the totally surgically implanted ones requiring a laminectomy.

Nevertheless, the long-term success rate is so great that Shealy still considers dorsal column stimulation to be a technique that is rarely indicated, and only in extremely desparate situations.

The same year that Shealy presented his first paper on the experimental results of dorsal column stimulation, Fordyce (1976) introduced the concept of behavioral modification or operant conditioning for management of pain. This concept will be discussed in the chapter on pain clinics.

In 1970, Shealy recognized that he was selecting only 6% of the patients sent to him for dorsal column stimulation, and began investigating the possibility of alternative solutions to pain management in the vast majority of such patients. In 1971 he visited Fordyce's program. Fordyce had treated approximately 100 patients with his two-month inpatient behavioral modification program, working with one to four patients at a time. Shealy returned from that visit to establish an intensive active behavioral modification program working with up to 25 patients at a time. In 1972, Shealy organized a national meeting on the management of pain, some 400 individuals attended that meeting; and as a result of that, several of the physicians set up similar multidisciplinary, comprehensive pain clinics, modeled after the Shealy system. Over the next few years, increasing numbers of physicians established various types of pain clinics.

In 1976, *Medical World News* presented a cover article, "Pain Clinics, Medicine's New Growth Industry." That article suggested that there were approximately 50 pain clinics in the country, 20 of which *Medical World News* considered "holistic," with the others based upon the Bonica model. Following that cover article, pain clinics indeed did become one of medicine's growth industries. By 1977, Bonica reported at the Walter Reed Pain Symposium that there were some 800 pain clinics in the country.

Shealy's (1976) active behavioral modification program was transformed in 1974 to a greater emphasis on biofeedback, autogenic training, and self-regulation technique as a major modality for changing behavior. Although there have been some refinements in techniques and technology during the past 10 years, there has been no further major innovation in the management of pain. Thus, as we enter the 1990s, quantum leaps in management of pain have been made in the last 25 years through the introduction of transcutaneous and percutaneous electrical nerve stimulation, to some extent implanted electrical stimulators, and through the use of biofeedback, autogenic training, and related techniques for behavioral modification. The implications and results of these techniques will be discussed in greater detail in the chapter on multidisciplinary pain clinics.

The innovations in pain management sparked by the gate control theory have led also to a number of new organizations and pain-related publications.

Some Major American-Based Organizations Related To Pain:

American Association for the Study of Headache
International Association for Study of Pain - 1974
American Pain Society
  Regional Pain Societies
  Eastern, Midwestern, etc.
American Academy of Pain Medicine
  (Originally American Academy of Algology)
American Academy of Pain Management

Some Major Publications Related To Pain:

Pain
Headache
Clinical Journal of Pain
Anesthesia & Analgesia—Current Research
Pain Practitioner

Chart 1. The History of Pain Treatment

2600 + B.C.
  Acupuncture
  Massage
  Exercise
  Opium
  Alcohol
  Herbs
  Witch Doctors
  Medicine Men
  Prayer
  Exorcism
  Sacrifices
  Religious Ceremonies

18th Century
  Mesmerism
  Electrotherapy (Crude)

19th Century
  Nitrous Oxide (into medical & dental field in 1863)
  Hypnosis
  Muller's Specificity Theory
  Morphine
  Codeine
  Aspirin (introduced in 1899 by Dreser)
  Diethyl Ether (1846)

Needle/Syringe
Cocaine (1884)
Opioid Narcotics
  Opium (1806 by Serturner)
  Codeine (1832 by Robiguet)
  Papaverine (1848 by Merck)
Local Anesthetics (Cocaine)
Physical Therapy
Hydrotherapy
Thermotherapy (Diathermy)
Mechanotherapy
X-Ray for Diagnosis & Therapy
Electrotherapy

20th Century
Procaine (introduced in 1905 by Einhorn)
Pattern Theory
Cordotomy
Lobotomy
Gate Control Theory
Dorsal Column Stimulation
TENS
Biofeedback
Operant Conditioning
Multidisciplinary Pain Clinics
Neurotomy/Neurectomy
Modern Anesthetics
Narcotic Agonists/Antagonists
Non-steroidal Anti-inflammatories
Steroids
Thalamic Stimulation

W. A. OLDS.
ELECTRICAL TREATMENT APPARATUS.
APPLICATION FILED AUG. 17, 1914.

1,207,614.

Patented Dec. 5, 1916.
2 SHEETS—SHEET 1.

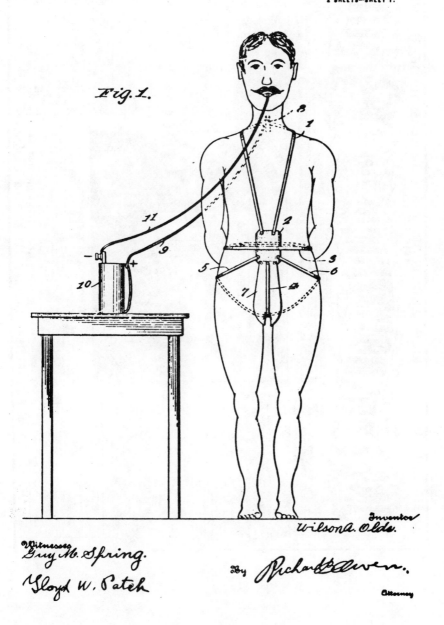

Fig. 1.

Witnesses
Guy M. Spring.
Lloyd W. Patch

Inventor
Wilson A. Olds.

By Richard B. Owen.

Attorney

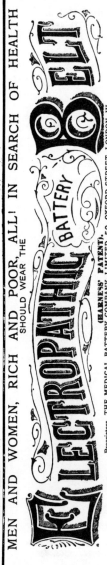

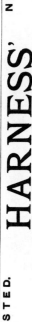
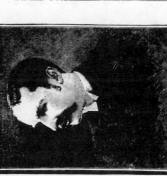

REFERENCES

Bonica, J. J. (1990). *The management of pain, Vol. 1.* (2nd ed.) p. 2. Philadelphia: Lea & Febiger.

Fordyce, W. (1976). *Behavioral models for chronic pain and illness.* St. Louis, MO: The C. V. Mosby Co.

Goldscheider, A. (1894). *Ueber den schmerz im physiologischer und klinischer hinsicht.* Berlin: Hirschwald.

Hardy, J. D., Wolff, H. G., & Goodell, H. (1952). *Pain sensations and reactions.* Baltimore: Williams & Wilkins.

Melzack, R., & Wall, P. D. (1965). Pain mechanisms: A new theory. *Science, 150*:871.

Nafe, J. P. (1934). The pressure, pain, and temperature senses. In C. A. Murchison (Ed.), *Handbook of general experimental psychology.* Worchester, MA: Clark University Press.

Nuprin Pain Report (1986).

Shealy, C. N., Tyner, C. F., & Taslitz, N. (1966). Physiological evidence of bilateral spinal projections of pain fibers in cats and monkeys. *Journal of Neurosurgery, 24*:708-713.

Shealy, C. N. (1966). The physiological substrate of pain. *Headache, 6*:101-108, October.

Shealy, C. N., Taslitz, N., Mortimer, J. T., & Becker, D. P. (1967). Electrical inhibition of pain: Experimental evaluation. *Anesthesia and Analgesia—Current Research. 46*:299-305.

Shealy, C. N., Mortimer, J. T., & Reswick, J. B. (1967). Electrical inhibition of pain by dorsal column stimulation: preliminary clinical report. *Anesthesia and Analgesia—Current Research. 46*:489-491.

Shealy, M. C., & Shealy, C. N. (1976). Behavioral techniques in the control of pain: A case for health maintenance vs. disease treatment. In Matisyohu Weisenberg & Bernard Tursky (Eds.), *Pain: New perspectives in therapy and research.* New York: Plenum Press.

Sinclair, D. C. (1955). Cutaneous sensation in the doctrine of specific nerve energy. *Brain, 78*:584.

von Frey, M. (1894). Ber. Verhandl. konig. sachs. Ges. Wiss. Leipzig. *Beitrage zur Physiologie des Schmerzsines, 46*:185, 188.

Weddell, G. (1955). Somesthesis in chemical senses. *Annual Review of Psychology, 6*: 119.

ANNOTATED BIBLIOGRAPHY

Abbe, R. (1911). Resection of posterior roots of spinal nerves to relieve pain, pain reflex, athetosis, and spastic paralysis - Dana's operation. *Medical Records, New York, 79*:377-381.
    The first spinal rhizotomies were done by Abbe.

Anstie, F. E. (1873). Papers on electrotherapy: No. 1 - On the relations of faradic electricity to pain. *The Practitioner: A Journal,* **pp. 2,351-2,360.**
Francis E. Anstie published an article on the relations of faradic electricity to pain in London in 1873.

Behan, Richard J. (1922). *Pain: It's origin, conduction, perception, and diagnostic significance.* **New York: Appleton and Co.**
This is a good early treatise.

Bonica, J. J. (1967). *Management of intractable pain.* **In E. L. Way (Ed.),** *Concepts of pain* **(pp. 155-167). Philadelphia: Davis.**
Bonica has emphasized the necessity for the use of a nerve block to determine if the surgical procedure would yield the desired results.

Bonica, J. J. (1976). Recent studies on the nature and management of acute pain. *Hospital Practice,* **January, 6-7.**
According to John Bonica, the use of narcotics as analgesics for nonsurgical pain and for surgical anesthesia goes back "2,000, 3,000 or 4,000 years." Morphine was isolated 170 years ago.

Bonica, J. J. (1990). *The management of pain, Vol. 1* **(2nd ed.). Philadelphia: Lea & Febiger.**
"There is only one pain that is easy to bear," said the French surgeon Rene Leriche, "and that is the pain of others."

Braunwald, E., Epstein, S. E., Glick, G., Wechsler, A. S., & Braunwald, W. S. (1967). Relief of angina pectoris by electrical stimulation of the carotid-sinus nerves. *New England Journal of Medicine, Vol. 227,* **pp. 1,278-1,283.**
Perhaps the first use of implanted stimulators for relief of pain was that of carotid sinus nerve stimulation which relieved the pain of angina.

Brockbank, W. (1954). *Ancient therapeutic arts.* **London: Heinemann.**
The Eber's Papyrus written about 1500 B.C. has one of the first written records of treatment of pain. For "suffering in the abdomen" they recommended an enema of oil and honey. It is interesting to me that at the Massachusetts General Hospital, when I was a resident, milk and molasses enemas were sometimes recommended.

Brockbank, W. (1954). *Ancient therapeutic arts.* **London: Heinemann.**
Cupping seems to have been practiced in primitive cultures for thousands of years, and Hippocrates mentions it as being practiced 400 years B.C. The American Indians used a buffalo horn for cupping.

Leeching is mentioned at least 200 years B.C., and was an important part of medical and lay healing technique of many centuries, in fact, it is still done in some third world countries. Blistering also seems to have been used for many years, and there are written accounts of the use of blistering appearing in the second century A.D.

Brockbank, W. (1954). *Ancient therapeutic arts*. London: Heinemann.

Hippocrates is quoted as having said, "Those diseases which medicines do not cure, iron cures (meaning the knife). Those which iron cannot cure, fire cures, and those which fire cannot cure to be reckoned wholly incurable."

Fordyce, W. E. (1976). *Behavioral methods for chronic pain and illness*. St. Louis: C. V. Mosby Company.

Fordyce created the concept of behavioral responses of operant conditioning as the major underlying causes for pain. The Fordyce concept is that pain is a learned or conditioned response to a given stimulus or "operant" condition. "Respondents can therefore be said to be controlled by antecedent stimuli. Operants, on the other hand, in contrast, are responsive to the influence of the consequences that systematically follow their occurrence. Operants can and do occur as a direct and automatic response to antecedent stimuli, as is true of respondents." In other words, punishment versus reward, benefits from particular behaviors determine whether or not they are learned and become part of the individual.

Fordyce, W. E. (1988). Pain and suffering: A reappraisal. *American Psychologist*, April, 276-283.

Fordyce has particularly emphasized the difference between pain and suffering.

Francois-Franck, C. A. (1899). Signification physiologique de la resection du sympathique dans la maladie de basedow, l'epilepsie, l'Idiotie et le glaucome. *Bull. Acad. Med. Paris*, *41*:565-594.

Sympathectomy for relief of pain was introduced by Francois-Franck.

Garrison, F. H. (1929). *History of medicine* (4th ed.). Philadelphia: Saunders.

The pattern theory has been supported by Weddell and Sinclair. A neurologist, Spiller, noted a patient with a tuberculoma of the anterior lateral quadrant of the spinal cord who lacked pain sensation on the opposite side of the body. He encouraged Frazier, a neurosurgeon in 1899 to perform a cordotomy. It was Frazier who also began sectioning roots of the fifth nerve for trigeminal neuralgia in 1901.

Hammond, B. J. (1965). *A history of electric therapy: Part one.* **World Medical Electronics.**
In 1551, Jerome Cardan differentiated between the electricity of amber and the magnetism of lode stone, and introduced a "fluid therapy of electricity which is accepted as marking the transition from supernational to physical accounts of the phenomenon."

Horsley, V., Taylor, J., & Colman, W. S. (1891). Remarks on the various surgical procedures device and the relief or cure of trigeminal neuralgia ("Tic Douloureux"). *British Medical Journal.* **Vol. 2:** 1,1139-1, 1143, 1891A; 2:1,191-1,193, 1891B; 2: 1,249-1,252, 1891C.
Victor Horsley, the great British neurosurgeon, introduced the concept of gasserian neurectomy in 1891.

Jenkner, F. L., & Schuhfried, F. (1981). Transdermal and transcutaneous electric nerve stimulation for pain: The search for an optimal wave form. *Applied Neurophsiology, 44* :5-6, pp. 330-337.
The question of the optimal wave form for electrical stimulation has never been adequately settled. Jenkner has emphasized what he considers to be an optimal wave form.

Kellaway, P. (unknown). *The part played by electric fish in the early history of bioelectricity and electrotherapy.* **McGill University, Montreal, Canada.**
This is a marvelous article on the role of the electric fish and was the William Osler Medal Essay. Comments that even in early days in this country electric fish were used and often kept in a tank on plantations to be used for pain control, and these were "much favored by the Indians and the Negros."

Letievant, J. J. E. (1873). *Traite des sections nerveuses: Physiologie pathologique, indications, procedes operatoires.* **Paris: Balliere.**
Apparently the first book on surgery pain was written by Letievant in 1873 and was primarily concerned with neurectomies for neuralgias of face and extremities.

Lytle, Loy D., Messing, R. B., Fisher, L., & Phebus, L. (1975). Effects of long-term corn consumption on brain serotonin and the response to electric shock. *Science, Nov. 190:* 692-694.
Hyperalgesic, which appears with tryptophan deficiency (serotonin deficiency), is well-discussed in this article.

Mann, F. (1971). *Acupuncture: The ancient chinese art of healing.* **London: William Heinemann.**

The oldest records of acupuncture date to bone etchings of 1600 B.C., and the first book on acupuncture was written about 200 B.C.

Medtronic Neuro Division (1983).

An extensive bibliography on transcutaneous electrical nerve stimulation was published by the Medtronic Neuro Division in March, 1983.

Melzack, R., & Wall, P. D. (1965). Pain mechanisms: A new theory. *Science, 150:***3699, November, pp. 971-979.**

Modern concepts of pain physiology began in 1894, with the specificity theory of von Frey. Von Frey felt that "pain is a specific modality like vision or hearing with its own central and peripheral apparatus." Goldscheider, on the other hand, maintained that "nerve impulse pattern for pain is initiated by intense stimulation of nonspecific receptors since there are no specific fibers and no specific endings."

Melzack, R., & Wall, P. D. (1965). Pain mechanisms: A new theory. *Science, 150:***3699, November, pp. 971-979.**

It was the advent of the gait control theory by Melzack and Wall which really revolutionized modern pain therapy. Their theory incorporates both physiological specialization as well as central summation and input control. Basically, they believe that at the level of the substantia gelatinosa in the spinal cord, input over the smallest fibers, C-fibers, is presymmetrically inhibited by information coming over the larger beta fibers. Beta fiber stimulation never creates a painful sensation, whereas unopposed C-fiber sensation is perceived as very agonizing pain.

Mitchell, S. W. (1872). *Injuries of nerves and their consequences.* **Philadelphia: Lippincott.**

"Perhaps few persons who are not physicians can realize the influence which long continued and unendurable pain may have upon both body and mind."

Mortimer, J. T. (1968). *Pain suppression in man by dorsal column electroanalgesia.* **Unpublished Ph.D. dissertation, School of Engineering Cleveland, Case Western Reserve University.**

The subject of pain has been likened by Mortimer to the fable of a blind man and an elephant. Each saw and interpreted the elephant only as that particular part of the subject with which the individual blind person had come in contact. Thus, pain has been viewed throughout much of history from a noncomprehensive point of view, each person and each discipline having a rather limited view of the whole.

Reynolds, D. V., & Sjoberg, A. E. (1971). (Eds.) *Neuroelectric research: Electroneuroprosthesis, electroanesthesia and non-convulsive electrotherapy.* Springfield, IL: Charles C. Thomas.
Kratzenstein, a German physicist, was probably the first modern scientist to report therapy with "electrification" in 1744. Interestingly he reported that it increased his pulse and allowed a better quality of sleep. He used it to treat partial paralysis as well.

Of course we all know the work of Benjamin Franklin, who was very cautious about interpretation. He stated, "I never saw any advantage from electricity in palsies that was permanent." In the late 1800s there was a great flurry of activity in electrotherapeutic. Rousell reported, "It is especially in the genital organs that electricity is truly marvelous. Impotence disappears, strength and desire of youth return, and the man, old before his time, whether by excesses or privations, with the aid of electrical fustigation, can become fifteen years younger." Machines as large as eight feet in diameter were used to create anelectrical static discharge. Out of this, of course, grew convulsive electroshock therapy. "Some treatments and instruments have been introduced as original as many as a dozen times since the early 1700s."

Schmidt, J. E. (1959). *Medical discoveries.* pp. 180. Springfield, IL: Charles C. Thomas.
Surgeons gradually moved higher and higher in the nervous system attempting to relieve pain with destructive procedures, and finally it was in 1950 that Mandel introduced the frontal lobotomy for the relief of intractable pain. It had been used, of course, over 10 years earlier for treatment for psychosis.

Shealy, C. N. (1974). Transcutaneous electrical nerve stimulation for control of pain. *Clinical Neurosurgery, 21* (0), pp. 269-77.

Shealy, C. N., & Mauer, D. (1974). Transcutaneous nerve stimulation for control of pain: A preliminary technical note. *Surgical Neurology, Vol. 2,* No. 1, Jan., pp. 45-47.

Smith, R. H. (1963). *Electrical anesthesia.* Springfield, IL: Charles C. Thomas.
"Safe anesthesia produced by application of electrical current has been a goal for over eighty years (in 1963!)." Russian electrosleep therapy was fully described in 1914 by Robinovitch. "Anesthesia produced by the application of electrical current has been called electronarcosis." Leduc, in 1902, published his early work with electronarcosis. He tried various frequencies of current, but mostly used 100 cycles per second of direct current square wave. Although he produced a rather cataplectic state in which the patients weren't able to move, they still were aware

of pain. Glen Smith reported successful electronarcosis in dogs over 200 times, in rhesus monkeys six times, and in the chimpanzee once.

Solomon, R. A., Vierstein, M. C., & Long, D. M. (1980). Reduction of postoperative pain and narcotic use by transuctaneous electrical nerve stimulation. (pp. 142-146). *Surgery,* **Feb.**
This is another good article to quote.

Spiller, W. G., & Martin, E. (1912). Treatment of persistent pain of organic origin in the lower part of the body by division of the anterolateral column of the spinal cord. *Journal of the American Medical Association, 158***:1,489-1,490.**
According to Sweet and White, in 1905 Spiller of Philadelphia discovered the problem with tuberculoma of pain, and Martin was the one to carry out the first successful cordotomy.

Tapio, D., & Hymes, A. C. (1987). *New frontiers in transcutaneous electrical nerve stimulation.* **Minnetonka, MN: LecTec Corporation.**
Electric eels were known by ancient Egyptians and Hippocrates as potentially useful for producing an electrical shock to control pain, but it was apparently Scribonius Largus who first the electric ray torpedic fish for treatment of both headache and gout, and recorded this in 46 A.D. William Gilbert was reported to have been the first to classify and generalize the phenomenon of electricity (1544-1603). Richard Lovett in *The Subtil Medium* proved in 1756 dozens of cures for many diseases using electricity. John Wesley, the founder of the Methodist church, was extremely enthusiastic about this treatment, and also described many examples of diseases "cured" with electrotherapy, including sciatica, headache, gout, pleuritic pain and angina pectoris. Between 1750 and 1780 there were 26 publications dealing with clinical electricity. John Birch, an English surgeon, used electrical current to control pain in 1772. Beginning in the early 1900s various electrical stimulators were sold to the public by door-to-door salesmen as well as in various catalogs. These instruments were very popular and came with all types of claims and cures, including curing cancer. The FDA banned the sale of such instruments in the early 1950s. In 1967, Shealy introduced the concept of dorsal column stimulation for control of pain, and that led to work with electromodulation.

Thorsteinsson, G., Stonnington, H. H., Stillwell, G. K., & Elveback, L. R. (1977). Transcutaneous electrical stimulation: A double-blind trial of its efficacy for pain. *Archives of Physical Medicine and Rehabilitation, 58***: 8-13.**
A number of double-blind studies have emphasized that transcutaneous electrical nerve stimulation is not a placebo.

U. S. Department of Health, Education, and Welfare (1968). National Insitutes of Health. *Pain:* **September.**
Two hundred years A.D. Galen advocated opium and mandragora as well as electrotherapy for control of pain. The first public demonstration of anesthesia on a patient was in 1846. The one important contribution to the management of pain was the development of the syringe and hypodermic needle (1845-1855). Cocaine was introduced into medical practice in 1884. Dr. William Halstead of Johns Hopkins discovered the principles of block anesthesia which was the injection of cocaine into a nerve trunk in 1884. Spinal anesthesia was introduced in 1898. In 1967, the National Institutes of General Medicine Sciences offered the first center grant to the University of Pennsylvania and in 1968 the second to Harvard University to develop "anesthesia research and training centers where teams of scientists in many disciplines worked together in studying basic molecular research to anesthesia techniques in the operating room."

White, J. C., & Sweet, W. H. (1955). *Pain: Its mechanisms and neurosurgical control.* **Springfield, IL: Charles C. Thomas.**
and
White, J. C., & Sweet, W. H. (1969). *Pain and the neurosurgeon: A forty year experience.* **Springfield, IL: Charles C. Thomas.**
In more modern times the classics were written by White and Sweet.

Wolff, H. G. (1963). *Headache: And other pain* **(2nd ed.). New York: Oxford University Press.**
Headache, one of the most common of major pain complaints was perhaps most well studied by Harold G. Wolff.

Section 2

THE ELEMENTS OF MULTIDISCIPLINARY PAIN MANAGEMENT INCLUDING CLASSIFICATION AND ASSESSMENT

Chapter 3

THE CLASSIFICATION OF PAIN

B. Eliot Cole, M.D.

Dr. Cole captures the importance of using a clear system for classifying pain. He reports that treatment options are linked to the type of pain involved and that an accurate pain classification system is essential for successful management. Accurate classification may in of itself help reduce a patient's suffering.

Within this chapter, Dr. Cole defines and discusses important major systems of taxonomy employed by clinicians who treat pain patients. The text on acute vs. chronic pain; benign vs. cancer pain; intensity and suffering; and real vs. psychogenic pains is interspersed with case examples. Dr. Cole argues in favor of a focus which blends somatic with psychosocial analyses and which also considers a review of the disruption that pain may cause the patient.

Chapter 3

THE CLASSIFICATION OF PAIN

B. Eliot Cole, M. D.

INTRODUCTION

Pain is an unpleasant sensory and emotional experience (Merskey, 1979), motivating patients to seek relief from it. Why bother to classify pain? Classifying pain is necessary for research and clinical purposes. To assess the pain complaint clinically the practitioner must be able to define the location, intensity, frequency, and duration. From this data, a working diagnosis is made and the pain is treated relative to broad categories. Researchers in the field of pain management work to expand the classification of pain, and to specifically tailor treatment for each diagnostic possibility. Clinicians and researchers must attempt to know the cause of the pain problem to understand how it is to be treated.

There is a need for the expanded classification of pain as long as patients continue to suffer from pains which we do not understand and which are inadequately treated. According to Wall (1989), pain classified by our ignorance about underlying mechanisms and therapy falls into three groups: pains where the cause is apparent but the treatment is inadequate (deep tissue disorders, peripheral nerve disorders, root and cord disorders), pains where the cause is not known but the treatment is adequate (Trigeminal neuralgia, tension headaches), and pains where the cause is not known and the treatment is inadequate (back pain, idiopathic pelvic and abdominal pain, migraine headache).

The classification of pain is a source of confusion for many clinicians, and as a result of this confusion a number of different classification systems are now commonly used by pain practitioners. Pain is classified according to the time course, the involved anatomy, the intensity, the type of patient, and the circumstances of the pathology. To be a successful pain practitioner one must be able to work with pain classifications encompassing all of these areas, and be capable of switching from one model to another. While the distinctions between one system and another may seem arbitrary, without some framework to categorize pain complaints, the unsophisticated clinician easily becomes lost in the pain behavior of the patient and the demand for quick solutions. Treatment options are linked to the type of pain involved, and accurate pain classification is essential for successful pain management. The pain conditions that the clinician cannot recognize, and accurately diagnose, cannot be satisfactorily treated.

At a more practical and human level, patients want to know if their pain will ever completely go away. Patients are frightened that their pain is attributable to unrecognized pathology and so search for the ultimate cure. Going from practitioner to practitioner serves to worsen the confusion, and the patient hopes that someone will be able to illuminate the difficulty. By being able to classify the pain into a recognizable and explainable syndrome, the pain practitioner, unlike the other clinicians, is able to offer some hope. Although treatment often does not yield a completely pain free state, understanding the basis for the pain, and knowing that some awful disease does not exist, provides significant relief from some of the suffering.

Case Example

Ms. W. was a forty-five-year-old woman who had seen a number of practitioners during the previous three years since her car accident. Physical therapy, massage therapy, acupuncture, and psychotherapy in isolation after thorough evaluation by neurologists, neurosurgeons, and orthopedic surgeons failed to produce lasting comfort. When she was referred to the pain clinic she was tense, angry, and argumentative. She was informed that she would never be completely pain free as a result of her well established myofascial pain, but could eventually resume her life if she entered a pain management program. She was surprised to learn that her pain condition had a name, was recognized by the physician as a benign process, and could respond to intradisciplinary treatment. Previous clinicians had recommended that she learn to live with the pain, but did not tell her how to do this. Although no specific therapy occurred during the evaluation in a conventional sense, she was relaxed and more comfortable when she left the office.

It is not always certain that pain can be conveniently classified into some system. Some patients will present with more than one pain problem over time, and can have the pains classified simultaneously into different categories. The chronic pain patient may experience acute painful episodes unrelated to the original pain condition, the chronic benign pain patient may develop cancer-related pain after years of marginal pain management, and the acute pain patient may experience a number of different aches and pains from the original pathophysiologic process, or as a consequence of the therapies to correct it.

ACUTE VERSUS CHRONIC PAIN

The duration of the pain process, the temporal perspective, is the most obvious distinction that is made when classifying pain. This temporal distinction is an important consideration for understanding the neurophysiology of pain (Crue, 1983). Acute pain is limited to pain of less than 30 days, while chronic pain persists for more than six months. Subacute pain describes the interval from the end of the first month to the beginning of the seventh month for continued pain. Recurrent acute pain defines a pain pattern that persists over an extended period of time, but recurs as isolated pain episodes. Chronic pain is further divided by the underlying etiology, into benign and cancer-related (Crue, 1983; Foley, 1985; Portenoy, 1988).

The primary distinction between acute and chronic pain regardless of the etiology is crucial. Acute pain is useful and serves a protective purpose. It warns of danger, limits utilization of injured or diseased body parts, and signals the departure of pathology when the limiting condition resolves. Without acute pain it is doubtful that most of us would be able to survive at all (Cousins, 1989). Chronic pain has little protective significance, persists despite normalization after injury or disease, and ultimately interferes with productive activity. The patient with chronic pain lives a full-time nightmare, where pain relief is constantly sought yet rarely obtained without professional help, and the pain controls the activities of daily living. Chronic benign pain occurs with or without adequate patient coping. The patients who cope with the chronic pain manage to live productive lives, while the patients who are not able to cope with their pain are disabled by the chronic suffering (Crue, 1983).

Acute pain is almost always self limited. When the condition resolves which produces the pain, or when the nociceptive input is blocked by a local anesthetic or altered by the use of peripheral or central analgesic medications, the pain leaves. The skin heals, the fractures mend, the inflammation subsides, and the nociceptive input stops, so the pain intensity fades away and disappears (Crue, 1983). The use of comfort measures such as applications of heat or cold, splinting, casting, or brief time limited analgesic medication all help to relieve this discomfort. Sentiments of concern and expected recovery from friends and family aid in the relief of pain for the acute pain sufferer.

Case Example

Mr. B. was a twenty-two-year-old downhill skier who sustained a shoulder dislocation in a fall. His shoulder was relocated in the field and he was placed in a shoulder immobilizer for one week. He was assured that his injury was not significant by his physician and would not interfere with his participation in an important race later in the season. After limited physical therapy to restore his range of motion and strength, he was able to resume competitive racing with no detectable difficulties.

The pain after surgery, postoperative pain, is a specific type of acute pain. It is often poorly managed because patients receive significantly less opioid analgesics than are ordered, the nursing staff are overly concerned about opioid addiction, analgesics are irrationally selected, and many physicians have inadequate knowledge about the pharmacology of analgesics (Waldman, 1990). Although postoperative pain is experienced by millions of patients throughout the world it is not recognized as producing harmful physiological or psychological effects (Cousins, 1989).

Chronic pain confuses most sufferers, because it dominates, depresses, and debilitates. If treated by using acute pain models, chronic pain may become more intense and the patient may experience increased disability and suffering. Instead of comfort measures, chronic pain is managed by the use of rehabilitative techniques when it is of a benign origin, or aggressive, supportive techniques when due to cancer.

Acute pain is reasonably managed and usually resolved by the efforts of a single practitioner. "Tincture of time," with injury or illness specific therapy, is the best remedy for acute pain. Chronic pain requires the coordinated efforts of a broadly based treatment team which can bring a number of physical and psychological strategies together. Chronic pain patients demand more effort and resources than a single, well meaning practitioner can provide. In isolation, the solo practitioner is unable to address the variety of problems that chronic pain causes, and so must resort to symptom management usually by over utilizing a single therapeutic approach.

Case Example

Ms. D. was a twenty-eight-year-old woman referred for the management of chronic, mechanical low back pain secondary to an industrial lifting injury. Her referring neurosurgeon who had been treating her unsuccessfully for three years became motivated to refer her to a pain management program when his partners began to complain about her drug seeking behavior when they were on call. A full review of her medical record revealed that she had received 3,900 oxycodone and acetaminophen tablets in the six months prior to referral. At the time of referral she was using twelve (12) to fifteen (15) of the oxycodone and acetaminophen analgesic tablets, sixty (60) milligrams of diazepam, and an uncertain number of butalbital, aspirin, and caffeine containing tablets every day to obtain pain relief. She was admitted to an outpatient chronic pain management program, and over six weeks was successfully detoxified from all medications. She returned to the work force after the program in a less physically demanding position.

Acute pain usually only briefly disables the patient during the recovery time, while chronic pain often prevents return to meaningful and gainful employment. Some chronic pain patients are not able to return to their former, high paying work due to pain-related limitations, and the unwillingness of employers who fear losing profits (Chapman & Brena, 1989). They are caught in the ridiculous position of having to maintain their disability rather than return to an entry level position with inadequate financial compensation for their needs. Legal entanglements cloud chronic benign pain problems and contribute to the inability to resolve the suffering. The desire for the best legal settlement, often the only reward for the pain problem, prevents the patients from full recovery in some cases.

It is sadly said that a sure sign that the pain problem is chronic is a letter of referral from one practitioner to another that begins with an apology. Chronic pain patients are so often viewed as angry, hostile, depressed, and manipulative, that they evoke feelings of anxiety, resentment, and desperation in the treating clinicians. A pain patient who requests that the results of the initial evaluation be sent to an attorney, should alert the pain practitioner of involvement in impending litigation. As some lawyers actually send patients for pain management assessments to strengthen the position for a claim of pain and suffering after and accident or injury, it is necessary to understand whose interests are being served by the evaluation. Patients and lawyers stand to gain more financially from a legal action if the patient does not recover from the injury (Chapman & Brena, 1989).

Subacute pain is possibly the last opportunity for a full restoration and a pain- free existence, much as acute pain, so must be recognized before the pain becomes chronic. Subacute pain is quite similar to acute pain in its etiological and nociceptive mechanisms (Crue, 1983). Once the pain has been established for more than six months, the likelihood of complete pain relief is small. The first 100 days of pain appear to respond fully to therapy and return the patients to near normality. Beyond the first 100 days, most patients still recover the majority of lost function, but do not feel fully restored or comfortable. By the time pain becomes subacute, the rehabilitative approach used for chronic pain is more appropriate than further acute pain management strategies.

Recurrent acute pain is the acute flare-up of peripheral tissue pathology due to an underlying chronic pathological entity and occurs with headaches, gastrointestinal motility disorders, degenerative disk and joint disease, collagen vascular disease and similar functional processes (Crue, 1983). Unlike chronic or subacute pain, recurrent acute pain implies discrete acute episodes which return over time. The dividing line between recurrent acute and subacute is often a judgement decision by the pain practitioner. Daily pain for several weeks is subacute pain, but several limited pain episodes over many months or years is typical of recurrent acute pain. The importance of recognizing recurrent acute pain is to apply a more comprehensive management approach of patient education, contingency planning, and family involvement than a single pain episode would ordinarily require.

BENIGN VERSUS CANCER PAIN

Pain persisting for more than six months, chronic pain, must be differentiated between cancer-related or that of a benign cause. Chronic cancer pain is generally managed for the patient, while benign pain is managed by the patient through education, empowerment, and rehabilitation. Cancer-related pain management, like acute pain management, focuses on the comfort of the patient, and involves a strategy of palliation. Palliative care involves the liberal use of medication, often opioid analgesics, with maximum comfort through symptom relief, but toxicity from therapy kept acceptable relative to the distress produced by the symptoms being addressed.

Chronic benign pain, the grist for most pain clinics, involves a number of different pathophysiologic problems which render the sufferer unable to enjoy life, but does not threaten to end life. This type of pain is described in relationship to an anatomical site, and engenders considerable anxiety. Myofascial pain, pain arising from muscle and connective tissue, accounts for a considerable amount of chronic benign pain, requires specific active therapy (stretching, trigger point injections) and corrective actions for pain relief (Travell & Simons, 1983).

Cancer pain is divided by the presumed pathophysiology into somatic, visceral, and deafferentation. This classification system focuses on the site of nociception (potential tissue damaging situations), being peripheral for somatic pain, intra-abdominal for visceral pain, and injury to afferent neural pathways for deafferentation. The pain which results from somatic processes is well localized, constant, aching or gnawing in character. The visceral pain is poorly localized by comparison, but is constant and aching in character, and is referred to cutaneous sites. Deafferentation pain is characterized by paroxysmal or burning dysésthesia, and is best managed with adjuvant medications, antidepressants, and anticonvulsants, not opioid analgesics like visceral and somatic pain (Foley, 1985).

Temporally, chronic cancer pain may worsen over time, due to the disease progression and from the various interventions (chemotherapy, radiotherapy, and surgery) used to treat the disease. The need for increasing doses of opioid analgesics is more often related to these situations, not to the rapid development of tolerance or medication abuse as many practitioners mistakenly believe. Chronic benign pain may also worsen over time, resulting in significant behavioral changes (pain behavior), and excessive use of analgesic medication.

It has been recommended by Foley (1979, 1985) to classify the cancer patients with pain into five groups: patients with acute cancer-related pain; patients with chronic cancer-related pain, due to either progression or therapy; patients with preexisting chronic benign pain and cancer-related pain, predisposed to illness behavior; patients with a chemical dependency history and cancer-related pain; actively dying patients who must be provided comfort measures (Portenoy, 1988). This system of classifying pain according to the type of patient involved allows for a rich psychosocial approach and prospective planning for the comprehensive needs of the patient, rather than narrowly focusing on a single dimension of the pain. It also explains some of the unusual situations that develop while treating cancer pain patients, such as the following:

Case Example

Mr. P. was a fifty-year-old gentleman with invasive head and neck squamous cell cancer. He had previously declined surgery but had radiation therapy one year before entering the hospice program with an ulcerated, foul-smelling neck mass. His pain was initially managed by his referring physician with acetaminophen and codeine elixir, six hundred (600) milligrams/sixty (60) milligrams every four (4) hours, and oral lidocaine two (2) percent viscous solution every four (4) hours as needed. While not appreciated at first, it became readily obvious that he had a long-standing alcohol abuse disorder. He regularly supplemented his gastric tube feedings with liberal quantities of vodka, beer, and coffee liquor. He alleged that he only used small amounts to cleanse the feeding tube, but was found to be frankly intoxicated on many occasions. When his pain became more difficult to control with codeine, after three months of hospice involvement, he was given morphine concentrate (twenty (20) milligrams/milliliter) via the gastric tube. He quickly began to abuse the morphine, and occasionally took as much as one hundred (100) to two (200) hundred milligrams at a time, when only twenty (20) to thirty (30) milligrams had been prescribed. He ultimately stopped abusing the alcohol beverages, but enjoyed the large doses of morphine at night when he wanted to sleep.

Few cancer pain patients exist in isolation, and most of these patients are cared for in some regard by concerned family members and friends. The support of the primary caregiver, with an emphasis on anticipatory bereavement, is an important element of hospice management. During the impending death of the cancer patient, the family members frequently become uncertain about their ability to provide continued care. To be able to keep the dying patient comfortable, unpleasant symptoms (nausea, vomiting, seizures, terminal restlessness) are aggressively controlled, and the caregiver is routinely provided support and respite breaks (Cole & Douglass, 1990).

INTENSITY AND SUFFERING

Benign pain is often rated along a continuum from mild to moderate to severe, but incapacitating and overwhelming become necessary qualifiers for cancer pain. The intensity of the pain is perhaps the least desirable system for classifying pain, as intensity varies for most pain patients over time, and is uniquely subjective. One pain patient might describe his pain experience as a ten, while another might feel that the same intensity of pain is only a five (using a zero to ten scale where zero signifies no pain at all and ten represents the worse pain one could ever imagine). Rather than focus on a specific amount of pain, it is more useful to look at the disruption that the pain causes the patient. Pain interfering with appetite, pleasurable activity, or sleep is more distressing than pain which leaves an otherwise intact life, regardless of the reported intensity. Over time, most patients adapt to the pain and demonstrate little or exaggerated pain behavior. Suffering, the response to the pain experience, is not necessarily linked to the intensity of the pain as much as it is to anxiety or depression (McCaffery & Beebe, 1989). One patient may suffer with modest levels of pain, while another is able to function despite high levels.

There is no way to know how much another person is in pain, and it is best to assume that the pain exists whenever a patient says it does, and is whatever the patient says it is (McCaffery & Beebe, 1989). Pain behavior is influenced and shaped by the environment, so the emphasis on function over intensity is critical for the rehabilitative approach to control chronic benign pain. Family members and significant others, by altering their response to the pain behavior are involved with helping the patient to manage the chronic pain.

REAL VERSUS PSYCHOGENIC PAIN

All pain is real to the patient, and little is to be accomplished by challenging the validity of the pain. Since pain is experienced in the mind and requires the interpretation of bodily sensations, there is a psychological overlay to every pain problem. It is artificial and absurd to try to divide pain into real or psychogenic types, especially when the distinction is based upon the treating practitioners ability to identify objective pathology. To understand the relationship between nociception and the psychological effects of acute and chronic pain, the practitioner must recognize emotional distress rather than pure nociception as a cause of pain, and understand that psychological mechanisms do intensify pain perception (Abram, 1985). An emotional reaction to pain does not mean that pain is caused by an emotional problem (McCaffery & Beebe, 1989).

Psychosomatic pain is unfortunately synonymous with imagined pain, yet this pain may be as severe and distressing as somatogenic pain (Abram, 1985). While the threshold, the point where pain is first noted, is fairly constant from person to person, the tolerance, what pain a person will endure is highly variable (Bowsher, 1983). Factors such as depression, anxiety, and motivation significantly influence the tolerance for pain, and may determine the amount of suffering and pain behavior generated. Secondary gain, any practical advantage resulting from the symptom of pain, is not malingering, the outright fabrication of pain, and does not mean that pain is psychogenic (McCaffery & Beebe, 1989).

The use of placebo medication or therapy to determine the reality of pain is highly deplorable. Since the ability to respond positively to a placebo has to do with the belief system of the patient, nothing about the reality of the pain will be learned from the use of sham therapies. The only accurate conclusion about a person who responds positively to a placebo is that he wants pain relief and that he trusts someone or something to help him (McCaffery & Beebe, 1989). Curiously, we give placebos to patients who are the least likely to respond to them, the patients we do not like, and who do not believe in our efforts. Rarely do we use placebos with the cooperative patients who could respond to them.

RESEARCH CLASSIFICATION

A complex pain classification system has been published by the International Association for the Study of Pain [IASP] (1986), and provides the clinician with descriptive lists about pain syndromes. This taxonomy defines pain syndromes, allows improved communication between clinicians and researchers, and leads to improved treatment options which are specific for each syndrome. A five axes coding scheme signifies the region of the pain, organ system, temporal characteristics and pattern of occurrence, patient's statement of intensity and duration since onset of pain, and the presumed etiology. Using the IASP classification of chronic pain the reader is able to obtain definition, site, main features, associated symptoms, laboratory findings, usual course, complications, social and physical disabilities, pathology, summary of essential features and diagnostic criteria, and differential diagnosis for most pain problems. Specific definitions with notes on usage are included, providing consistency in describing pain itself.

The IASP system is evolving and may be widely accepted over time. Presently, it is not readily utilized by clinicians or payment sources in the

United States. It is the best effort at codification available at this time. The IASP classification system allows pain syndrome diagnoses with inclusion, not exclusion criteria. Pain syndromes are diagnosed by what they are, not what they are not. Patients want to know what they have, not told to live with what their clinicians cannot diagnose.

CONCLUSION

Pain has plagued humanity as long as humans have existed. To attempt to remedy the suffering, and relieve the pain, accurate assessment and diagnosis must occur. Although many pain syndromes do not presently have specific therapies, by classifying pain into certain categories it is now possible to design treatment approaches to benefit most of our patients, and over time, hopefully, we will help the others.

REFERENCES

Abram, S. E. (1985). Pain pathways and mechanisms. *Seminars in Anesthesia, 4,* 267-274.

Bowsher, D. (1983). Pain mechanisms in man. *Resident and Staff Physician, 29,* 26-34.

Chapman, S. L., & Brena, S. F. (1989). Pain and litigation. In P. D. Wall & R. Melzack (Eds.), *Textbook of pain,* (2nd ed.), (pp. 1032-1041). Edinburgh: Churchill Livingstone.

Cole, B. E., & Douglass, M. C. (1990). Hospice, cancer pain management and symptom control. In R. S. Weiner (Ed.), *Innovations in pain management: A practical guide for clinicians.* Orlando, FL: Paul M. Deutsch Press.

Cousins, M. J. (1989). Acute and postoperative pain. In P. D. Wall & R. Melzack (Eds.), *Textbook of pain,* (2nd ed.), (pp. 284-305). Edinburgh: Churchill Livingstone.

Crue, B. L. (1983). The neurophysiology and taxonomy of pain. In S. F. Brena & S. L. Chapman (Eds.), *Management of patients with chronic pain,* (pp. 21-31). Jamaica, NY: Spectrum Publications.

Foley, K. M. (1979). Pain syndromes in patients with cancer. In J. J. Bonica & V. Ventafridda (Eds.), *Advances in pain research and therapy,* Vol. 2, (pp. 59-75). New York: Raven Press.

Foley, K. M. (1985). The treatment of cancer pain. *The New England Journal of Medicine, 313,* 84-95.

International Association for the Study of Pain (1986). Classification of chronic pain: Descriptions of chronic pain syndromes and definitions of pain terms. Pain, *supplement 3,* S1-S225.

McCaffery, M., & Beebe, A. (1989). *Pain, clinical manual for nursing practice.* St. Louis, MO: C. V. Mosby Company.

Merskey, H. (1979). Pain terms: A list with definitions and notes on usage. *Pain, 6,* 249-252.

Portenoy, R. K. (1988). Practical aspects of pain control in the patient with cancer. *Ca—A Cancer Journal for Clinicians, 38,* 327-352.

Travell, J. G. & Simons, D. G. (1983). *Myofascial pain and dysfunction: A trigger point manual.* Baltimore, MD: Williams & Wilkins.

Waldman, S. D. (1990). Acute and postoperative pain management—An idea ripe for the times. *Pain Practitioner, 2,* 4, 9-10.

Wall, P. D., (1989). Introduction. In P. D. Wall & R. Melzack (Eds.), *Textbook of pain,* (2nd ed.), (pp. 1-18). Edinburgh: Churchill Livingstone.

Chapter 4

MULTIDISCIPLINARY PAIN CLINICS

Current Status

C. Norman Shealy, M. D., Ph. D.
Roger K. Cady, M. D.

Doctors Shealy and Cady trace the movement within the pain field which has led to the multidisciplinary pain clinic. The Shealy Institute for Comprehensive Health Care is cited as an example of one of the original pain clinic models. The authors state that management of chronic pain began in earnest as a result of three innovations. These include: (1) Dr. John Bonica's efforts to promote an interdisciplinary team approach to pain control, (2) the Wall-Melzack theory for gate control of pain, and (3) Dr. Fordyce's emphasis on behavior modification.

Following a review of the developments leading up to today's pain management program, the authors then share elements crucial for pain evaluation, composition of team staffing, and modern interventions. The authors conclude that today there are many models of pain clinics ranging from specialized programs engaged in nerve blocks only, to those which provide comprehensive services. A final section describes the cost-effectiveness of comprehensive pain treatment.

Chapter 4

MULTIDISCIPLINARY PAIN CLINICS

Current Status

C. Norman Shealy, M. D., Ph. D., D. Sc.
Roger K. Cady, M. D.

The management of chronic pain began to evolve from the witch doctor approach (exorcism, drugs, and ablative surgery) to the modern concept as the result of three innovations:

1. Dr. John Bonica's concept of a multidisciplinary, interdisciplinary team approach to pain management.
2. The Wall-Melzack theory for gate control of pain.
3. Fordyce's behavioral modification or operant conditioning concept.

Bonica's concept of a multidisciplinary, interdisciplinary clinic began following World War II, and evolved over a period of 10 years or so. As late as 1960, the clinic that he had founded at the University of Washington was the major such clinic in this country, but a few other university centers were beginning to follow his model. This model is called the nerve block drug-cut psychiatry clinic because it was originally run entirely by anesthesiologists and led to an unfortunate sequence of events. Even though a group of up to 15 or 20 different health specialists were represented in the weekly reviews of patients, the initial major approach was to look at the patient who was perceived as having a reasonable physical cause of pain and as a potential anatomical specimen where one could do a peripheral or differential spinal nerve block, relieve the pain, or send the pain to the neurosurgeon for ablation of that appropriate pain pathway.

The failure of destructive neurosurgery is what led to the development of transcutaneous and dorsal column stimulation, because the only types of pain which respond to ablation successfully in the long-run are cancer pain, trigeminal neuralgia, and facet joint pain. In virtually all other situations, long-term success from neurosurgical destructive procedures is roughly less than 10 per cent.. Thus, the patients tend to have nerve blocks and destructive procedures, sometimes a second set of nerve blocks and destructive procedures, to be tried on a wide variety of drugs, and at that point told that it's, "All in your head", and sent to a psychiatrist.

Many physicians tended to believe up until at least the mid-1970s that if patients did not respond to surgical ablative surgery and hard drugs, then they must be "crazy" or seriously psychologically disturbed. On more than one occasion Shealy was told by a psychiatrist, "When you have taken care of the physical component of the pain, send the patient to me and I will take care of the psychological part." But Shealy never saw a patient with chronic pain helped by a psychiatrist. The major approach of psychiatrists has been to make patients feel either guilty that they are being an imposition on their family or society, or angry at someone. This approach simply does not work.

On the other hand, the basic concept of a true multidisciplinary, inter-disciplinary team is currently the most valid one. The model that Shealy evolved is very different from that at the University of Washington, where the primary approach has also evolved from just nerve blocks and cutting to what he would call a somewhat more comprehensive approach. At the present time in Seattle, patients have pain education, physical therapy, occupational therapy, vocational counseling, individual psychotherapy, and a modicum of relaxation therapy. The University of Washington program considers itself likely to be successful when the patient is suffering from physician-prescribed inappropriate medications, physical deactivation, depression, superstitious behaviors and beliefs about the body, and reasonable outcome goals. The educational program at the Clinic has gradually taken on many of Fordyce's concepts, as described later.

Although Bonica is responsible for the concept of a major pain clinic, Wall and Melzack's gate control theory sparked more innovation in the management of pain than any other concept in history. As a direct result of Wall and Melzack's theory, Shealy was prompted to develop dorsal column stimulation and transcutaneous electrical nerve stimulation which, by 1971, led him to start the first holistic comprehensive multimodal, multidisciplinary pain management clinic. The details of the gate control theory have already been covered in the chapter on the history of pain management.

Fordyce's concept of pain as an operant or conditioned response also has been critically important in the development of today's pain clinics. Fordyce (1976) emphasized that the "reinforcing consequences" provided by family, friends, and acquaintances, when an individual suffers from pain, often reinforce pain behavior. Individuals who have been deprived of social recognition and nurturing at a subconscious level often find the tremendous attention that they receive when they suffer from chronic illness to provide them a long-neglected nurturing-type environment. This reinforcement pattern must be brought to the patient's attention and often more forcefully to the attention of the spouse or other family members if the chronic cycle of an invalid pain status is to be broken.

In 1965, having been sent a copy of the gate control theory of pain prior to its publication, Shealy visited Pat Wall and then theorized that the most effective way to influence the gate was to stimulate the dorsal column of the spinal cord since at that anatomical level the beta fibers are separated from the C-fibers, the only place in the body where that is a significant anatomical fact. This led Shealy to the development of both dorsal column stimulation, the first patient being implanted in 1967, and at the same time the concept that transcutaneous electrical nerve stimulation would be more effective in a wider variety of people than would the implanted device.

Because of the tremendous number of patients, sent to Shealy for dorsal column stimulation, who were not candidates for the procedure because of psychological (operant or behavioral) aspects of their illness, in 1971 Shealy opened the first non-university pain clinic and the first pain clinic which offered a truly holistic approach to the concept of pain. From the beginning the policy was that they would include any safe modality, but look also at all of the social, environmental, physical, emotional, chemical, and spiritual stresses in the individual's life. The treatment program evolved from an inpatient treatment program to an outpatient model.

Starting in 1971, Shealy's program, with an inpatient active behavioral modification program rather than a passive behavioral modification program, lasted an average of 32 days of inpatient management with 25 patients in a special unit where the nurses were trained to ignore pain behavior or pain complaints. The patients were advised in advance that this would be the approach. An extremely active day was planned. The patients began at 7 o'clock in the morning following breakfast in an ambulatory dining area. During the day they were scheduled from morning until at least 7 o'clock in the evening, and often until 9 o'clock in the evening. They were assigned to walk the hall, given a number of laps with increasing laps each day, to ride a stationary bicycle for increasing minutes, and to do various other physical exercise activities. Five days a week they went to a swimming pool where they had one hour of water calisthenics. Five days a week they went to occupational therapy for an hour. Each patient had vigorous slapping massage of the area of their pain for at least five minutes four times a day, followed by at least a five minute ice rubdown of the area of pain. They had generalized mechnical vibratory massage 15 minutes four times a day, were in a whirlpool twice a day, and had a hands-on total body massage every other day.

Transcutaneous electrical nerve stimulation and acupuncture were an intimate part of pain management in this clinic from the beginning, and for the first year "group therapy" was handled by a psychiatrist. At the end of that time, having attended one of the group therapy sessions, group therapy was discontinued as Shealy felt that it had negative reinforcing qualities to it. Instead, he then introduced autogenic training 30 minutes twice a day, and began to introduce temperature, EEG, and EMG biofeedback.

By the end of the first year, Shealy had treated over 400 patients of whom approximately 6 per cent had had dorsal column stimulators inserted, and 1 per cent had had peripheral nerve implanted stimulators.

At the end of 32 days, the average hospital stay, 75 per cent of the patients were off drugs, markedly improved in their pain complaints and behaviors, and had a significant increase in physical activity. Over the next year and a half, reliance upon stress reduction and cognitive educational aspects increased, and during this time Shealy developed the concept of Biogenics®. The Biogenics® retraining component of Shealy's (Shealy, 1978) pain management program became so prominent that in 1974 the inpatient program was closed and for the last 16 years Shealy has run only an outpatient pain management program. Today, most clinicians consider it inappropriate to hospitalize chronic pain patients for anything other than drug withdrawal or severe psychiatric problems.

PAIN MANAGEMENT FOR THE 1990s

The single most important factor in managing chronic pain is evaluation of the patient. This must include the following:

1. A comprehensive history of the patient's pain problem including:
    onset
    predisposing factor
    drug history
    surgical history
    family history
    social interactions
    Symptom Index
    Pain Profile (at the end of this chapter)
    Total Life Stress (at the end of this chapter)

2. A review of all diagnostic tests.

3. A comprehensive physical and neuromuscular examination including:
    particular attention to the sacrum, posture,
    and spinal mechanics.

4. Special tests which might be needed include:
    myelogram
    CAT scan
    MRI
    EMG and sensory nerve conduction studies
    neuropsychological tests

psychological tests including:
California Personality Inventory (CPI)
Minnesota Multiphasic Personality
Inventory (MMPI)
Myer-Briggs Type Indicator (MBTI)
evaluation by physical therapist
evaluation by a psychologist

5. The minimum team needed for comprehensive pain management includes:
Physician (M.D. or D.O.)
R.N.
Psychologist, Psychotherapist, or someone with a Master's in Social Work
Physical Therapist

6. Once it is ascertained that the patient does not have a problem which needs primary surgery or medical drug management, the following modes of therapy need to be considered:
Educational Approaches
Physical Approaches
Pharmacological Approaches
Nutritional and Chemical Approaches
Psychological and Spiritual Approaches

Educational Approaches of critical importance to the patient are the following:

Understanding the anatomy and physiology of pain and appropriateness of surgical versus drug therapy.

Thorough understanding of stress:
Physical
Chemical
Emotional
Spiritual

An understanding of the concept of retraining the nervous system (Biogenics®).
Understanding the dynamics of interpersonal relationships.

Physical Approaches:
acupuncture
nerve blocks of
muscle trigger points
facet joints
sacroiliac joints
caudals (rarely)

intercostal blocks (rarely)
miscellaneous:
    occipital
    supraorbital
    infraorbital
    mental nerves

Transcutaneous electrical nerve stimulation
Use of at least two or three different types of devices:
Cranial electrical stimulation
Percutaneous electrical nerve stimulation
  (medium and intense current)

Soft tissue mobilization
    myofascial massage
    strain/counterstrain
    manipulative techniques
    vibratory massage
    mechanical massage
    heat
    ice

Exercise
    limbering
    aerobic
    muscle strengthening
    work hardening

Psychological Approaches:
    pragmatic
    ractical
    spiritually-oriented

Chemical Approaches:
    Possible therapeutic implications include:
    Dilantin
    Elavil or other antidepressant drugs
    Mexitil (especially for sensory deprivation pain)

Nutritional Approaches:
Special attention to vitamin C, vitamin B6 and magnesium (all deficient in a majority of patients)

BIOGENICS
The backbone of Shealy's self-regulation training program is Biogenics®. Biogenics® incorporates the work of a number of individuals including Dr. Elmer Green, Roberto Assagioli, Edmond Jacobson, Emil Coue,

Carl Jung, and, of course, J. H. Schultz. Essentially, many of these individuals have touched on aspects that interrelate to one another. As Shealy began synthesizing the techniques of self-regulation, the following steps were most emphasized:

Positive attitude.
A belief in self (that "I can do it"). Biofeedback proves this.
Relaxation.
Conscious control of sensation (Balancing Body Feelings).
> Individuals are taught the following:
> Balancing Body Feelings techniques:
>> Talking to the body.
>> Feeling the localizing pulsation of heartbeat.
>> Imaging.
>> Loving the body.
>> Tensing and relaxing.
>> Breathing through the body.
>> Collecting and releasing.
>> Circulating the electrical energy.
>> Expanding the electromagnetic energy field.
>> Induction of anesthesia mentally.

Balancing emotions:
> Recognizing that all distress is the result of fear of loss of:
>> life
>> health
>> money
>> love
>> moral values

Logically and internally recognizing that the only solutions are:
> assertion to correct the problem
> divorcing an unacceptable problem with joy
> accepting and forgiving (going for sainthood).

Programming goals (organ specific phrases).
Spiritual attunement.

Since some 90 per cent of individuals state that they believe in life after death, God, and living the Golden Rule, this universal belief is incorporated into teaching. Individuals are exposed to philosophical concepts to develop the transcendent will or the will of the soul, starting with the concept that all individuals have basic needs and desires in addition to those necessary for survival. The major part of cognitive understanding relates to accepting that pain, mostly psychologically aggravated, is the result of unfulfilled desires or failure to accept things as they are.

Ultimately, individuals must learn that there are a limited number of situations which can be totally changed,and that one should put effort into those which can be changed and learn total emotional-psychological detachment from those aspects of life which cannot be changed; in other words, to be at peace with the unchangable aspects of life. At the same time they are taught to control pain through the Biogenics techniques of Balancing Body Feelings.

Obviously there are many models of pain clinics. Some current clinics specialize only in doing nerve blocks, especially caudal nerve blocks, others primarily emphasize transcutaneous electrical nerve stimulation, and some emphasize more physical therapy approaches. All of these techniques are valuable in managing chronic pain. The indications for specific physical approaches such as acupuncture, nerve blocks, etc., are beyond the province of this particular chapter. References to some of the technology can be found at the end of this chapter.

COST-EFFECTIVENESS OF COMPREHENSIVE PAIN TREATMENT

No discussion of pain clinics would be adequate without attention to the catch-word of today, cost-effectiveness. Shealy's study in 1984 is one of the few that have been published.

At the Shealy Institute over 7,000 patients have been evaluated and/or treated intensely in a 13-day comprehensive program. At the present time, only 10 to 15 per cent of patients evaluated enter the intense program. Most of the others are satisfactorily managed with one or two modalities of treatment with occasional follow-up visits. Sixty per cent of those who enter intense therapy have had unsuccessful back surgery; 10 per cent have back pain without prior surgery; 10 per cent have headaches; the remainder have a wide variety of post-traumatic, post-surgical metabolic or degenerative pain syndromes. Sixty per cent are women; 40 per cent are men. They have ranged in age from 8 to 90 years with most patients between 35 and 67 years old. Approximately 20 per cent have had worker's compensation injuries.

Patients have been incapacitated from one to seven plus years. Medical expenses have ranged from $10,000 to $450,000 with average medical expenses of over $10,000.

RESULTS FOLLOWING COMPREHENSIVE TREATMENT

In any given year, five to seven per cent of patients who enter the program fail to complete it. About one per cent are sent home because of open resistance to therapy. The others who drop out do so because they "don't believe in it." Almost all of these drop-outs are male smokers and are either worker's compensation or medicaid patients.

Of the 94 per cent who complete the program, follow-up at six months and two to three years, data from 800 patients; (600 followed two + years; 200 followed six months) consistently reveal that:

- 35 per cent return to work
- 90 per cent are off all drugs except aspirin or acetaminophen
- 70 per cent are improved 50 to 100 per cent (at 6 months 72 per cent are greatly improved; over the next two years this decreases to 70 per cent)
- 30 per cent who do not improve greatly almost invariably did not practice the techniques taught
- 5 per cent had a facet rhizotom
- 25 per cent continued use of TENS for at least six months
- Pain intensity is reduced an average of 70 per cent
- Percent of time pain is present is reduced an average of 65 per cent
- Mood is improved in 90 per cent of patients
- A majority have significant stress illness such as hypertension, diabetes, peptic ulcer, etc.
- Less than 5 per cent have additional surgical procedures after treatment
- Drug expenses after therapy are reduced 85 per cent
- Hospitalization after therapy is reduced 90 per cent
- Total medical expenses are reduced after therapy 80 to 85 per cent
- Cost of the treatment ranges from $3,500 to $6,000, and rarely more, depending upon need for hospitalization, for drug withdrawal, etc.

In 1972, Fordyce reported that his average patient had had prior expenses of $50,000. His program, at that time, cost $5,000. Most pain clinics today charge from $5,000 to $35,000. Fordyce estimated that society would break even if only 10 per cent of his patients returned to work. If one takes into account the income produced by those who return to work, even less than 10 per cent work-return success would produce a break even for society.

Presently, with prior medical expenses often exceeding $60,000 average, and an average cost of less than $5,000 for the comprehensive treatment program, society breaks even if only 8 per cent return to work. Since 35 per cent of Shealy's patients return to work, the cost-effectiveness is at least 3.4 to 1. Since total medical expenses are reduced by well over 75 per cent, the cost of the comprehensive rehabilitation program is recouped in less than six months. In medical costs alone, in just a two-year period, the cost-effectiveness is 4 to 1. That is, "society" saves, within two years, four times as much money as the cost of the treatment program. When the added benefit of 35 per cent return to work is considered, the cost-effectiveness is even greater than 4 to 1.

The data reported here apply only to treatment at the Shealy Institute for Comprehensive Health Care and cannot be extrapolated to other pain treatment programs or modalities (Shealy, 1976).

THE OUTLOOK FOR THE FUTURE: CERTIFICATION OF PAIN CLINICS

In 1983, CARF (Commission for Accreditation of Rehabilitation Facilities) instituted a program of accreditation of both outpatient and inpatient pain clinics. Since then, five states have introduced varying forms of legislation that require pain clinics to be accredited to receive either regular insurance or worker's compensation insurance reimbursement for pain treatment. Nevertheless, estimates of the total number of pain clinics in the United States range from 3,000 up, and less than 200 such clinics are currently certified by CARF. There are no formal residency training programs. Most individuals who run pain clinics today are either anesthesiologists, neurosurgeons, family physicians, psychiatrists, or orthopedists. Many of these have trained themselves, a few have spent various periods of time working in established pain clinics before setting up their own models. As the increasing numbers of pain clinics develop, it is obvious that not only is a certification for clinics essential, but a certification for the professionals working in those clinics is necessary. That particular issue is being addressed by the American Academy of Pain Management through its current Board certification process.

Pain Profile

On the columns below, grade yourself (circle your choice):

Pain Intensity (Severity)	0	5	10	15	20	25	30	35	40	45	50	55	60	65	70	75	80	85	90	95	100
Decrease in Physical Activity	0	5	10	15	20	25	30	35	40	45	50	55	60	65	70	75	80	85	90	95	100
Percent of Time Pain Felt	0	5	10	15	20	25	30	35	40	45	50	55	60	65	70	75	80	85	90	95	100
Effect on Mood	0	5	10	15	20	25	30	35	40	45	50	55	60	65	70	75	80	85	90	95	100
Drugs Consumed	0	5	10	15	20	25	30	35	40	45	50	55	60	65	70	75	80	85	90	95	100
Effect on Sexual Activity	0	5	10	15	20	25	30	35	40	45	50	55	60	65	70	75	80	85	90	95	100
Overall Well-being	0	5	10	15	20	25	30	35	40	45	50	55	60	65	70	75	80	85	90	95	100
Overall Energy	0	5	10	15	20	25	30	35	40	45	50	55	60	65	70	75	80	85	90	95	100

Pain Intensity: 100 = intolerable, excruciating, horrible.

Physical Activity: 100% restricted = bedridden. 75% restricted = up and about, but very little.
50% restricted = can't work, up and take care of myself, must rest frequently.
25% restricted = must rest every 4 to 6 hours, light work exhausted me, can't do *fun* activities.
0 = normal, I do any physical activity I choose.

Effect on Mood: 0 = normal; 100 = totally withdrawn, panicked, overwhelmingly depressed.

Drugs Consumed: Doctor will do this. Mark all drugs you take on reverse side of this page or separate sheet.

Sexual Function: 0 = no activity; 100 = perfectly normal activity.

Overall Feeling of Well-being: 0 = terrible; 100 = best anybody could feel.

Overall Energy: 0 = can't get up or get going; 100 = most I've ever experienced.

Name _____ Date _____

Drug Usage

Aspirin, Tylenol, etc.	up to 10 per day	10
	up to 20 per day	25
Valium, Ativan, diazepams	up to 20 mg per day	25
	up to 40 mg per day	50
	over 40 mg per day	75
Librium	up to 20 mg per day	25
	up to 40 mg per day	50
	over 40 mg per day	75
Phenothiazines, Serax, Thorazine, etc.	up to 20 mg per day	25
	up to 40 mg per day	50
	over 40 mg per day	75
Tricyclic antidepressants: Elavil (10 mg), Vivactil (5 mg.) Tofranil (10 mg), Aventyl	up to 4 per day	25
	4 to 8 per day	30
	8 to 12 per day	40
	over 12 per day	50
Monamine Oxidizers (antidepressants) Nardil, etc., Mild to moderate addicting, Codeine (30 to 60 mg), Percodan, Talwin tablets, Darvon, Darvocette, Stadol, Nubain, Barbiturates (30 to 60 mg)	up to 4 per day	60
	4 to 8 per day	75
	over 8 per day	90
Demerol, Injectable Talwin, Morphine, Dilaudid	up to 4 doses per day	75
	up to 8 doses per day	90
	over 8 doses per day	100
Sleeping Medicines	up to 1 per day	25
	2 per day	50
	over 2 per day	60
Dilantin		50
Prolixin		50

TOTAL =

(Narcotics full count, all others ½ count when added to other drugs on these lists)

PERSONAL STRESS ASSESSMENT
Total Life Stress Test

Name_____ Date _____

Read your stress points on the lines in the right-hand margin, and indicate subtotals in the boxes at the end of each section. Then add your subtotals to determine your total score.

A. DIETARY STRESS
Average Daily Sugar Consumption

Sugar added to food or drink	1 point per 5 teaspoons	____
Sweet roll, piece of pie/cake, brownie, other dessert	1 point each	____
Coke or can of pop; candy bar	2 points each	____
Banana split, commercial milk shake, sundae, etc.	5 points each	____
White flour (white bread, spaghetti, etc.)	5 points	____

Average Daily Salt Consumption

Little or no "added" salt	0 points	____
Few salty foods (pretzels, potato chips, etc.)	0 points	____
Moderate "added" salt and/or salty foods at least once per day	3 points	____
Heavy salt user, regularly (use of "table salt"and/or salty foods at least twice per day)	10 points	____

Average Daily Caffeine Consumption

Coffee	½ point each cup	____
Tea	½ point each cup	____
Cola drink or Mountain Dew®	1 point each cup	____
2 Anacin® or APC tabs	½ point per dose	____
Caffeine Benzoate tablets (NoDoz®, Vivarin®, etc.)	2 points each	____

Average Weekly Eating Out

2-4 times per week	3 points	____
5-10 times per week	6 points	____
More than 10 times per week	10 points	____
	DIETARY SUBTOTAL	⬚ A

B. ENVIRONMENTAL STRESS
Drinking Water

Chlorinated only	1 point	____
Chlorinated and fluoridated	2 points	____

Soil and Air Pollution

Live within 10 miles of city of 500,000 or more	10 points	____
Live within 10 miles of city of 250,000 or more	5 points	____
Live within 10 miles of city of 50,000 or more	2 points	____
Live in the country but use pesticides, herbicides and/or chemical fertilizer	10 points	____

Soil and Air Pollution

Exposed to cigarette smoke of someone
else more than 1 hour per day   5 points   ____

ENVIRONMENTAL SUBTOTAL [____] B

C. CHEMICAL STRESS
Drugs (any amount of usage)

Antidepressants	1 point	____
Tranquilizers	3 points	____
Sleeping pills	3 points	____
Narcotics	5 points	____
Other pain relievers	3 points	____

Nicotine

3-10 cigarettes per day	5 points	____
11-20 cigarettes per day	15 points	____
21-30 cigarettes per day	20 points	____
31-40 cigarettes per day	35 points	____
Over 40 cigarettes per day	40 points	____
Cigar(s) per day	1 point each	____
Pipeful(s) of tobacco per day	1 point each	____
Chewing tobacco — "chews" per day	1 point each	____

Average Daily Alcohol Consumption

1 oz. whiskey, gin, vodka, etc.	2 points each	____
8 oz. beer	2 points each	____
4-6 oz. glass of wine	2 points each	____

CHEMICAL SUBTOTAL [____] C

D. PHYSICAL STRESS
Weight

Underweight more than 10 lbs.	5 points	____
10 to 15 lbs. overweight	5 points	____
16 to 25 lbs. overweight	10 points	____
26 to 40 lbs. overweight	25 points	____
More than 40 lbs. overweight	40 points	____

Activity

Adequate exercise,* 3 days or more per week	0 points	____
Some physical exercise, 1 or 2 days per week	15 points	____
No regular exercise	40 points	____

Work Stress

Sit most of the day	3 points	____
Industrial/factory worker	3 points	____
Overnight travel more than once a week	5 points	____
Work more than 50 hours per week	2 points per hour over 50	____
Work varying shifts	10 points	____
Work night shift	5 points	____

PHYSICAL SUBTOTAL [____] D

*Adequate means doubling heartbeat and/or sweating minimum of 30 minutes per time.

E. Holmes-Rahe Social Readjustment Rating*

(Circle the mean values that correspond with life events listed below which you have experienced during the past 12 months.)

Death of spouse	100
Divorce	73
Marital separation	65
Jail term	63
Death of close family member	63
Personal injury or illness	53
Marriage	50
Fired at work	47
Marital reconciliation	45
Retirement	45
Change in health of family member	44
Pregnancy	40
Sexual difficulties	39
Gain of new family member	39
Business readjustment	39
Change in financial state	38
Death of close friend	37
Change to different line of work	36
Change in number of arguments with spouse	35
Mortgage over $20,000	31
Foreclosure of mortgage or loan	30
Change in responsibilities at work	29
Son or daughter leaving home	29
Trouble with in-laws	29
Outstanding personal achievement	28
Spouse begin or stop work	26
Begin or end school	25
Change in living conditions	24
Revision of personal habits	23
Trouble with boss	20
Change in work hours or conditions	20
Change in residence	20
Change in schools	19
Change in recreation	19
Change in church activities	18
Change in social activities	17
Mortgage or loan less than $20,000	16
Change in sleeping habits	15
Change in eating habits	15
Vacation, especially if away from home	13
Christmas, or other major holiday stress	12
Minor violations of the law	11

(Add the mean values to get the Holmes-Rahe total. Then refer to the conversion table to determine your number of points.)

F. EMOTIONAL STRESS

Sleep

Less than 7 hours per night	3 points	＿＿
Usually 7 or 8 hours per night	0 points	＿＿
More than 8 hours per night	2 points	＿＿

Relaxation

Relax only during sleep	10 points	＿＿
Relax or meditate at least 20 minutes per day	0 points	＿＿

Frustration at work

Enjoy work	0 points	＿＿
Mildly frustrated by job	1 point	＿＿
Moderately frustrated by job	3 points	＿＿
Very frustrated by job	5 points	＿＿

Marital Status

Married, happily	0 points	＿＿
Married, moderately unhappy	2 points	＿＿
Married, very unhappy	5 points	＿＿
Unmarried man over 30	5 points	＿＿
Unmarried woman over 30	2 points	＿＿

Usual Mood

Happy, well adjusted	0 points	＿＿
Moderately angry, depressed or frustrated	10 points	＿＿
Very angry, depressed or frustrated	20 points	＿＿

**Any Other Major Stress Not Mentioned Above
You Judge Intensity (Specify):**

＿＿＿＿＿＿＿＿＿＿＿＿＿＿＿＿   (10 to 40 points)   ＿＿

EMOTIONAL SUBTOTAL ☐ F

Add A ＿＿ + B ＿＿ + C ＿＿

+ D ＿＿ + E ＿＿ + F ＿＿ = ☐

YOUR PERSONAL STRESS ASSESSMENT SCORE

If your score exceeds 25 points, you probably will feel better if you reduce your stress; greater than 50 points, you definitely need to eliminate stress in your life.

Circle your stressor with the highest number of points and work first to eliminate it; then circle your next greatest stressor, overcome it; and so on.

Conversion Table

Your number of points:	Holmes-Rahe less than	Anything over 351 = 40 +
0	60	
1	110	
2	160	
3	170	
4	180	
5	190	
6	200	
7	210	
8	220	
9	230	
10	240	
11	250	
12	260	
13	265	
14	270	
15	275	
16	280	
17	285	
18	290	
19	295	
20	300	
21	305	
22	310	
23	315	
24	320	
25	325	
26	330	
27	335	
28	340	
29	345	
30	350	

HOLMES-RAHE SOCIAL READJUSTMENT RATING (CONVERTED) ☐ E

*The Social Readjustment Rating Scale: See Holmes, T.H. and Rahe, R.H.: The social readjustment rating scale. *Journal of Psychosomatic Research, 11*:213–218, 1967, for complete wording of these items. Reproduced with permission of the authors and publisher.

REFERENCES

Fordyce, W. (1976). *Behavioral methods for chronic pain and illness.* St. Louis, MO: The C.V. Mosby Co.

Shealy, C. N. (1978). Biofeedback training in the physician's office: Transfer of pain clinic advances to primary care. *Wisconsin Medical Journal,* Vol. 77, April.

Shealy, C. N. *Biogenics: A synthesis of biofeedback and autogenic technics for control of pain.* (pp. 69-74). In Leon R. Pomeroy (Ed.) *New dynamics of preventative medicine,* Vol. 5. Medical progress through innovation.

Shealy, C. N. (1986). *Biogenics® health maintenance.* Fair Grove, MO: Self-Health Systems.

Shealy, C. N. (1984). Cost-effectiveness of comprehensive pain treatment. *Insurance Adjustor,* March.

Shealy, C. N. (1976). *The pain game.* Millbrae, CA: Celestial Arts.

Section 3
THE TREATMENT OF COMMONLY OCCURING PAIN SYNDROMES

Chapter 5
ASSESSMENT AND DIAGNOSTIC TECHNIQUES

Richard S. Materson, M. D.

Richard S. Materson, M. D. gives both his personal philosophy and methods gleaned after 25 years of practice for assessment of acute and chronic pain. Building upon an adequate history and appropriate physical examination, Dr. Materson goes on to describe a flexible algorithm for deciding the use of examinations, imaging, electro-diagnostic, and psychosocial data.

The author argues that adequate time must be devoted to the assessment of a chronic pain patient's presenting problems to ensure a proper intervention strategy. Key elements that comprise an intake history are described. Following the history, a physical examination with possible ancillary testing, form the basis of a clinical diagnosis and treatment plan.

Chapter 5

ASSESSMENT AND DIAGNOSTIC TECHNIQUES

Richard S. Materson, M. D.

I shall attempt to share with the reader my personal philosophy and techniques derived from both close attention to the medical literature and 25 years of clinical experience in Physical Medicine and Rehabilitation dealing with acute and chronic pain patients.

There have been a number of attempts to define "pain" and that which is currently internationally approved taxonomy from the International Association for the Study of Pain (IASP) is, "...an unpleasant sensory and emotional experience associated with actual or potential tissue damage or described in terms of such damage (de Jong, 1980)."

I believe that a patient describing a pain experience in the terms implied above, regardless of whether or not there is a findable pathophysiologic mechanism, or whether or not there is evidence of tissue damage, is experiencing pain and deserves my attention, assessment, and proper selection of diagnostic techniques and proper treatment. Patients come to physicians for relief of pain, not simply "diagnosis" and are not at all helped by being told, in the absence of findable organic disease that "its in your head," a statement made all too often which is clearly of negative therapeutic value and a leading destroyer of physician-patient relationships.

Those patients with an acute pain experience seem to be vastly different in their presentation, diagnosis, ease of relating the pain and its effects to specific actual or potential tissue damage, remediation with direct and simple means, and less psychosocially and environmentally driven than chronic pain patients in which the pain syndrome itself becomes the disease; the role of psychosocial and environmental factors are dominant, and in which the relationship of the pain to a pathophysiologic cause is often hazy at best and nearly always out of proportion to the "objective" physical findings, with less direct and often multi-dimensional treatment required. I agree with Bonica's (1990) plea to not artificially define chronic pain as that occurring six months post onset but rather "... as pain that persists a month beyond the usual course of an acute disease or a reasonable time for an injury to heal, or is that associated with a chronic pathological process that causes continuous pain or the pain recurs at intervals for months or years."

The approach to acute and chronic pain is so different, the latter demanding a much more extensive interview, and broadening of inquiry in the psychosocial, vocational, cognitive, and environmental domains, that the clinician must be mindful of these definitions to avoid errors of omission in appropriate investigation. For the purposes of this chapter I will deal primarily with chronic pain patients.

How then should the clinician procede? I believe that accurate assessment is the key to good pain management. Therefore, a personal schema should be developed which, like an algorithm, allows for a practical decision tree with each yes/no checkpoint, that is at once flexible and practical for various situations and yet comprehensive enough to get the job satisfactorily done. It must be sensitive to all elements of the pain syndrome including nociception, pain, suffering, and pain behavior (Loeser, 1982).

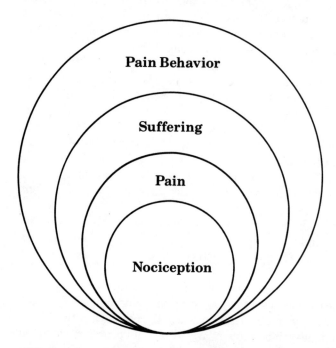

Fig. 1. The four concepts in Loeser's concept of pain. From Loeser, J. D. (1982). Concepts of pain. In M. Stanton-Hicks & R. Boas (Eds.), *Chronic low back pain*. New York: Raven Press. Reproduced with permission.

For assessment I believe the following items must be included:

1. Adequate pain history
2. Appropriate physical examination
3. Necessary laboratory exams
4. X-ray and other diagnostic imaging
5. Electrodiagnostic testing/Thermography as indicated
6. Psychosocial data
7. Articulation of patient's goals

Experience shows that most chronic patients seeking help from a pain specialist (algologist) have already experienced prior contacts with the health care system which may have been less than fruitful, or even frustrating and disappointing. Trust in physicians is often at a low ebb. Therefore, establishment of a positive, caring, empathetic relationship is of paramount importance. A calm manner; flexible history-taking technique; concise, accurate description of the process you will take the patient through; and assurance that you will take the necessary time and steps to come to a satisfactory outcome is required. Many pain centers use a screening technique which allows review of past medical records, discussion with the referring physician or agency for details of the case, a complete pharmaceutical history, and previous treatment history before the patient is seen. Some also obtain benefit from a pain questionnaire (Melzack, 1975) filled out by the patient in advance, a one- or two-week diary of the patient's life including time sitting, walking, standing, and reclining, with major activity and medications used, including the dose and frequency, correlated with the patient's estimate of pain level (Chapman & Syrjala, 1990). Such advance information can provide a much more complete picture of the patient's pain, suffering, and pain behavior than a simple interview which often is driven by the patient's most recent symptoms and less accurate memory of events. Further, advance data can be obtained from the spouse and/or significant others in the patient's life.

Whether or not one chooses to form a pre-visit information system, the interview itself must not be replaced by the pre-visit data. In practical terms, that means that the first interview and examination is likely to be quite thorough and therefore, time-consuming and demands adequate time scheduling. For the process alone for the first visit, one and a half hours is most often necessary, and to review all the data and prepare a report and do necessary paperwork, two hours is usual. In my opinion, the most serious error made by most physicians is inadequate scheduling of time.

An adequate pain history has the following elements:

1. Date of onset
2. Circumstances of onset

   3. Velocity of onset and graph of pain intensity versus time
   4. What improves the pain? What worsens it?
   5. What behavioral changes and changes in function are
      attributed to the pain?
      Are there identifiable secondary gains/losses?
   6. Pain drawing and patient-rated pain intensity measure(s)
   7. Diagnostic history to date
   8. Treatment history including self-treatment
   9. Pharmaceutical history
  10. Other medical history, including allergy
  11. Substance abuse/excesses
  12. Psychosocial data

A pain history without psychosocial data is like a tree without leaves! Psychosocial history will be covered in detail later in this chapter.

Establishment of the date of onset is critical to the process of sorting out diagnostic possibilities and determining the course of the process. Was the pain sudden in onset? Related to a specific event? If mechanically induced, what were the forces and vectors and timing of their influence on the body? Is there evidence of repetitive trauma and the disease a consequence of accumulative effect? If an illness or injury, has there been unusual complication? Delay in healing? Deviation from expected disease natural history? Was there anything unusual about the circumstances at onset?

I find it useful to have the patient help me create a graph denoting the onset and then intensity of the pain related to time. In this manner, exacerbations and remissions, peaks and valleys, nocturnal or other time-locked patterns are discovered and inquiries regarding activity at the time of pain increase or decrease or the effect of activity/rest can be understood easily on the graph. One can also help the patient to make important observations about the effect of medicine, physical treatment, self-remedy, stress, and vocational requirements on the pain syndrome. During the course of this inquiry one can learn what changes in lifestyle, behavior, mood, anxiety level, appetite, sleep pattern, familial, and other social relationships have occurred in relationship to the pain both as possible cause and effect.

As the history taking procedes, and the patient is more comfortable with the totality of the inquiry, questions regarding secondary gain and loss can be admixed. Does the patient now get something which he would not otherwise have were it not for the pain? Or, equally importantly, what is taken from this patient that would remain were it not for the pain? Ego, pride, sexual identity , job promotion or demotion, sports and recreational activities, as well as monetary issues must be explored. What insurance benefits have been applied for or received? Is there unemployment compensation? What changes have been necessary in the roles of family or friends or co-workers because of the patient's pain?

I remember a long ago lecture during my residency given by Professor Sedgewick Mead of Vallejo, California on the entymology of pain vocabulary and the language of pain. Most of the adverbs, adjectives, and nouns used to describe pain derive from external sources of body injury most of which likely never have actually been experienced by most patients except in their mind's eye. Consider pressure, rasping, crushing, mauling, lancinating, burning, sticking, jabbing, and similar words. No wonder that different patients describe their pain in such different ways. Those with rich imagery histories, the intellectual and well-read will have a greater choice of words and use them more readily than the stoic, inhibited, concrete, less well-read, or educated person. Further, each patient will likely be influenced by his culture, society, and his parents methods for both pain description and pain reaction. Patients anatomic sophistication varies widely, or cultural inhibitions may interfere with proper anatomic referral such as "hip" for buttocks, "chest" for breast, "stomach" for vaginal or rectal. Awareness of these variations will make the algologist take a detailed history using such phrases as "show me" or "point to it" or "tell me in another way" to clarify and increase accuracy.

A pain drawing is often helpful. Done on a front and back drawing of the human form, not only location, but type of pain experienced, size, intensity, temperature, and color, track of movement from one place to the other can be drawn with symbols and/or color to represent the imagery of the pain. Perhaps the most widely tested and used is the McGill Pain Questionnaire (Melzack, 1975). Melzack uses the five following words expressing pain intensity for selection by the patient:

1. Mild
2. Discomforting
3. Distressing
4. Horrible
5. Excruciating

He uses groups of adjectives describing sensory experience of pain, affective, evaluative, and miscellaneous groups such as:

1. Flickering, Quivering, Pulsing, Throbbing, Beating, Pounding
2. Jumping, Flashing, Shooting
3. Pricking, Boring, Drilling, Stabbing, Lancinating
9. Dull, Sore, Hurting, Aching, Heavy
11. Tiring, Exhausting
18. Tight, Numb, Drawing, Squeezing, Tearing

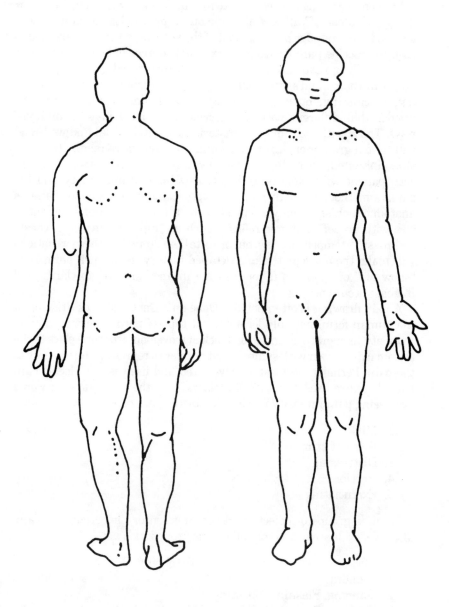

Fig. 2 From Melzack, R. (1975). *The McGill Pain Questionnaire: Major properties and scoring methods.* Pain, 1:275. Reproduced with permission.

and pain changes with time:

1. Continuous, Steady, Constant
2. Rythmic, Periodic, Intermittent
3. Brief, Momentary, Transient

Numerical Rating Scale:
Instructions: Choose a number from 0 to 10 which indicates how strong your pain is right now.

No pain at all = 0 1 2 3 4 5 6 7 8 9 10 = The worst pain imaginable

Visual Analog Scale:
Instructions: Mark on the line below how strong your pain is right now.

No pain at all _____

The worst pain imaginable _____

Category Scale:
Instructions: Choose the word below which best describes how your pain feels right now.

Mild   Discomforting   Distressing   Horrible   Excruciating

Pain Relief Scale:
Instructions: Mark on the line below the amount of relief you have from your pain right now compared to yesterday. (Another comparison may be used.)

No relief 0% _____

Complete relief 100% _____

Fig. 3. *Single dimension self-report measures. Measurement of pain.* From Chapman and Syrjala. (1990). In John Bonica (Ed.), *The management of pain.* Philadelphia: Lea & Febiger. Reproduced with permission.

He also asks the patient to list which word represents the worst toothache the patient ever had; the worst headache, and the worst stomachache to invite comparisons with the current process and the patient's degree of imagery.

Other authors have suggested modifications or used other scales. A 10- to 100-point scale with zero for no pain and 10 or 100 dependent upon the scale used for the worst pain imaginable is helpful. In my experience, most patients accept the 100-point scale, but those who have trouble with it can often select with reliability from a $1.00 scale with $1.00 representing the worst pain possible—how many cents worth of pain do you have? Repeat measures during the course of illness and treatment measure

When filling out each daily diary, please keep track of time by rounding off to the nearest 15, 30, 45, 60 minutes.
Record the amount and type of medications taken in the appropriate time slot.
Record the intensity of the pain for each hour you are awake. Use a scale 0–10 (0 = no pain, 10 = unbearable).

Tuesday   Date   4-2-85

	SITTING		WALKING & STANDING		RECLINING		MEDICATIONS		PAIN LEVEL
	Major Activity	Time	Major Activity	Time	Activity	Time	Amount	Type	(0-10)
1 AM					Sleep	60			
2 AM					Sleep	60			
3 AM					Sleep	60			
4 AM					Sleep	60			
5 AM					Sleep	60			
6 AM					Sleep	60			
7 AM					Sleep	60			
8 AM	Eating	15	Cooking	15	Sleep	30	2	Tylenol #3	6
9 AM	Reading	60							3
10 AM	TV	60					2	Tylenol (325 mg)	1
11 AM	TV	60							0
12 AM					Rest, TV	60			0

Time	Activity	Sitting	Activity	Walking	Activity	Reclining	Dose	Medication	Pain
1 PM	Eating	30	Cooking	30					2
2 PM	TV	45	Laundry	15					3
3 PM	Reading	60						2	Tylenol (325 mg)	3
4 PM	Visiting	45	Ironing	15					1
5 PM	TV	30			Rest	30	2	Tylenol #3	4
6 PM	Eating	30	Cooking	30					1
7 PM	TV	45	Dishes	15					0
8 PM	Telephone	15	Cleaning	15	Rest, TV	30			6
9 PM					Rest, TV	60	5 mg	Valium	6
10 PM					Reading	60			0
11 PM					Sleep	60			
12 PM					Sleep	60			
		SITTING $8\frac{1}{2}$		WALKING $2\frac{1}{4}$		RECLINING $13\frac{1}{2}$			

Pain Scale: 0 = No pain
10 = Unbearable

Hours sitting + hours walking + hours reclining = 24 hours)

Fig. 4. *Activity Diary.* From Chapman and Syrjala (1990). *Measurement of pain.* In John Bonica (Ed.), *The management of pain.* Philadelphia: Lea & Febiger. Reproduced with permission.

response and can be correlated with a scale for relief of pain or improvement of function with 0 for no pain relief or function increase and 100 for complete relief or normal function. Positive changes shared with the patient are used as encouragement and to allay anxiety and to establish an internal locus of pain control.

History-taking is incomplete without a complete present and past medical history, review of systems, review of previous testing and treatment, and an accurate pharmaceutical history. The latter is best served by having the patient bring his or her present and past medication containers, but also looking at pharmaceutical receipts. It is not unusual for a patient to be taking medications given at different times by the same doctor, or by different doctors, adding one drug but not dropping another. The hazards of polypharmacy can only be discovered with a careful history. The pharmacy history time is nearly ideal for extending the conversation to other substances taken, food and or alcohol abuse/excess, and any treatment for the same. The clever historian will piece together a working hypothesis and let the history confirm or rule out suspected disorders. As in all of medicine, if you don't think of it…you'll miss it, so ask yourself constantly, is there anything else I've missed? There are as many rules about the conditions of history taking as there are historians. I prefer my patient to be comfortable. If pain relief is needed to go on with a long history session I provide it in the form of physical relief (ice, heat, massage , posture change); or mild analgesic or anti-anxiety medication. The patient may sit, stand, or lie down and change as often as he or she wishes. Another person can be present with the condition that the patient's history is what I'm after, and that I'll take verifying history or another opinion later. While I do not permit young children or infants to be present in most circumstances, we do provide a day care center to avoid the distraction. If the history-taking is too prolonged it may be tiring for the patient and may require two or, rarely, more appointments.

THE PHYSICAL EXAMINATION

The physical examination process takes place with the first contacts with the patient. Posture, gait smoothness or lack thereof, specific limps, quality of handshake, eye contact, abnormal autonomic activity, i.e., gooseflesh, sweating, blushing, pupillary dilatation, and other signs of tension such as fidgetiness, automatisms, or bitten fingernails should be noted. These observations can be considered "the exam before the exam" and are most critical to the whole picture. Particularly important is the observation of significant exam feature changes in the "formal physical exam" from the "exam before the exam." Such changes suggest pain augmentation and must be explained, however, they are not per se evidence of malingering. These changes are particularly important when the formal physical exam findings are sparse or out of proportion to the subjective complaints.

I have made a habit of asking my patients during the physical examination process of their observations of the findings of previous examiners as contrasted with my findings. A surprisingly high percentage allege that the previous examiner has not had the patient disrobe, or has left out a significant number of what to me are basic sophomore-level medical school examination rituals. I stress that the patient must be undressed, but comfortable and with modesty protected without sacrifice of a thorough medical exam of all pertinent parts. Presence of a nurse or medical assistant is mandatory during the physical examination of a disrobed patient of the opposite sex of the examiner. I often read "pelvic deferred" or similar words in charts and I question "deferred" till when? Gynecologic pathology in women, and testicular pathology in men represents easily diagnosed and treatable causes of pain which are inexcusable to miss because of lack of adequate examination. Therefore , if one does not feel equipped or competent to perform the genital area exams, defer to a definite time and examiner and take responsibility to see that you review the consultant's report.

The physical examination itself is designed to answer the clinical diagnostic hypothesis you made when you completed the history-taking process. It is used to rule in or out the various diagnostic possibilities and to observe the patient's reaction to the examination process. As the exam features unfold, new possibilities come to mind, and must, be in turn, ruled in or out. Here again, if you don't think of a diagnostic possibility, you may miss it. The more experienced the clinician, the more comprehensive, yet efficient, is the process of physical examination. The words "show me" liberally scattered throughout the examination indicate a properly conducted examination.

I believe that the physical examination is also a good teaching tool for the patient and helps develop a closer physician-patient relationship and fosters mutual respect. Tell the patient, briefly, what you are doing, why you are doing it, and what your observations are in a nonthreatening manner during the process of the exam. Remarks on weight, height, blood pressure, respirations and pulse characteristics, and other findings which bear on the patient's general health are helpful, even if not directly related to the painful process, and assure the patient of your interest in preventive health care. In doing the exam this way you can solicit the patient's trust and facilitate relaxation before you directly approach the painful area. While this chapter cannot be a physical diagnosis textbook some highlights will be mentioned. Observation of vital signs, mental status, gait, posture, and station are critical. Are significant asymmetries of muscle, bone, or other structure present? Remember the ophthalmologic examination. . .the eye is the window to disease. The carefully done oral examination will be rewarding in identifying many causes of cranial pain. Especially look for malocclusion, bruxisms, dental carries and gum disorders, temporo-mandibular dysfunctions, and oral evidence of systemic disease.

Much musculo-skeletal pain derives from pathology about the head and neck which may be manifested on physical examination by observation of range of motion, muscle symmetry, manual muscle testing, body posture, presence of scoliosis or other pathological curvatures, arm length discrepancies, and careful search for muscle trigger areas or for "latent triggers," the latter of which are identified by their tenderness on palpation and classic referral areas and "jump sign". I prefer to use the polio-proven voluntary muscle testing grades of "Normal, Good, Fair, Poor, Trace, and Absent" using " + " and " – " with each grade to allow more specific levels of strength or weakness. Examination for proximal strength deficits is frequently neglected. Observation of forward abduction of the arms holding them parallel in front of the body without and then with resistance and looking for scapular winging checks the serratus anterior, while the arms held obliquely in front and overhead as in a "blessing the masses" posture checks the trapezius and deltoid muscles

In the lower extremity stepping up and down steps or squatting and arising check the hip extensors and knee extensors, principally the gluteus maximus and quadraceps; standing on one foot and leveling the pelvis checks the lateral hip stabilizers especially the gluteus medius, and toe and heel stands look at the posterior and anterior compartment muscles of the leg. Following directions carefully, the balance necessary to carry these activities on are also carefully observed.

Both "active" (patient self-performed) and "passive" (examiner moves the part without the assistance of the patient) range of motion studies of joint movements are necessary. In the painful or pain-anxious, "active self-assisted" range of motion is often helpful during which a patient actively moves a segment as far as comfort and/or fear allow, and then slowly, gently adds his or her own passive help to complete a range of motion test. This technique doubles as a range of motion preserving exercise format.

A comprehensive neurological examination is necessary including observations of the skin (for neurological disease manifestations), mental status, neuro-opthalmologic, coordination, motor performance alterations, disturbances of muscle tone, bulk, symmetry, presence or absence of spasticity, rigidity, tremor, or other involuntary motor disorder, sensory testing for all modalities, special senses including vision and hearing, autonomic nervous function, and deep tendon reflex testing. For grading the latter I prefer the Mayo Clinic technique in which "0" is normal and diminished reflexes are recorded " – 1" to " – 4" with " – 4" flaccid and " – 1" minimally reduced with " – 2" and " – 3" as in-between grades. For reflex augmentation , grade " + 4" represents sustained clonus, " + 3" unsustained clonus and " + 1" and " + 2" slight to moderate increases. Absolute values and asymmetries are both important as are "overflows" in which the tendon jerk afferrant response enters one root, but overflows and is represented in another root often while its own motor root is blocked. The latter often represents a combination of upper and lower motor deficits.

In addition to the routine testing mentioned above, a thorough examination of viscera, lymphatics, cardiovascular, and pulmonary systems are necessary to rule out systemic causes of pain syndrome not the least of which is mitotic disease, diabetes, and vascular disease all commonly associated with pain.

Those pain syndromes associated with mechanics, especially spinal disorders demand the use of the "show me" know how. Show me what you were doing when the pain came on. Show me the movement that makes it hurt. Assume the painful posture. Show me how you relieve the pain. Show me how you would lift this imaginary 100-pound box. Show me how you would open that valve. Show me your golf swing. And so on.

When the history and physical examination are completed, the clinical diagnosis is confirmed or revised in most instances, and then, what remains is nailing the diagnosis down with necessary ancillary testing.

ANCILLARY TESTING

Clinical medicine offers many modern choices to follow-up diagnostic impressions to clarify and expand upon the history and physical. With a mind toward careful selectivity to produce the maximum yield and yet at the same time be cost-conscious, the algologist can select most often from the following:

Necessary Laboratory Examination
Blood
Urine
Biopsy material
Nails/Hair exam for metals; drug use

X-ray and Other Diagnostic Imaging
Standard X-ray
Bone scans
Doppler ultrasound imaging
Contrast studies, i.e., myelography
Computerized Axial Tomography
Magnetic Resonance Imaging (MRI)
Thermography

Electrodiagnostic Testing
   Needle electromyography
   Traditional nerve conduction studies
   Late wave studies
   "H" reflex
   "F" wave
   Blink reflex
   Cortical-evoked potentials
   Somatosensory
   Visual
   Brain Stem Auditory

The blood studies range from those in hematology in which anemia or abnormality in blood cell size and configuration, and maturation, presence of appropriate platelets and white cell morphology all can lead to diagnosis, to specific simple clinical chemistry such as blood and/ or urine sugar levels looking at glucose metabolism abnormalities. Today, immunologic testing is useful in auto-immune diseases, viral states, rheumatologic disorders, and the vasculidities. While there is argument regarding hair analysis for cocaine and narcotic use, it has long been well-regarded in heavy metal poisonings. Specific metabolities can be measured in disorders such as porphuria. Renal and hepatic disorders are often easily identified with blood chemistries, and specific genetic disorders can be identified with chromasomal studies. When a tissue diagnosis is possible, biopsy material is the route to take. To be sure, not every test can be conducted, so the algologist must make informed choices and play clinical hunches keeping in mind the statistics regarding the diseases he or she is investigating, and searching for the rare when indicated.

Radiology has improved both in its application of routine studies with closer control of ionizing radiation with proper tubes and shielding and image intensifiers, and in high-resolution films, subtraction techniques to look at bone and soft tissue based on the relative radiodensity of the structures involved. Multiplanar tomography allows a slice and focus technique for helping sort out abnormalities location in a three-dimensional volume with a two-dimentional test. Nevertheless, the hazards of cumulative radiation dosimetry must be carefully weighed, and "routine" chest and spine films are no longer acceptable, now requiring justification.

Still newer techniques, such as nuclear scanning, add great dimension to testing from cardio-pulmonary to bone, joint, and visceral studies. Doppler ultrasound, used in "A" and "B" mode can look at such diverse areas as intrauterine, cardiac valve, and arterial and venous flow, cranial and visceral, or other tissue masses without the dangers of ionizing radiation.

There are still times when contrast studies such as myelography, today done with easily dispersible water-soluble dyes, remain the study of choice as investigating spinal cord tumors, or in angiography or intra-venous pyleography, however radiation dosimetry remains a major consideration. Contrast material study, when added to newer imaging techniques, such as computerized axial tomography and magnetic resonance imaging, is thought by some to add data to spinal and disc evaluations unequaled by either study alone.

Magnetic Resonance Imaging (MRI), a study of radio frequency emissions from atomic subparticles altered in their movements by a large magnetic field, continues to improve with experience with different spin weights and recording techniques ever decreasing the time to record the exam and increasing the resolution of the image. It may eventually replace CAT scanning (a computer-assisted ionizing radiation technique) nearly altogether, offering instead a nonionizing radiation detailed three-dimensional look at tissues previously only seen in two dimensions. Magnet size reduction, and cooling efficiency increases have made MRI units more reasonable in size and portable, enabling more efficient use and spreading their considerable cost among various users. Still, many patients become claustrophobic in the units even when pre-tranquilized, and patients with internal metal susceptible to magnet-induced movement are precluded from using the technique. Positron Emission Tomography (PET) scanning is still primarily a university center, highly expensive technology not often available outside of research institutions, but has the potential to demonstrate neural substrate activity and will be particularly useful in the study of activity of neural transmitters and the organic basis of emotional and cognitive aspects of pain. Different institutions possess varying "generation" scanners and the experience of radiologists varies, so that the physician is encouraged to investigate both where and by whom the study is best conducted, and consult the radiologist regarding the most appropriate and cost-efficient technique to arrive at a correct diagnosis. Communication of good clinical data to the radiologist is critical and cannot be overemphasized. One must be cognizant that in all new techniques time is required to determine true norms and then deviation from the norm. MRI and CAT scans have offered such a huge volume of sensitive anatomic data in the aging spine that many consider the findings of the degenerative cascade of aging "over read" and of less clinical use than at first suspected. As normative age-related data and pathologic difference data accumulate, by wedding imaging, electrophysiologic, and clinical data, the proper role of each will become clearer.

Another imaging technique, looking at skin temperature reflective in controlled circumstances of autonomic nervous system function and dysfunction, via sweat and vascular regulatory mechanisms, is thermography. Done either by the liquid crystal contact technique, or by the more expensive and comprehensive tele-electronic infrared system, measures of skin temperatures and "isotherms" are recorded for comparison with norms and with asymptomatic sides to assist in diagnosis of primarily sensory radiculopathy or neuropathy and neurovascular disorders. I find this technique of unparalleled assistance in the early detection of reflex sympathetic dystrophy and the follow-up of proper treatment as well as the earliest detector of reoccurrence. Others have noted its usefulness in cranial neuralgia, vascular extremity disorders including observation for over-tight casts in unconscious or uncooperative patients, and as a detector of bony pathology such as periostitis, fractures and tumor, and of cervical or lumbar radiculopathy with disturbance of thermotome symmetry. The original declaration that thermography was a picture of "pain" is, of course, untrue and netted the technique a dubious disdain as it was overused, abused, and overcharged for. However, the technique is a measure of somatosensory and somatosympathetic system dysfuntion and in the hands of experienced and ethical practitioners takes its place among the other listed diagnostic techniques available to the algologist.

Similar to imaging techniques which look primarily at structure, the electrodiagnostic medicine armamentarium, which looks primarily at physiology or function can be called into play when central and peripheral neurologic system or muscle disorders are suspected. There is little discomfort with needle technology in an advanced stage, and today's disposable needle markedly decreases the risk of slow virus and AIDS transmission. The reliability of the clinical diagnostic examination is only as good as the education, training, and experience of the electromyographer who determines the proper combination of electrodiagnostic tests related to answering the clinical hypothesis. Obviously the better the communication between the electomyographer and the algologist, the more readily the problem is answered. An electromyographer certified by the American Board of Electrodiagnostic Medicine, and a member of the American Association of Electrodiagnostic Medicine is often a better choice than an electromyographer without those credentials.

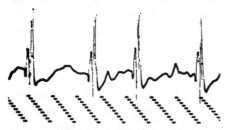

Fig. 5. Reduced recruitment in severe axonal neuropathy. (Monopolar needle in ext. dig. 1.) Note firing rate is 36 Hz. (Caliber: Each slanted line = 10 msec. Height = 200uV.) From Johnson, E. W. (1988). *Practical electromyography.* Baltimore: Williams & Wilkins. Reproduced with permission.

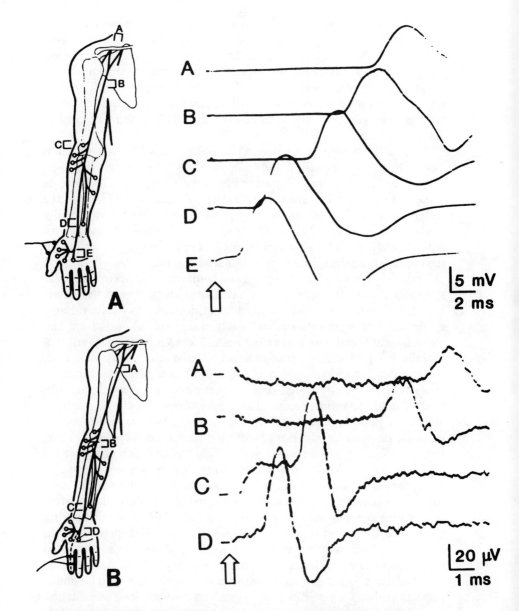

Fig. 6. (A) Motor nerve conduction study of the median nerve. The sites of stimulation include Erb's point (A), axilla (B), elbow (C), wrist (D), and palm (E). Compound muscle action potentials are recorded percutaneously from the thenar eminence. (B) Sensory nerve conduction study of the median nerve. The sites of stimulation include the axilla (A), elbow (B), wrist (C), and palm (D). Digital potentials are recorded antidromically, using the ring electrodes placed around the second digit. From Kimura, J. (1983). *Electrodiagnosis in diseases of the nerve and muscle* (2nd ed.). Philadelphia: F. A. Davis. Reproduced with permission.

Specific neuropathies including those which present as mononeuropathy multiplex or entrapments can be observed when combining needle EMG with nerve conduction testing. The value of nerve conduction velocity, specific latencies across known anatomical segments, the amplitude, duration, and configuration of the evoked motor (M) or sensory (S) potential and when used and compared with asymtomatic side and/or normative data. contribute to identification of neuropathology and with clinical data to diagnosis.

"H" and "F" waves can be used to look at proximal nerve segmental dysfunction and plexopathy or radiculopathy. The "H" reflex involves measurement of afferent large diameter fiber conduction from the limb, its synapse to anterior horn cell, and conduction along motor fibers to the tested muscle. The "F" wave propagates a stimulus antidromically towards the spinal cord along motor nerve fiber, involves Renshaw or other "backfiring" of the motor neuron, and orthodromic propagation of the impulse from the spinal cord to the peripheral muscle tested. Like the "H" wave the propagation is long arc and bi-directional making the measurement of value in such multi-segmental myelinopathies as those seen in renal disease, and proximal myelinopathies such as Guillain-Barre syndrome. The blink reflex allows study of that reflex's ipsilateral and contralateral polysynaptic distribution and looks at both afferrent cranial nerve V and efferrent cranial nerve VII and interneuron functions.

Computer technology and multiple stimulation with measurement over peripheral nerve, spinal cord, and cranium has allowed measurement of small potentials produced form measurements of fields of a large number of neural generators which can be readily identified and analyzed for presence or absence of expected peaks, amplitudes of peaks, interpeak latency, asymmetries, and the like. Stimulation of peripheral nerve, dermatomal segments innervated by specific sensory nerve produce predictable somatosensory-evoked potentials. Auditory clicks varying in amplitude and frequency are used to produce brain stem auditory-evoked responses, and visual bright flashes or alternating checkerboard field stimulation produces visual-evoked potentials. In each case, deficits may be identified by knowing the commonly expected peaks produced along the anatomic pathway, and searching for deviations from the norm. Disorders such as disseminated sclerosis, with its multi-segmental involvement can produce deficits on such long arc studies. Somatosensory-evoked potentials are also useful in interoperative monitoring to protect against neural tissue damage. Several textbooks are available to assist the reader. Some of my favorites are referenced (Chiappa, 1990; Johnson, 1988; Kimura, 1983).

In summary, the algologist by this time will have completed the history and physical examination and formed a clinical hypothesis, verified the diagnosis by selection of appropriate laboratory tests, the anatomy of the lesion through imaging, and the pathophysiology through electrophysiologic and thermographic data. To understand the pain perception and the functional disharmony caused by whatever diagnosis requires more than anatomy and physiology. It requires knowledge of the psychosocial profile of the patient before any reasonable treatment plan can be considered.

Psychosocial Data Notes
   Behavior often reproduces itself
   View the patient from each of his/her roles
   Identify pain-contingent behaviors/outcomes
   Look for internal versus external locus of pain control
   Search for disharmonies: home/job/religious/financial
   Sexual history is critical
   Quantify the degree of pain suffering
   Estimate degree of pain augmentation
   Role of formal psychometric testing

   In the obstetrical suite one can often find experienced nurses who predict the degree of pain behavior and pain suffering from the labor pain experience based on a patient's race, religion, and most importantly, cultural background. They have learned these behaviors are often culturally nurtured. We learn our socially acceptable pain behavior from our parents. Of course individual behavior cannot always be predicted by group-typified characteristics, but how parents and the patient's culture conditioned a patient is important.

   Further, the algologist will find useful the patient's previous pain experiences and the reaction to them. That data is included in the McGill Pain Questionnaire as the standard dictum that behavior reproduces itself is often true for pain. The examiner will have to survey the patient from his or her various roles in life looking to see if or how the pain has affected those roles. Acute pain is often accompanied by a transient decrease in responsibility, a regression of expectation for performance toward the immature from the mature, towards passivity and loss of control from activity and self-control, toward being cared for from being the care giver, from the traditional "masculine role" toward the more "feminine role." As pain becomes chronic, the syndrome associated with it often is exemplified by maintenance of these more regressed behaviors. While acute pain has a physiologically useful role in tissue protection and survival, chronic pain never plays a useful physiologic role, and retards behaviors which can effect happiness and function increase necessary for normal role-playing. Therefore, by examining each of the roles the patient plays, both prior to the onset of the pain syndrome and after it, one can better deal with the measurable effects and previous psychosocial pathologies. It is of no surprise that persons with previous psychosocial pathologies experience more frequent and more devastating chronic pain syndromes.

Further pain can cause very heightened anxiety which in and of itself augments pain perception, and long-time fear of pain and chronic suffering typically leads to depression and maladaptive behaviors.

One must observe for those behaviors and responses which are pain-contingent: relief of responsibility, additional sympathy or demonstrations of affection, medication consumption, posture assumption, sexual dysfunction or disinterest, acting out against or avoidance of spouse and or children, employers, teachers, insurers, and others, receipt of otherwise unearned income, such as workman's compensation or disability insurance. There are, of course, others which are negative: loss of self-esteem, loss of consortium, loss of job, disrespect from family and friends, and mistrust and other negatives from the "system" representatives. Fordyce (Fordyce, 1976; Fordyce, Roberts, & Sternbach, 1985), has led in the identification and use of operant conditioning techniques to change pain contingent-behaviors and his experience is worthy of attention.

Critically important is the patient's view of whether or not the pain is within his control or external to him and therefore, out of his control, making him a victim. Regaining an internal locus of control is critical to learning techniques to modulate pain and gain control of pain behavior. The anxieties associated with pain can lead to phobic and avoidance behaviors such as kinesiophobia (fear of movement), which must be identified to be treated, and which often persist long after the original conditioning stimulus is history.

Regardless of the timing of appearance before or after the onset of the pain syndrome, life disharmonies at home, the job, with finances, and with religious concepts tend to worsen during pain syndromes and demand identification and resolution within the totality of the pain syndrome complex. Psychosocial problems which could be supressed or managed prior to pain syndrome onset become terrible barriers to progress unless specifically identified as problems and specifically worked out. This medical "holism" is critical to success but often denied by insurance adjusters in the mistaken belief that the physical domain is their only responsibility and that the psychological somehow is the patient's own responsibility. This tends to slow the resolution of maladaptive behavior at the start and allows the behavior to become chronic and ingrained and the treatment time necessary for resolution prolonged. In chronic pain, an understanding and enlightened insurance adjuster is a critically important team member. Unfortunately, abuses of psychosocial measures and exhorbitant, seemingly endless, excessive charges have led to bona fide suspicion of the unproven program.

Sexual dysfunction is ubiquitous in chronic pain sufferers and its absence would raise my suspicion of the syndrome if absent. Since sexual dysfuntion rarely affects only the patient, spousal, and or "significant other," history is important. The poor communication fostered by the role changes, short tempers, frustration and anxious depression rarely have any but negative effects on lovemaking, and once this negativism appears it rarely, in my experience, self-corrects. Yet, not dealt with it, remains as a major impediment to chronic pain syndrome effective treatment which is often hidden and unresearched and can act like a silent cancer, confounding other treatment until removed. Sensitivity is a must in dealing with the issue; however, straightforward discussion is better in my experience than incomplete and veiled references and questioning.

The McGill format pays attention to pain suffering quantification and enables a reasonable estimation of pain augmentation. It should be often emphasized that we are dealing here with chronic pain unassociated with mitotic disease (so called "benign" chronic pain although no chronic pain is truely benign) Those chronic pain syndromes associated with mitosis must be identified and treated in their own unique way including, as necessary, narcotic pharmacolgic relief in proper dose and frequency, anxiety and sleep disturbance relief. For the nonmitotic chronic pain sufferer, most observors believe that abusable substances are best avoided although Ronald Melzack (1990) advocates lower-dose-higher frequency narcotics orally as safe and effective without major problems of addiction. Since the pain experience is remembered, many programs offer imagery techniques to describe it in size, color, temperature, shape, and radiation as a deliberate cognitive treatment, closely observing change (for the better from the memorized version), and deconditioning the suffering response and pain behavior associated with it.

Psychometric testing can be quite helpful in dealing with these psychosocial questions, in learning previous behavioral patterns, and in planning effective treatment. The Minnesota Multiphasic Personality Inventory (MMPI) (Hatthaway & McKinley, 1967), Millon Behavioral Health Inventory (MBHI), and the Derogatis self-reported inventory (Deragotis, Rickels, & Rock, 1976) are those formal tests I have found most helpful in my practice. They are easily completed, lend themselves to computer scoring, and have wide-based experiences in pain populations with extensive normative data. The tests must be carefully explained to the patient. Language or non-North American cultural exclusions must be applied. The data refect anxiety, depression, somatic concern, internal or external locus of control, indices which raise suspicion for addictive or antisocial behaviors, and reality distortions. The tests require high school-level vocabulary skills and a willingness to self-complete without coaching. They are supplemented by professional psychological interviews and other appropriate testing. Many patients will also require intelligence-testing, cognitive testing, perceptual motor testing, and vocational testing to complete their profile before and during treatment.

Perhaps the most important aspect of assessment is the development of an understanding of patient goals.

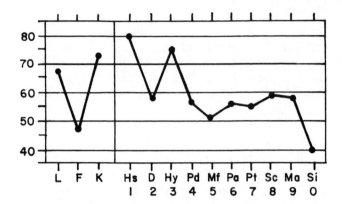

Fig. 7. "Conversion V" MMPI profile, obtained from a 39-year-old man with job-related chest and shoulder pains. There was a large behavioral component to his pain problem, as evidenced by his wife's assumption of his household responsibilities and worker's compensation equal to his former salary. From Chapman and Syrjala. (1990). *Measurement of pain.* In John Bonica (Ed.), *The management of pain.* Philadelphia: Lea & Febiger. Reproduced with permission.

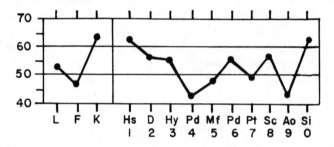

Fig. 8. Normal profile, obtained from a 69-year-old woman with chronic upper back pain. This patient was not found to have problems with depression or excessive medication use, but was deactivated secondary to pain. From Chapman and Syrjala. (1990). *Measurement of pain.* In John Bonica (Ed.), *The manangement of pain.* Philadelphia: Lea & Febiger. Reproduced with permission.

PATIENT GOALS

- Critical to management
- Identify in writing
- Develop time-frame for reaching

Many chronic pain patients are lost. They find it impossible to list specific goals except vague "take my pain away" verbiage. The algologist must explain the results of the assessment to the patient, and within that context work to develop very simple, clearly measurable series of short-term goals and some broader long-term goals which might be reached by attainment of the short-term goals in orderly fashion. The goals must be in writing and provide a means of measurement. I will walk 150 yards by Tuesday. I will stay out of bed two additional hours per day by the first of the month. I will demonstrate proper lifting techniques at the completion of back school. I will not drink any alcohol as of now. I will reduce my cigarettes by one per day till I smoke none next Wednesday. I will return to widget-making four hours per day sitting on July 1st. Be sure the goals are reasonable and attainable so that profuse reward can be given for making them and new higher goals may be set. They must be the patient's goals, not the examiner's, although the examiner may influence them.

Finally, your brilliant ideas, conceived after completion of the above steps, and the patient's informed consent, equal a good management plan. This will be a plan based on easily measurable goals formulated in writing with your help by the patient. The outcome of a good assessment and diagnostic plan is a good management plan.

REFERENCES

Bonica, J. (1990). *Definitions and taxonomy of pain.* (p. 19). In J. Bonica (Ed.), *The management of pain.* Philadelphia: Lea and Febiger.

Chapman, C. R., & Syrjala, K. (1990). *Measurement of pain.* (p. 587). In John Bonica (Ed.), *Measurement of pain.* Philadelphia: Lea and Febiger.

Chiappa, K. (1990). *Evoked potentials in clinical medicine,* 2nd ed. New York: Raven Press.

de Jong, R. H. (1980). Defining pain terms. *JAMA, 244*:143.

Derogatis, I.R., Rickels, K., & Rock, A. F. (1976). The SCL-90 and the MMPI, a step in the validation of a new self-report scale. *British Journal of Psychology, 128*:280.

Fordyce, W. E. (1976). *Behavioral methods in chronic pain and illness.* St. Louis: C. V. Mosby.

Fordyce, W., Roberts, A, & Sternbach, R. (1985). Behavioral management of chronic pain: A response to critics. *Pain, 22*:113.

Hathaway, S. R. & McKinley, J. C. (1967). *The Minnesota Multiphasic Personality Inventory Manual.* New York: The Psychological Corporation.

Johnson, E. (1988). *Practical electromyography.* Baltimore: Williams and Wilkins.

Kimura, J. (1983). *Electrodiagnosis in diseases of nerve and muscle,* 2nd ed. Philadelphia: F. A. Davis.

Loeser, J. D. (1982). *Concepts of pain.* In M. Stanton-Hicks & R. Boas (Eds.), Chronic low back pain. New York: Raven Press.

Melzack, R. (1990). On the treatment of pain. *Scientific American, 262*:31.

Melzack, R. (1975). *Pain.*

Melzack, R. (1975). The McGill pain questionnaire: Major properties and scoring methods. *Pain, 1*:275.

Chapter 6

THE PSYCHIATRIST'S ROLE IN PAIN MANAGEMENT

Nelson Hendler, M. D., M. S.

Nelson Hendler, M.D. reports that a psychiatrist involved in pain management engages in many roles; e.g., diagnostician, pharmacologist, sociologist, psychotherapist and, at times, a patient advocate. Doctor Hendler describes three approaches employed by the psychiatrist. These include: the medical model, the psychiatric model, and the integrated response model. A family systems theory explanation from which the patient finds fulfillment by his/her symptoms from family members is also discussed. The concept of learned helplessness and the need for the therapist to assist the patient regain control of life events is reviewed.

Doctor Hendler divides chronic pain patients into four groups: (1) objective pain patient; (2) exaggerating pain patient; (3) an undetermined pain patient; and (4) affective or associative pain patient. Treatment may consist of psychotherapy, biofeedback, family therapy, group psychotherapy, medication, and hypnosis. These methods are reviewed as a specialized treatment for pain management.

Reprinted, with changes, from *The Anaesthesiologist's Guide to Pain Management,* Carol Warfield (Ed.). Dordrecht, The Netherlands: Kluwer Academic Publishers.

Chapter 6

THE PSYCHIATRIST'S ROLE IN PAIN MANAGEMENT

Nelson Hendler, M. D., M. S.

The role of a psychiatrist in chronic pain management is multiple. He or she must be a diagnostician, a pharmacologist, a sociologist, a psychotherapist, and even, on occasion, a patient advocate. Therefore, by definition, the psychiatrist must have an eclectic orientation, and be broadly schooled in all forms of diagnostic and therapeutic interventions.

There are at least three approaches to chronic pain that a psychiatrist may use. Each has its own advantages and disadvantages:

The Medical Model. Using this paradigm, pain is defined as a manifestation of a disease. This approach lends clarity to the problems of pain, and offers predictive capabilities for outcome. It may offer a cure where none existed before. As an example, "pain in the back and the leg" is a description, but "a herniated disc with radiculopathy" is a diagnosis. Surgery on the disc may cure the pain. However, should the surgery not work, or should there be psychological problems or social problems compounding recovery, response to surgery may not be as predicted.

The Psychiatric Model. Using this approach, a psychiatrist tries to establish a psychiatric diagnosis to explain behavior of a pain patient who is troublesome or not responding in the predicted fashion. Using this tact, personality disorders, affective disorders, or anxiety traits that might be the source of a patient's complaints are identified and treated. Unfortunately, the use of psychiatric intervention in this fashion very often leads to an "either-or" type of thinking, with psychiatric diagnosis being established to the exclusion of medical diagnosis. A person with a histrionic personality disorder, who has surgical excision of a disc, and doesn't get well, may run afoul of the system. His or her lack of recovery is ascribed to "secondary gain" or "dependency needs," but not to retained disc material missed by the first surgery.

The Integrated Response Model. Using this model, the psychiatrist tries to establish both medical and psychiatric diagnoses, not only from the point in time at which a patient is seen, but also based on the historical perspective of the patient, i.e., the "pre-morbid" or "pre-pain" personality. In this fashion, one can determine the appropriateness of response to pain, and to treatment. This approach is time-consuming and involves a multidisciplinary approach, with multi-level diagnoses, and integration of material. In this model, both medical and psychiatric diagnoses can exist.

Adherence to the medical model is often found within pain treatment centers, or in clinical practices, that utilize only medical evaluation of the patient. The absence of a psychiatric or psychological professional, to assist in evaluation and diagnosis, limits the evaluation of the chronic pain patient to only medical assessment. It disregards the possibility that a patient may have psychiatric problems, as the result of chronic pain, which can lead to diagnostic oversights. Indeed, there are some authors who feel that the incidence of depression, in association with chronic pain, is remarkably high (Krishnan, France, Pelton, McCann, Davidson, & Bruno, 1985; Hendler, 1984; Pilowsky & Bassett, 1982). On the other hand, other authors have advanced the theory that chronic pain may be a manifestation of an underlying depression (Engel, 1959; Maruta, Swanson, & Swanson, 1976). Therefore, the medical assessment of chronic pain, without psychiatric assessment, (to determine the pre-existing personality characteristics, and motivations, which may lead to an exaggerated response to chronic pain, or may, in fact, lead to the expression of psychiatric disease as a chronic pain process) would compromise any medical diagnostic endeavor. By the same token, severe and chronic illness certainly produces depression, and other associated psychiatric disorders, which would benefit from therapeutic intervention. The use of a purely medical model can not be endorsed.

Likewise, the purely psychiatric model suffers from many of the same problems. In a most thorough review of the problem, Dr. Charles Ford (1986) discusses what has been called the "somatizing disorders." In this article, Ford discussed the concept of the sick role, which allows the ill person to be released from regular duties and obligations. He further differentiates illness from disease, describing the latter as objectively measured, while illness discusses the change in functioning of an individual. He further clarifies the point, indicating that disease can occur in the absence of illness, while conversely, illness can occur in the absence of disease. Doctor Ford further describes somatization as "the process by which an individual uses the body, or bodily symptoms, for psychological purpose or personal gain." However, Ford does concede that somatization can occur in the presence of demonstrable physical disease, with amplification of the response to a real physical disorder. Ford then lists nine reasons why people somatize: (1) To avoid unpleasant tasks, or to achieve primary or secondary gains, in the form of payment; (2) to solve family problems; (3) to allow an individual to focus on physical symptoms, rather than psychological problems; (4) as a form of communication of displeasure; (5) as a way of expressing oneself when they are not capable of expressing themselves otherwise; (6) a culturally-determined response; (7) using a physical symptom, because is it more culturally acceptable than a psychiatric one; (8) focusing on physical problems, that are manifestations of underlying stress; (9) utilizing a fashionable diagnosis to explain underlying/ psychiatric disease, such as hypoglycemia. Ford further feels that patients may utilize somatic symptoms instead of expressing depression, and further indicates that these depressions are unrecognized. Anxiety may also manifest as a somatic complaint, which he also felt was undiagnosed. According to Ford, "chronic pain syndromes are one of the more common forms of somatization." He also includes disability syndromes under the description of somatizing disorders. He describes hard-working individuals, who have an accident, and then fall apart. This inability to function allows the individual to have support and secondary gains, and allow an underlying dependency to become manifest.

In a superb review article, Dr. Dennis Turk and Dr. Herta Flor (1984) reviewed the psychological models contributing to chronic back pain. In this article, they discuss theoretical constructs, which explain the transition from acute to chronic back pain, with the exception of the psychoanalytic approach. In this approach, unexplained back pain is considered a conversion neurosis, or a manifestation of underlying tension, manifesting as increased muscle activity, and spasm. Using this model, various authors have suggested that pain of unexplained origin should be treated as depression, with the use of antidepressant drugs. Another explanation for unexplained back pain advances the family systems theory. In this approach, the basis idea is that "symptoms of the patient fulfill the emotional needs of other family members." They suggest that the sick role is used for conflict avoidance. Another theory that is advanced is the observational learning theory based on cognitive behavioral assumptions. In this model, the patient expresses feelings of helplessness and hopelessness, and a loss of control of his environment. Another theory, originally advanced by Flor, discusses the diathesis-stress model of chronic back pain. In this model, biopsychosocial interactions lead to the development of chronic back pain. This is an attempt to integrate the physical, psychological, and social factors which lead to the development of illness. In this diathesis-stress model, hyperactivity of the back muscles may be due to (1) "the existence of a response stereotypy (diathesis) involving the back muscles, (2) recurrent or very intense adverse situations perceived as stressful, and/or (3) inadequate coping abilities of the individual."

Another attempt to explain pain of unknown etiology utilizes the diagnostic manual of the American Psychiatric Association. Reich, Rosenblatt, and Tupin (1983) attempt to explain the use of this diagnostic system for chronic pain patients. In this article, the authors indicate that attempts to categorize chronic pain patients "merely in terms of the prime physical complaints has obvious shortcomings." They describe the five categories, or axes, in the DSM-III manual, which correspond to five major areas of concern: Axis I, used to describe thought disorders, such as schizophrenia, and/or manic depressive disease, and drug abuse problems; Axis II, used to describe personality characteristics; Axis III, used to describe medical diagnoses, or physical complaints; Axis IV, used to describe the severity of psychosocial stress; and Axis V, used to describe the highest level of functioning the past year. Reich and his group feel that an entire category of diagnoses, "The Somatiform Disorders," can be used to categorize chronic pain patients, in whom there is a strong psychological component, that could explain a pain unexplained by physical diagnosis. The major diagnosis within this group is "psychogenic pain disorder." The criteria for utilizing this diagnosis is (1) the absence of appropriate physical findings, and (2) the presence of psychological factors, which may explain the etiology of the complaint. Attendant to this diagnosis is a variety of subjective assessments, such as the severity of the pain, the inability of the pain to conform with anatomical distribution, and, perhaps the most subjective assessment of all, that the severity of the pain be out of proportion to what one might anticipate. Further diagnostic categories under the somatiform disorders are hypochondriasis, and conversion disorders. In the former, the patient is concerned with the development of a severe, debilitating illness, despite the lack of objective findings. In this instance, the patient's concerns are considered inordinate, since the organic complaint was not substantiated. In conversion disorders, the physical condition suggests an underlying organic disease, but the basis of the illness is purely psychological. The authors then offer several examples of DSM-III diagnoses, in which the predominant feature of Axis III, that is the physical axis, is the use of words "inconsistent with physical findings," "pain, etiology unknown," and prior surgeries "with residual pain." The authors advocate the use of DSM-III taxonomy, since it has achieved better reliability than previous psychiatric diagnostic systems. The kappa value for somatization disorders is 0.66, indicating a reasonable degree of reproduceability. However, the validity of these diagnoses remain in question.

The third approach to diagnosing chronic pain patients, utilizing an integrated response model, avoids the diagnostic dualism of the previous two models. In this model, an attempt is made to study the normal response to chronic pain, in a previously well-adjusted individual, and using these responses as a benchmark, against which other responses can be measured. Only by thoroughly understanding the normal patterns of response can one determine what is abnormal. It is for this same reason that a medical student studies anatomy before he studies pathology, or physiology before one studies pathophysiology. It also attempts to integrate responses, taking into account physical, psychological, and environmental factors, including sociological and legal considerations. One such attempt at integration has been advanced by Richard Black, M.D. (1982). In his chapter, Dr. Black asserts that a patient with a chronic pain syndrome must be assessed simultaneously for physical, mental, and environmental factors. He feels that sociological and economic factors rarely get considered, except where litigation is involved. He delineates six factors that should be considered when evaluating a chronic pain patient: (1) somatogenic, referring to the physical perception of the pain, divided into both an acute and chronic complaint; (2) anxiety, divided into the psychological state versus the personality traits of the individual; (3) depression, divided into biochemical depression, reactive depression, depression secondary to the use of medications (but, unfortunately, not including any history about pre-existing depressions, prior to the acquisition of the pain); (4) social factors, divided into problems at work and problems at home; (5) gains, divided into financial gains and personal gains; and (6) cultural factors, which would allow varying degrees of expression of a patient's pain. While not complete, this paradigm does offer some useful suggestions. First and foremost, Dr. Black does recognize the fact that certain psychological problems, in chronic pain states, are transient, while other psychological problems are part of the personality characteristics of the individual, and probably preceded the acquisition of the pain. He is one of the first authors to raise the question of cause-effect relationships. This is an often-neglected consideration, since most articles about psychological components of chronic pain fail to take into consideration the pre-morbid state of the individual, i.e., what was the person like before they had chronic pain?

In an effort to further clarify this issue, Hendler and Talo (1989) offer a diagnostic system, which takes into consideration (1) the pre-morbid (pre-pain) adjustment of the individual (pathological or well-adjusted), (2) the response to the pain (pathological or appropriate), and (3) the actual physical diagnosis (the presence or absence of objective findings). Central to his formulation are two basic concepts: (1) chronic pain can create psychological problems in a previously well-adjusted individual, and (2) regardless of the pre-morbid (pre-pain) personality characteristics, if a person has a normal response to chronic pain, then the chance of a valid, organic basis for the complaint of pain is quite high. This would be true, even in the absence of objective laboratory studies, or physical findings. Restated for emphasis, if a patient's response to pain is appropriate, but there are no objective physical findings, it is incumbent upon the physician to keep looking for the source of the patient's complaint.

Hendler (1981) has divided the chronic pain patients into four groups, based on the three factors mentioned above, i.e., (1) pre-morbid adjustment, (2) response to pain, and (3) the presence or absence of objective physical findings on laboratory studies or physical examination. These four categories are: (1) objective pain patient, defined as an individual with (a) good pre-morbid adjustment, (b) normal response to chronic pain, and (c) a definable organic lesion; (2) exaggerating pain patient, defined as an individual with (a) psychopathology as part of a pre-morbid adjustment, (b) an unusual response to pain, in that there might be an absence of anxiety, or depression, and (c) minimal organic findings; (3) an undetermined pain patient, defined as an individual with (a) good pre-morbid adjustment, (b) a normal response to pain, and (c) an absence of objective physical findings or physical examination (it is this individual who warrants further investigation); (4) affective or associative pain patient, defined as an individual with (a) a poor pre-morbid adjustment, (b) an unusual response to chronic pain, and (c) a total absence of objective physical findings or positive laboratory studies.

By studying the normal response to chronic pain, one can then compare any patient against a known standard. In this case, the objective pain patient serves as the "normal" model against which all other responses to chronic pain should be judged. The objective pain patient has a good pre-morbid adjustment, which can be defined as (1) a good work record, (2) a stable family background, (3) a negative psychiatric history, with no previous suicide attempts, or depression, (4) the absence of alcohol or drug abuse, (5) a good marital history, (6) lack of financial difficulties prior to the pain, (7) a good sexual adjustment, (8) no sleep difficulties, (9) no radical changes in weight, other than conscious attempts to change it, (10) the absence of any arrests or sociopathic behavior (Hendler, 1982). Hendler further expands upon the objective pain patient, indicating that this individual goes through four stages, in response to the chronic pain. The acute stage, anywhere from 0 to 2 months, is when the individual expects to get well, and has no psychological problems. Psychological testing administered during this time is within normal limits. In the sub-acute stage, anywhere from 2 to 6 months, the individual begins to experience somatic concerns, and might have elevated Scales 1 and 3 on the MMPI. In the chronic stage of chronic pain, anywhere from 6 months to 8 years after the acquisition of the pain, the previously well-adjusted individual then develops depression, and has elevated Scales 1, 2, and 3 on the MMPI, with Scale 2 (Depression) being higher than Scales 1 and 3 (Hypochondriasis and Hysteria). Anywhere from 3 to 12 years after the acquisition of the pain, the patient enters the sub-chronic stage of chronic pain, during which time the depression resolves, but Hypochondriacal and Hysterical Scales of the MMPI remain elevated, as one might expect, because the patient still has somatic concerns.

If all of the above occurs in an individual with a definable organic lesion, with positive objective testing, then one categorizes this type of patient as an objective pain patient. If all of the above psychological features are present, but no objective testing is positive, then one considers this individual an undetermined pain patient, who still needs further medical investigation (Hendler, 1981).

In order to facilitate diagnosis, using the four categories described above, Hendler and his coworkers have devised the "Mensana Clinic Back Pain Test" (Hendler, Mollett, Viernstein, Schroeder, Rybock, Campbell, Levin, & Long, 1985). Using a simple, 15-question screening test, chronic pain patients can be divided into the four diagnostic categories, described by Hendler. The screening test had good predictive values, since women scoring in the objective pain patient category (17 points or less) had positive findings on EMG, nerve conduction velocity studies, thermography, CT scan, myleogram, or X-ray, 77% of the time. If women scored in the exaggerating pain patient category (21 points or greater), none of the 53 women studied had objective physical findings. This is in counterdistinction to the MMPI, which had a great deal of scatter, with only the Depression Scale correlating at all with the absence or presence of physical findings. Hendler and his colleagues (1985) also published results for the predictive volume of his test for men, showing that, in 31 men there was a 91% chance of organic pathology if the patient scored in the objective pain patient range. Overall, the predictive value of the test was 85% (Hendler, Mollett, Talo, & Levin, 1988). The usefulness of the four diagnostic categories for chronic pain patients is highlighted by the ability to predict the presence or absence of objective physical findings, based on (1) pre-morbid adjustment, (2) response to chronic pain, and (3) description of the pain itself. The fact that the MMPI, which measures personality traits, was not a useful predictor of physical abnormalities, lends support to the belief that personality characteristics and physical abnormalities are independent events, which reduces the accuracy of the current DSM-III diagnostic manual, for validating the complaints of pain (Hendler and Talo, 1989).

The preceding lengthy preamble, regarding the psychiatric diagnosis is critical to defining the role of a psychiatrist in treating chronic pain patients. It is essential to have a diagnosis of an individual, before instituting the therapy. By offering a clinician a variety of diagnostic systems from which he or she can choose, then the selection of appropriate therapy becomes a less formidable task. Whether one strictly adheres to DSM-III diagnoses, or less conventional diagnostic systems, is a matter of which system gives the best results in the hands of a particular practitioner. This should facilitate selection of an appropriate therapy. While there are many types of psychotherapy available, treatment results are not well documented for any of the forms of therapy. This chapter will deal with the more conventional modalities, i.e., (1) individual psychotherapy, (2) biofeedback, (3) family therapy, (4) group psychotherapy, (5) pharmacotherapy, (6) narcosynthesis, and (7) hypnosis.

PSYCHOTHERAPY

There are very few reports in the psychiatric and medical literature which support the contention that individual psychotherapy is a useful treatment for chronic back problems, or pain of any sort. For the purpose of definition, one should consider psychotherapy as an individual session, conducted between a patient and a therapist, without the use of specialized techniques, such as hypnosis, biofeedback, or narcosynthesis. Likewise, group psychotherapy or conditioning therapy are separate and distinct from individual, insight-oriented, dynamatic psychotherapy. When one imposes these parameters on the definition of psychotherapy, reports on its efficacy are sparse indeed. However, there are some components of individual psychotherapy that have therapeutic benefit, even though it is difficult to substantiate their efficacy. Rutrick (1981) reports that psychotherapy can be effective, if the therapist directs his activity towards understanding the "psychosomatic" personality, described as individuals who have (a) difficulty with psychological thinking, (b) expressing emotion, and (c) being impulsive. In his abstract, Rutrick suggests that character analysis is a critical element of psychotherapy, and "is necessary to assure real emotional insight, and effect integretation." He suggests that "digestible interpretations" would encourage learning of what component of the pain is thought to be psychological. Furthermore, he suggests using countertransference, and relationships in the patient's life to help freer expression of emotions. Dr. Rutrick concludes that psychotherapy can overcome major emotional obstacles, and facilitate the acceptance of chronic pain, and functioning, despite the presence of chronic pain. He indicates that psychotherapy can generate improved self-esteem, and relationships between individuals in the patient's life. He attributes this to the re-ordering of "narcissistic forces," meaning the patient is encouraged to reprioritize their goals and perceptions about themselves. Unfortunately, there is no substantive data associated with this report, and it is largely anecdotal, utilizing case reports for illustration.

Very often, psychotherapy is administered, in conjunction with other modalities of therapy. As such, "eclectic studies, employing numbers of interventions provide some evidence for the usefulness of comprehensive treatment programs. However, the lack of control groups, the lack of a comprehensive pain assessment and the uncertainty about the effective components do not allow definite conclusions to be drawn. Here too, a wide variety of patients have been treated with a lack of or widely divergent sample descriptions. It needs to be determined which patients profit from what treatment. Component analysis of eclectic and cognitive-behavioral treatments are needed to determine the effective interventions and thus reduce cost and treatment time and enhance the effectiveness of the treatment (Turk & Flor, 1984).

One element of psychotherapy, which is present whether an individual therapist recognizes it or not, is the component of modeling. This process occurs when patients observe another person with chronic pain, who is functioning despite their physical damage. This other individual serves as a model for the patient's behavior, and straddles the bridge between individual psychotherapy, and behavioral therapy. Some therapists have used videotapes of patients in pain coping with their problem, while others have used a directive approach, actually instructing a patient about what behaviors are acceptable, and which are not (Webb, 1983).

BIOFEEDBACK

The use of biofeedback as a modality for assisting patients with chronic pain has created much controversy. Some authors feel that biofeedback does not offer any advantage over relaxation techniques, and attributed its efficacy to its placebo effect (Webb, 1983). Other authors have conducted a more comprehensive review, and conclude that EMG biofeedback may be a promising treatment modality for chronic back pain (Turk & Flor, 1984). In their most evenhanded review of biofeedback techniques, Turk and Flor report only the results of EMG biofeedback. This modality seems to have the most usefulness for patients with muscle tension-type pain. In their review, Turk and Flor found that there were three types of reports in the literature: (1) anecdotal or systematic case studies, (2) group outcome or comparison studies, or (3) controlled group studies. The efficacy of EMG biofeedback was further complicated by the fact that in a review of over 20 articles, all researches, save one, utilize concomitant medication, and not biofeedback exclusively. In the two controlled studies, reviewed by Turk and Flor, both showed strong effects of EMG biofeedback on reducing pain and tension levels. In one study, a decrease in 60% in pain intensity and duration, as suffered by the patient, was noted. As expected, as muscle tension levels drop, pain intensity also drops. However, interestingly, at three month follow-up, even though muscle tension increased, pain reduction was maintained. In the other study reviewed, EMG biofeedback was compared to medical treatment, and "pseudotherapy." In this study, conducted by Flor and her co-workers, they found that EMG biofeedback was more efficacious than pseudotherapy and control groups receiving just medical treatment alone. They noted that EMG readings decreased, and the patients sought less medical attention, when utilizing EMG biofeedback. Turk and Flor conclude that muscle relaxation alone does not necessarily contribute to the beneficial effects of EMG biofeedback, but rather a cognitive process is important. Hendler and his co-workers attribute EMG biofeedback effectiveness to another factor. In their study, they found two groups of patients: (a) those who responded to biofeedback, and (b) those who did not respond to biofeedback (Hendler, Derogatis, Avella, & Long). In this study, 13 patients were evaluated, using EMG biofeedback. Six of the 13 reported that they had less pain on at least 4 out of 5 days of EMG biofeedback training, but 11 of the 13 were unable to alter EMG biofeedback in the affected muscle group. EMG relaxation consisted of reduction of muscle tension in the forehead. Therefore, one might conclude that specific muscle relaxation was not the therapeutic component of the EMG biofeedback. There were no significant differences between either the starting EMG muscle tension levels, or the final levels, between the two groups. However, the response rate, that is 6 out of 13, was double what one might expect from a placebo effect alone on a consistent basis (Hendler & Fernandez, 1980). The difference between the two groups was thought to be the stage at which the patient was in their chronic pain process, i.e., whether they were in the acute stage, subacute stage, chronic stage, or subchronic stage. The difference between the patients who responded, and those who didn't respond, was the presence of depression in the responders. Those who did not respond, did not have elevated depression scales, using the SCL-90.

Other components that may contribute to efficacy of biofeedback therapy is the issue of the patient's motivation or preparedness for change (Large, 1985). Large utilized a measure for "illness attitudes" in an effort to determine which patients might respond to therapeutic interventions. They used an illness behavior questionnaire, developed by Pilowsky and Spence, and expanded upon this, by using a repertory grid technique, which has been described by Bannister and his co-workers. Seven of the 18 patients did not experience overall relief of symptoms, while 11 of the subjects did. In this report by Large, 48 ratings were analyzed to determine the discrepancy between how a patient perceived him or herself, and the patient wished they would be. Correlating these findings with response to biofeedback showed that people who were dissatisfied with their condition, i.e., chronic and persistent pain, were more likely to respond well to biofeedback.

FAMILY THERAPY

The role of the family in the maintenance of chronic pain behavior may be one factor to consider when dealing with treatment failures. The poorest outcome among patients with chronic pain was found in families with the greatest degree of agreement when rating the severity of the patient's pain (Webb, 1983). Webb interprets this as "tertiary gain," indicating that the pain is maintained because of the psychological importance to another family member. A more likely explanation is the fact that a person with severe debilitating disease would have difficulty concealing the deficit from the family members and they would be in agreement with his assessment of the pain. Webb describes family studies in which it is clear that the spouse and children of patients with chronic pain experience distress, as might be expected. This is particularly true in families where the patient is unemployed, while less so in families where the patient is retired. Webb (1983) feels that families can reinforce the pain and worsen the prognosis.

A more empathic study involved that of the spouse of a chronic pain sufferer. Two nurses (Rowat & Knafl, 1985) studied the impact of pain on 40 spouses of chronic suffers (21 males and 19 females). Rowat and Knafl found that 60% of the spouses were uncertain as to the cause or persistence of the pain in their partner. Additionally, 83% of the spouses reported experiencing emotional, physical, or social disturbances, that they directly attributed to the pain in their spouse. Sixty-nine per cent of the spouses felt that they were experiencing emotional difficulties as a result of their partner's pain. The most frequent forms of emotional disturbance were sadness or depression, fear, irritability, and nervousness. Forty per cent of the spouses reported that there was a sense of helplessness, since they were unable to effect any change their partner's pain, and they were uncertain as how to proceed with doing so. They expressed feelings of loss of control. Seventy-five per cent of the spouses felt that they could delineate which factors influence their mate's pain, such as increased activity which reduced or increased the pain, and medications reducing the pain. Rowat and Knafl (1985) divided the spouses into two groups: (1) high distress spouses, and (2) low distress spouses. The high distress spouses reported feeling stress within the physical, emotional, and social dimensions of their lives. They experienced disturbances of sleep, appetite, physical symptoms, attention, anxiety, fear, sadness, isolation, and loss of freedom. They felt trapped in their relationship. Interestingly, 50% of the high distress spouses ranked their mate's pain higher on the McGill Pain Questionnaire than the patient himself did. In counterdistinction, the low distress spouses denied any major disturbance in their personal life or family life as a result of chronic pain. The major distinction between the low distress spouse was the fact that their mate had only been in pain for an average of 6.85 years while the high distress group had experienced pain as part of their marital relationship for 12.5 years. Also, only 3 of 13 patients were unemployed in the low stress spouse group, while 7 of 12 patients were unemployed in the high stress spouse group. From this study, the authors conclude that the uncertainty of the pain, uncertainty of the family life, uncertainty of pain management, and spousal distress were all factors which contributed to their own distress. Of particular note is the fact that the high distress spouse group was unable to recognize factors which influenced the pain experience by their partners. Perhaps this one element of loss of control over a particular situation contributed to the distress that they were contributing. The authors certainly make a strong point for including family members in the psychotherapy of chronic pain patients.

In a very fine review article, a pair of authors (Payne & Norfleet, 1986) examine the factors influencing family relationships, and feel that certain family characteristics and behaviors contribute to the problem of chronic pain, as well as influencing outcome. In their review, Payne and Norfleet (1986) found that some authors believe that there might be a relationship between the maintenance of pain and a large family size. The rationale for this is obvious. In a large family, one of the only ways to get attention and to reduce tension, would be the expression of disability, or invalidism. Some authors have even reported that the majority of their patients come from families with four or more children. Birth order was also considered as a factor influencing the complaint of pain. One author found the youngest or the oldest child complained, while another author found that the complaint of pain might more effectively reduce tension for younger children in large families. These findings have not been supported by other authors. Socioeconomic status also may influence the expression of pain. The fact that a majority of pain patients come from blue collar workers has been interpreted as the inability of working class people to express emotional conflict, thereby using somatizing terms. Of course, one must take into account that there are probably more blue collar workers than there are professionals, and its the blue collar workers who have the manually strenuous jobs that put them at higher risk. Other equivocally substantiated theories have been offered, such as the quality of relationships with parents, early loss of a family member, incidence of pain or illness in the family and location of the pain corresponding to that of the family member. Depression in the family member has also been explained in psychodynamatic terms, which are equally as difficult to substantiate. No doubt, patients with chronic pain have reduced sexual activity and poor sexual adjustment, which may contribute to a poor marital relationship. Unfortunately, the majority of studies in this area discuss only the patient, as they appear at the time that they are seen by the physician, without adequate historical perspective. One questions whether or not marital difficulties develop as the result of the chronic pain, or if marital difficulties predated the chronic pain, and the chronic pain became a convenient excuse to avoid further sexual contact. When chronic pain patients with depression were compared to patients with just depression, the former group had a more disturbed marital relationship than the latter. In another study, pain patients with no documented organic lesion were found to have more frequent "upsets, blows, conflicting interests, or separations," than those patients with definable organic lesions. Payne and Norfleet (1986) further report that 91% of couples interviewed at the Chronic Pain Treatment Center reported sexual problems, and a decline in their social lives, since the onset of their pain problem. This was confirmed by other researchers. The authors conclude that studies on marital relationships involving chronic pain patients consistently indicate high rates of sexual and marital maladjustment, even in previously stable relationships. However, they also advance the notion that the family may maintain the pain of an individual patient. Based on Payne's and Norfleet's review of the literature, they feel there are four factors that contribute to the persistence of chronic pain in a patient: (1) the patient's pain is an expression of dysfunction within the family system and it is easier to utilize the complaint of pain, rather than say there are difficulties with relationships, (2) the family acts as a reinforcer for pain behavior, by nurturing and caring for the injured member, (3) the patient may use the symptom of pain to control his family members and is reinforced when this works, and (4) the stresses of family life may produce physiological effects, which predispose an individual to stress and disease.

The review article considers the three approaches to family therapy: (1) behavioral, (2) transactional, and (3) systems approach of structural family therapy. The behavioral approach has been discussed in previous chapters in this volume. The transactional approach tries to make family members aware of the ways a patient can use pain for psychological "payoffs" and how they might foil these attempts. The systems approach model deals with the family as an organization, and tries to change the structure, so that no one family member has to take the sick role. Most articles report that family therapy is a combination of behavioral, transactional, and systems approach. Unfortunately, it is quite difficult to assess the efficacy of family therapy. However, follow-up studies, designed to reassess the recurrence of symptoms are the best way that one has of determining efficacy. One study coming from the Northwest Pain Center, compared 25 successful patients with 25 patients who did not maintain gains made at the pain treatment center. Interestingly, they found that there were more divorced or separated people in this success group, while the failure group had done little to change the patterns of behavior in their environment. They concluded that the role of the family for maintaining pain behavior contributed to the failures. Payne and Norfleet (1986) conclude that family members contribute to treatment outcome by reinforcing or not reinforcing pain behavior. They suggest that if a patient has a family who is appropriately supportive and has learned to not reinforce pain behavior, the chance of success with pain treatment is greatly improved. If family members have not participated in the program, or resist change to their own behavior, then the family member with pain will probably persist. When compared to these resistent family groups, a single pain patient will probably have a better chance at success even though they do not have family support.

GROUP PSYCHOTHERAPY

Group psychotherapy has been adjunctive treatment for patients with terminal disease, rheumatoid arthritis, and chronic, intractable benign pain. These three groups of patients share four common features: (1) they have not had success with conventional therapy, (2) they feel isolated and a burden to their family and friends, (3) they are angry at physicians, and disappointed about treatment failure, and (4) they have reactive depressions, frustration, and reduced physical activity (Hendler, Viernstein, Shallanberger, & Long, 1981). Group therapy can be utilized on both an inpatient and outpatient basis, although the structure and format for these two groups is somewhat different (Hendler, 1984). In the inpatient setting, the patient is involved in group therapy for only a relatively short period of time—usually 8 to 12 sessions. In this context, the group psychotherapy format more closely resembles a mixture of educational and free-interaction group psychotherapy, with a focus on more of the depressive components of the chronic pain process. The most common themes of inpatient groups deal with depression and frustration: (1) the feeling that treatment in a pain treatment center is a last resort, (2) expression of displeasure and anger towards physicians for not being helped, (3) a willingness to do anything to get rid of the pain, (4) a feeling of helplessness and guilt, compounded by feelings of inadequacy, and frustration, because of an inability to function with the pain, (5) indications about a relationship between the patient and their family which clearly indicate whether the family is supportive of the patient's behavior, or in conflict with it, (6) a questioning of religious faith, and the selection process (why me?), (7) explorations regarding feelings of dependency, (8) resentment towards the disbelief of family members, physicians, and associates, and (9) a fear about the origin of the pain, and its progression (Hendler, Viernstein, Shallanberger, & Long, 1981). These same authors then described outpatient group therapy which was more protracted, and allowed exploration of different themes: (1) feelings of physical inabilities, or handicaps, (2) resentment towards vocational rehabilitation, (3) difficulty readjusting life goals, (4) concern about other group members, (5) frustration regarding the slowness of the process of rehabilitation, and (6) fear regarding the loss of a spouse because of the chronic pain.

As with all forms of psychotherapy, it is difficult to access the efficacy of group treatment. However, Ford (1984) has utilized an objective measure of efficacy, i.e., the amount of medical care sought by patients prior to and after group psychotherapy, and has reviewed the literature on this topic. Ford offers a cogent argument for psychotherapy, if it is able to produce the number of medical visits, on a cost-effective basis, if for no other reason. Various authors reported between a 50-75% reduction in medical clinic visits, while patients with somatic illness were undergoing group psychotherapy concomitantly. Ford's own experience was not quite as dramatic, but he attributes this to patients belonging to a low socio-economic group, and underscores the need for very long-term group treatment, before any benefit was noted. The most important benefit to a patient seemed to be in the area of gaining control over their life. Other authors have advanced the notion that "peer modeling," and "interaction with other group members" allows the patient to more freely express their emotions, learn new coping methods, and to be more verbal when soliciting help (Gamsa, Braha, & Catchlove, 1985). While these authors conclude that group psychotherapy is a useful adjunct to their chronic pain treatment program, they do not offer any objective evidence. Hendler and his co-workers studied patients assigned to group therapy, or individual therapy (Hendler, Viernstein, Shallanberger, & Long, 1981). In their study, 8 of the 11 patients assigned to group therapy had remained in therapy, and 7 of the 8 had abstained from narcotic and hypnotic use. This was contrasted to a group of 12 patients, 7 of whom continued to use hypnotics, narcotics, or benzodiazepines, from other physicians. At the end of three months, 6 of the 12 had discontinued sessions. A much more comprehensive report (Hall, Hall, & Gardnar, 1979), compared the efficacy of combined group therapy and tricyclic antidepressants versus supportive individual therapy, analytically oriented therapy, and management by surgical specialists, using narcotics or antidepressants. Using the Zung Rating Scales as an indication of the severity of depression, Hall's group found that group psychotherapy, combined with tricyclic antidepressants, was the most efficacious modality of therapy, while individual psychotherapy, and surgical management, using narcotics or antidepressants, were least effective.

Although it is difficult to accurately assess the efficacy of group therapy, and many reports do not have objective measures of outcome, the technique is cost-effective, and provides a degree of modeling and social reinforcement, that is not available from other forms of therapy. The effectiveness of other self-help groups, such as Alcoholics Anonymous, would lend credence to the contention that group therapy is an effective modality for treating chronic pain patients.

NARCOSYNTHESIS

There have been many articles in the psychiatric literature, as well as in the chronic pain literature, which suggest that many of the undiagnosed chronic pain problems are really conversion reactions, or hysterical conversion disorders. Most of these articles are unsubstantiated, or deal with single cases, or a few cases, after which the authors attempt to apply their limited experience to the broad range of chronic pain patients. In reality, a number of conversion disorders presenting as chronic pain problems is probably very small. In this author's experience, after treating over 4,000 chronic pain patients, both at the Chronic Pain Treatment Center of Johns Hopkins Hospital, while under the direction of the Department of Neurosurgery, and at Mensana Clinic, over the past 11 years, the incidence of hysterical conversion disorders was three cases. Of course, these cases are quite memorable, and represented enormous therapeutic challenges.

One has to be quite careful in making the diagnosis of hysterical conversion reaction. In one of the classic studies, Slater (1965) did a nine year follow-up study on 85 people originally diagnosed as having hysterical conversion reaction, that had been seen at Queens Square Hospital in London. At the time of follow-up, only 19 of the 85 patients were free of symptoms. Of these 85 patients, seven were found to have recurrent endogenous depression, two were schizophrenic, three had undetected neoplasms, and of the four that committed suicide, two of them had atypical myopathy, and disseminated sclerosis. Each died of natural causes. Two of the patients were found to have trigeminal neuralgia, and one woman was finally diagnosed as having thoracic outlet syndrome. Three people were finally diagnosed as having early, previously undetected, dementia, while one woman, who had pain in the right shoulder and arm, was later diagnosed as having Takayasu's syndrome. The rest had a multiplicity of organic diseases, including epilepsy, vestibular lesions, and total block of the spinal cord. Of the 85 patients with the original diagnosis of "hysteria" meaning conversion reaction, only seven were really found to have an acute psychogenic reaction resulting in a formation of a conversion symptom, while 14 were diagnosed as having Briquet's syndrome which is a polysomatic hysterical neurosis more compatible with hypochondriasis, or somatizing disorders.

In a most thorough review of the literature, encompassing nearly a 50-year period of time, at Johns Hopkins Hospital, Stephens and Kamp (1962) found that the incidence of hysterical conversion reaction at a psychiatric hospital (Phipps Clinic of Johns Hopkins Hospital) was approximately 2% of all psychiatric admissions. Therefore, one must be quite cautious in assigning the diagnosis of conversion neurosis, or hysterical conversion disorder. Additionally, many clinicians have difficulty differentiating between histrionic personality disorders, and a hysterical personality disorder, resulting in many somatic complaints, which has been called Briquet's syndrome. These two disorders are different than a hysterical conversion reaction, since the last of these three disorders can occur in a previously well-adjusted individual, subjected to extreme stress (Hendler, 1981). A review of histrionic personality disorders versus hysterical, polysomatic Briquet syndrome versus hysterical conversion reactions versus malingering can be found in Hendler's book, *The Diagnosis and Nonsurgical Management of Chronic Pain,* (1981). Also, Hendler and Talo (1989) published a chapter, in which the differential diagnosis of these disorders is summarized.

If hysterical conversion reaction is suspected in the diagnosis, amobarbital narcosynthesis can be quite useful in assisting in the diagnosis. One of the leading proponents of this technique, Dr. Walters, of the University of California School of Medicine, has recommended dosages between 200-500 mg, taking a patient through surgical plains of anesthesia, including loss of corneal reflex which produces full relaxation of "psychogenic tissue pain" (Walters, 1973). Indeed, using too small a dose of amobarbital may contribute to many of the failures associated with lack of effectiveness of this technique (Hendler, Filtzer, Talo, Panzetta, & Long, 1987). In fact, Hendler and his group specifically found that a diagnostic failure, using Amobarbital narcosynthesis, was directly related to inadequate dosage of the Amytal, (dosage range 200 mg–250 mg). When the dosage was increased to 450 mg–600 mg, effective narcosynthesis was obtained (Hendler, Filtzer, Talo, Panzetta, & Long, 1987).

HYPNOSIS

When considering hypnosis for the patient in pain, one must make a distinction between acute pain, and chronic pain. There is no question that hypnosis is an effective treatment for acute pain problems. Scott (1974) has discussed the usefulness of hypnotic technique for treating badly burned patients, and for surgical candidates. However, even Scott admits that the effectiveness of this technique is variable, and unreliable. In theory, hypnosis can be used to treat the patient with acute pain, by altering his or her perception of the amount of time the pain is experienced. In this fashion, Teitelbaum (1965) has proposed hypnosis can be used for hypnoanalgesia, and calls this phenomenon "Time Distortion."

For chronic pain states, generalized relaxation therapy, as described by Jacobson (1964) seems to be quite useful. As with biofeedback, hypnotic relaxation techniques seem to work best with chronic pain patients who have myofascial pain or chronic muscle tension. Unfortunately, it is difficult to assess the efficacy of hypnosis, especially in chronic pain states. But the technique does not lend itself to controlled studies. "The question of the efficacy of hypnosis with chronic back pain awaits controlled empirical research (Turk & Flor, 1984)." The major objection to hypnosis lies in the fact that it might provide temporary relief for the patient with chronic pain, but long-term relief has not been adequately documented. However, hypnosis may be a useful diagnosis tool for uncovering underlying hysterical conversion reactions, although it may be less reliable than narcosynthesis, which has been previously discussed.

DIAGNOSIS AND TREATMENT OF DEPRESSION

No discussion about the psychotherapy of chronic pain patients would be complete without a thorough understanding of depression associated with chronic pain. One of the major difficulties one encounters in diagnosing chronic pain patients with depression pertains to the etiology of the depression. France and Krishnan (1985) make a distinction between despondency, or grief reaction in response to serious physical disease and depression, stating that despondency is similar to grief reaction, and must be differentiated from depression in chronic pain states (Krishnan, France, Pelton, McCann, Davidson, & Urban, 1985). France and his co-workers feel that one may differentiate various subtypes of depression in chronic low back patients, and distinguish (a) major depression, (b) minor depression, (c) intermittent depression, (d) chronic low back pain patients without depression. One way of making this distinction is the use of the dexamethasone suppression test as a biological marker of depression. The current Chairman of the Department of Psychiatry at Duke University, Bernard Carroll, first advanced the notion of elevated plasma cortisol, resistent to suppression by dexamethasone, in severe depressive illness (Carroll, Martin, & Davies, 1968). Subsequent to this original article in 1968, Dr. Carroll and his co-workers published extensively about the use of the "dexamethasone suppression test." Randall France, formerly of Duke University, and now at University of Utah, studied a group of 80 chronic back pain patients, with and without depression, by using the dexamethasone suppression test (DST) (France & Krishnan, 1985). France and his co-workers selected a uniform group of chronic low back pain patients, i.e., those with chronic low back pain associated with organic pathology, and divided them into two groups, based on the presence of absence of major depression, using DSM-III criteria. They then examined the cortisol response to dexamethasone in each group. Of this group of 80 patients, 35 patients were diagnosed as having major depression, which 45 patients did not satisfy the criteria for major depression. However, of these 45 patients who did not have major depression, 10 satisfied the criteria for dysthymic disorder. In the group of patients with the diagnosis of major depression, 14 of the 35 had a positive dexamethasone suppression test, while none of the 45 patients who did not have major affective disorder had a positive dexamethasone suppression test. Again, of this group of 45 patients, 10 of them were diagnosed as having a dysthymic disorder, which might be more appropriately described as a reactive depression. France very appropriately concludes that the abnormal dexamethasone suppression test is in response to a major depressive disorder, and not to chronic pain itself. Additionally, France notes that the incidence of abnormal cortisol response to dexamethasone is higher in depressed patients, without organic findings. As a conclusion, France and his co-workers state that the "difference in the rate of non-suppression in chronic back pain patients with and without depression, suggests that the notion of conceptualizing chronic back pain as a variant of depression or as a marked (sic) (masked) depression might be an oversimplification (France & Krishnan)."

In another study of 63 patients, conducted at the University of Washington Pain Clinic, 49% of the sample met the DSM-III criteria for major depression (Haley, Turner, & Romano, 1985). In this study, depressed patients did not differ significantly from nondepressed patients in the ratio male versus female, use of narcotics, use of sedative-hypnotics, or antidepressant medication, number of years in chronic pain, age, or number of surgeries. However, for women, depression was more closely related to subjective reports of pain, while in men, depression was more closely related to impairment of activity. In a review of 454 chronic pain patients, at Columbia-Presbyterian Medical Center, Department of Anesthesiology Pain Treatment Service, 100 patients were selected at random, and eventually 82 patients were contacted by telephone, for long-term followup of a subsample of the original number of patients (Dworkin, Richlin, Handlin, & Brand, 1986). In evaluating the original 454 chronic pain patients, 79 of these patients were found to be depressed, while 375 were not considered depressed. Between the two groups, there was no significant difference in the percentage of males, females, age, marital status, education, or compensation. The only significant differences existed between the percentage of patients undergoing litigation or being employed. The depressed patients had a higher percentage of litigation, and a lower percentage of employment, when compared to nondepressed chronic pain patients. When compared to pain-related characteristics, chronic pain patients with depression more often had constant pain, and a higher self-reported scale of pain than the nondepressed patients. In nondepressed patients, significant variables contributing to the ability to predict treatment outcome were number of treatment visits, compensation, number of previous therapies, and the location of pain. In depressed patients, the predictors of treatment outcome were employment and duration of pain.

Atkinson and his group in San Diego have defined three subgroups of chronic pain patients based on MMPI scores and the type of depression they experience (Atkinson, Ingram, Kremer, & Saccuzzo, 1986). Using Research Diagnostic Criteria, Atkinson and his co-workers found that 44% of the 52 patients examined had major depression, 19% had minor depression, 13% had other psychiatric disorders, and 22% had no mental disorder. Patients with a major depression were found to have a discrete

MMPI profile, with Scales F, Hs, D, Hy, Pd, Pa, Pt, Sc, Ma, and Si being significantly higher, and Scale K being significantly lower than the other three groups. The best predictors were Scales Sc, Pt, and D. When the patients were divided by clinical characteristics of somatization, depression, or hypochondriasis, patients with major depression fell into three depression MMPI profile group (2, 1, 3, for rank order elevation of MMPI scales or D, Hs, Hy). Despite these distinctions there was "an even distribution of objective evidence for pain across all MMPI subgroups." This supports the contention that Hendler and his co-workers have long maintained, i.e., the MMPI cannot predict the validity of the complaint of pain, and patients with psychiatric problems can also have real physical problems at the same time (Hendler, Mollett, Viernstein, Schroeder, Rybock, Campbell, Levin, & Long, 1985).

By using a psychiatric diagnostic system for delineating the various types of depression in chronic pain patients, and adhering rigorously to DSM-III diagnostic criteria, one can identify a group of chronic pain patients, that would respond to interventions for depression. There is no doubt that the use of antidepressant medication in the chronic pain patients with major depression would prove the most efficacious modality of therapy. In order to appropriately prescribe medication, physicians should understand the pharmacological contributions to normal sleep, pain perception, anxiety, and depression. In a review of the literature, Hendler (1982) describes the common pharmacological substrate of normal sleep, pain perception, and antidepressant activity within the central nervous system, as being elevation of serotonin levels. Therefore, drugs that enhance serotonin activity within the central nervous system are beneficial, and these include tricyclic antidepressants, as well as the newer bicyclic and tetracyclic antidepressants. Thus, an antidepressant, given at bedtime, may promote natural sleep, reduce the perception of pain, and reduce anxiety and depression. Dosage should be individually tailored, to suit the patient's age, and tolerance for medication, but as a starting dose, one might recommend 50-100 mg of amitriptyline, or doxepin, in patients who are both anxious and depressed, while one might consider using nortriptyline or desipramine at dosages between 25 and 75 mg, in patients who are depressed, and report lack of energy, or a feeling of sluggishness. Dosage can be escalated, by 25-50 mg increments, depending on the patient's response to the medication. It should be noted that the anti-anxiety effects of medication usually occur within the first two days, as does enhancement of sleep. However, it may take two to four weeks before the antidepressant effects of these medications are fully appreciated. If the use of antidepressants does not prove productive by the end of four weeks, therapeutic monitoring, using serum levels, will allow adjustment of the dosage into the proper range.

The use of specialized treatments for depression, such as monoamine oxidase inhibitors, or electroconvulsive therapy, is best left in the hand of psychiatrists, and the selection of patients for these types of therapies should be done only after psychiatric consultation has been obtained.

RESULTS

Describing pain patients is like blind men describing an elephant. Each clinic, each physician, each hospital, sees a different type of patient. Therefore, in order to access results properly, the demographics of the chronic pain patient population, under study, must be defined. On this point, the literature is in shambles. Even more chaotic is the reporting of results.

Few, if any individual psychiatrists, have published any results documenting the efficacy of their intervention. Reporting is hampered by the absence of objective criteria for improvement. What parameters should be measured to determine if a patient has benefitted from the intervention of a psychiatrist? How do you measure pain? Is pain relief or improved activity the desired goal? Can they exist independently? How long has the patient had pain? Is litigation involved?

Hendler and Talo (1989) reviewed the literature of chronic pain clinics that had published results of treating their pain patient population. Most clinics were either multidisciplinary or behavior modification clinics. Of note, one year after discharge from the clinic, most clinics reported that only 25% of their patients had maintained the improved level of activity they had experienced at discharge from the clinic. Pain relief ranged from slight to great in only 33% to 63% of the patients. That is to say, only about half the patients got any relief, even slight relief, and only 25% maintained any improvement in their level of activity (Hendler & Talo, 1989). Using a more objective set of criteria, Hendler (1989) reviewed 60 patients who had been diagnosed and treated at Mensana Clinic. All 60 of the patients were involved in litigation, and had been out of work an average of 4.9 years! By all accounts, this group of patients is considered to be difficult to treat because of the involvement of litigation and the chronicity of their problem. Ninety per cent of the patients had no difficulty discontinuing narcotics, hypnotics, and/or tranquilizers. Only 50% had pain relief, but 91% improved their sleep and level of activity. However, the most startling statistic was the number of undiagnosed surgical problems. Fifty per cent of the patients were referred on for further surgery (one to four additional operations) because they had not been properly diagnosed before referral (Hendler, 1989). Referral diagnosis was very often a vague or descriptive one, in 41% of the cases (25 /60), with such terms as "psychogenic pain," "pain neurosis," "low back pain," "chronic muscle strain," etc., being used, instead of any attempt at diagnosis. Since 96% of the referrals came from orthopedic or neurosurgeons, the failure to diagnose surgically correctable lesions is especially troubling. This was not a local or regional phenomenon, since 75% of Mensana Clinic patients come from around the country, from 25 states, and eight foreign countries, so far. Therefore, the need to accurately diagnose patients, both medically and psychiatrically is of paramount concern for the psychiatrist. The psychiatrist cannot rely upon the medical diagnosis of nonpsychiatric physicians. If he or she feels the patient merits further diagnostic evaluations, it is incumbent upon the psychiatrist to order additional diagnostic studies and to obtain consultation with top quality surgical colleagues.

THE PSYCHIATRIST AS EDUCATOR

Patients with chronic pain are frightened, because, very often, they do not know or understand what is wrong with them. Once an accurate diagnosis has been established, the psychiatrist should explain, in simple, concise terms, the anatomic origin of the pain problem, the options for treatment, the expected treatment outcome, and alternatives to treatment. Chronic pain is a devastating problem, but once a patient is fully informed about his or her options, anxiety is reduced, because the patient has been given an active role in the decision-making process. Patients appreciate this involvement, and respond in a positive fashion. Little has been written about the educator role for a psychiatrist, but, in the author's opinion, it is one of the most beneficial interventions he performs.

PSYCHOLOGICAL TESTS

Simply put, if a psychiatrist wants to measure personality traits, then he or she should use the MMPI or the Millon. If one wishes to measure psychological states, then the SCL-90, Beck Depression Test, Stress Vector Analysis, and Holmes Rahe Life Events tests should be used. In order to measure the validity of the complaint of pain, only the Mensana Clinic Back Pain Test (see end of chapter) is designed to do so, independent of pre-existing personality traits, or psychological states.

SUMMARY

Psychotherapy of chronic pain patients is a difficult task at best. In part, the process is complicated by the lack of precision of diagnosis within the realm of psychiatry, but also within the realm of medicine. For this reason, chronic pain patients engender controversy. Improved treatment may be achieved by improved precision of diagnosis, both in the medical and psychiatric realms. Unfortunately, the efficacy of psychotherapy is difficult to establish, but improved levels of functioning, less depression, better family relationships, and improvements in sleep, and pain levels, all can be achieved with appropriate interventions. Most importantly, the psychiatrist should serve as an objective observer and recorder of patient complaints and be a diagnostician. Without accurate diagnosis, all treatments are doomed to fail.

Screening Test
MENSANA CLINIC BACK PAIN TEST
(Clinician Administered)

(This test is designed to determine the validity of the complaint of pain in patients who have pain in their back, neck, arms or legs, for 6 months or longer. The pain must be constant in at least one site, and is *not* valid for headaches, intestinal disorders, face pain, or for patients with pain less than 6 months. It should not be given to a patient to answer, but should be clinician administered.)

Instructions: Each question is asked by an examiner, and the patient is given points according to the response that he makes. The number of points to be awarded for the various responses is shown in the column at the right. At the end of the test, the examiner calculates the total number of points. The results are interpreted as explained in the **Key.**

Points

1. **How did the pain that you now experience occur?**
   (a) Sudden onset with accident or definable event   0
   (b) Slow, progressive onset without acute
       exacerbation   1
   (c) Slow, progressive onset with acute exacerbation
       without accident or event   2
   (d) Sudden onset without an accident or definable
       event   3

2. **Where do you experience the pain?**
   (a) One site, specific, well-defined, consistent with
       anatomical distribution   0
   (b) More than one site, each well-defined and
       consistent with anatomical distribution   1
   (c) One site, inconsistent with anatomical
       considerations, or not well-defined   2
   (d) Vague description, more than one site, of which
       one is inconsistent with anatomical considerations,
       or not well-defined or anatomically explainable   3

Points

3. **Do you ever have trouble falling asleep at night, or are you ever awakened from sleep?**
If the answer is "no," score 3 points and go to question 4. If the answer is "yes," proceed:

   What keeps you from falling asleep, or what awakens you from sleep?

3A. (a) Trouble falling asleep every night due to pain   0
   (b) Trouble falling asleep due to pain more than three times a week   1
   (c) Trouble falling asleep due to pain less than three times a week   2
   (d) No trouble falling asleep due to pain   3
   (e) Trouble falling asleep which is not related to pain   4

3B. (a) Awakened by pain every night   0
   (b) Awakened from sleep by pain more than three times a week   1
   (c) Not awakened from sleep by pain more than twice a week   2
   (d) Not awakened from sleep by pain   3
   (e) Restless sleep, or early morning awakening with or without being able to return to sleep, both unrelated to pain   4

4. **Does weather have any effect on your pain?**
   (a) The pain is always worse in both cold *and* damp weather   0
   (b) The pain is always worse with damp weather *or* with cold weather   1
   (c) The pain is occasionally worse with cold or damp weather   2
   (d) The weather has no effect on the pain   3

5. **How would you describe the type of pain that you have?**
   (a) Burning; or sharp, shooting pain; or pins and needles; or coldness; or numbness   0
   (b) Dull, aching pain, with occasional sharp, shooting pains not helped by heat; or, the patient is experiencing hyperesthesia   1
   (c) Spasm-type pain, tension-type pain, or numbness over the area, relieved by massage or heat 2
   (d) Nagging or bothersome pain   3

(e) Excruciating, overwhelming, or unbearable pain,
     relieved by massage or heat   4

6. How frequently do you have your pain?
(a) The pain is constant   0
(b) The pain is nearly constant, occurring 50%–80%
     of the time   1
(c) The pain is intermittent, occurring 25%–50%
     of the time   2
(d) The pain is only occasionally present, occurring
     less than 25% of the time   3

**7. Does movement or position have any effect on
the pain?**
(a) The pain is unrelieved by position change or rest,
     and there have been previous operations for the pain   0
(b) The pain is worsened by use, standing, or walking;
     and is relieved by lying down or resting the part   1
(c) Position change and use have variable effects on
     the pain   2
(d) The pain is not altered by use or position change, and
     there have been no previous operations for the pain   3

8. What medications have you used in the past month?
(a) No medications at all   0
(b) Use of non-narcotic pain relievers; non-benzodiazepine
     tranquilizers; or use of antidepressants   1
(c) Less than three-times-a-week use of a narcotic,
     hypnotic, or benzodiazepine   2
(d) Greater than four-times-a-week use of a narcotic,
     hypnotic, or benzodiazepine   3

**9. What hobbies do you have, and can you still
participate in them?**
(a) Unable to participate in any hobbies that were
     formerly enjoyed   0
(b) Reduced number of hobbies or activities relating to
     a hobby   1
(c) Still able to participate in hobbies but with some
     discomfort   2
(d) Participate in hobbies as before   3

**10. How frequently did you have sex and orgasms
before the pain, and how frequently do you have
sex and orgasms now?**

(a^1) Sexual contact, prior to pain, three to four times a
week, with no difficulty with orgasm; now sexual
contact is 50% or less than previously, and coitus
is interrupted by pain　　　　　　　　　　　　0

(a^2) (For people over 45) Sexual contact twice a week,
with a 50% reduction in frequency since the pain　　0

(a^3) (For people over 60) Sexual contact once a week,
with a 50% reduction in frequency of coitus since
the onset of pain　　　　　　　　　　　　　　　0

(b) Pre-pain adjustment as defined above $(a^1$-$a^3)$, with
no difficulty with orgasm; now loss of interest in
sex and/or difficulty with orgasm or erection　　　1

(c) No change in sexual activity now as opposed to
before the onset of pain　　　　　　　　　　　　2

(d) Unable to have sexual contact since the onset of
pain, and difficulty with orgasm or erection *prior
to* the pain　　　　　　　　　　　　　　　　　3

(e) No sexual contact prior to the pain, or absence of
orgasm *prior to* the pain　　　　　　　　　　　4

11. Are you still working or doing your household chores?

(a) Works every day at the same pre-pain job or same
level of household duties　　　　　　　　　　　0

(b) Works every day but the job is not the same as
pre-pain job, with reduced responsibility or
physical activity　　　　　　　　　　　　　　　1

(c) Works sporadically or does a reduced amount
of household chores　　　　　　　　　　　　　　2

(d) Not at work, or all household chores are now performed by others　　　　　　　　　　　　　　　3

12. What is your income now compared with before your injury or the onset of pain, and what are your sources of income?

(a) Any one of the following answers scores　　　　　0
　　1. Experiencing financial difficulty with family
　　　income 50% or less than previously
　　2. Was retired and is still retired
　　3. Patient is still working and is not having
　　　financial difficulties

(b) Experiencing financial difficulty with family
income only 50%–75% of the pre-pain income　　　1

(c) Patient unable to work, and receives some
compensation so that the family income is at
least 75% of the pre-pain income　　　　　　　　2

(d) Patient unable to work and receives no compensation,
but the spouse works and family income is still 75%
of the pre-pain income   3

(e) Patient doesn't work, yet the income from disability
or other compensation sources is 80% or more of
gross pay before the pain; the spouse does not work   4

13. **Are you suing anyone, or is anyone suing you, or
do you have an attorney helping you with compensation or disability payments?**

(a) No suit pending, and does not have an attorney   0

(b) Litigation is pending, but is not related to the pain   1

(c) The pain is being sued as the result of an accident   2

(d) Litigation is pending or workmen's compensation
case with a lawyer involved   3

14. **If you had three wishes for anything in the world,
what would you wish for?**

(a) "Get rid of the pain" is the only wish   0

(b) "Get rid of the pain" is one of the three wishes   1

(c) Doesn't mention getting rid of the pain, but has
specific wishes usually of a personal nature such as
for more money, a better relationship with spouse or
children, etc.   2

(d) Does not mention pain, but offers general, non-
personal wishes such as for world peace   3

15. **Have you ever been depressed or thought of
suicide?**

(a) Admits to depression; or has a history of depression
secondary to pain and associated with crying spells
and thoughts of suicide   0

(b) Admits to depression, guilt, and anger secondary to
the pain   1

(c) Prior history of depression before the pain or a
financial or personal loss prior to the pain; now
admits to some depression   2

(d) Denies depression, crying spells, or "feeling blue"   3

(e) History of a suicide attempt prior to the onset
of pain   4

POINT TOTAL

Key to the Mensana Clinic Back Pain Test

A score of 17 points or less suggests that the patient is an objective
pain patient and is reporting a normal response to chronic pain. One may

proceed surgically if indicated, and usually finds the patient quite willing to participate in all modalities of therapy, including exercise and psychotherapy. Occasionally, a person with conversion reaction or post-traumatic neurosis will score less than 17 points; this is because subjective distress is being experienced on an unconscious level. Persons scoring 14 points or less can be considered objective pain patients with more certainty than those at the upper range.

A score of 18–20 points suggests that the patient has features of an objective pain patient as well as of an exaggerating pain patient. This implies that a person with a poor premorbid adjustment has an organic lesion that has produced the normal response to pain; however, because of the person's poor pre-pain adjustment, the chronic pain produces a more extreme response than would otherwise occur.

A score of 21–31 points suggests that the patient is an exaggerating pain patient. Surgical or other interventions may be carried out with caution. This type of patient usually has a premorbid (pre-pain) personality that may increase his likelihood of using or benefiting from the complaint of chronic pain. The patient may show improvement after treatment in a chronic pain treatment center, where the main emphasis is placed on an attitude change toward the chronic pain.

A score of 32 points or more suggests that a psychiatric consultation is needed. These patients freely admit to a great many pre-pain problems, and show considerable difficulty in coping with the chronic pain they now experience. Surgical or other interventions should not be carried out without prior approval of a psychiatric consultant. Severe depression, suicide, and psychosis are potential problems in this group of affective pain patients.

GRADING GUIDE FOR THE MENSANA CLINIC BACK PAIN TEST

©Nelson Hendler, M.D., M.S. — 1983

QUESTION 1

The answer to this question should be self-explanatory. If the patient is vague in determining the date of the onset of the pain, or in the progression of the pain, assume that this is a slow, progressive onset. However, if the person is definitely certain about the date, but the type of activity that they were doing, that is, lying in bed, watching television, reading a newspaper, etc., is not the type of activity that normally would result in injury to the back, grade this as a sudden onset without accident or definable event. The only counterindication for this scoring would be pain that is a result of the onset of a stroke or other vascular accident, which obviously would be of sudden onset with accident or definable event. Strokes could occur while engaging in non-strenuous activity. Please confirm with a physician if any doubts arise.

QUESTION 2

Where do you experience the pain? This is best correlated with physicians' opinion. Typically, pain in the back or pain in the back radiating down one or both legs is consistent with one site, and anatomical distribution. However, if pain is experienced in both the left arm and the right leg, this is inconsistent with anatomical distribution, but one must question further. Conceivably, one could experience pain in the left leg, or weakness in the left leg, fall, and, as a result of this, try to brace the fall by extending the right arm, thereby sustaining injury in 2 sites, that is, the left leg and right arm. This would be consistent with more than one site, each well defined. Persons who report that they hurt all over should be questioned further. If they still are unable to clarify the site of their pain, then they should be given the 3 point score for a "vague description, at more than one site."

QUESTION 3A AND 3B

Question 3a and 3b should be scored as one question. It is a three-part question. The first says: Do you have trouble falling asleep? If the answer is no, then go to the second part, which is: Do you ever awake from sleep? If the answer is still no, then the patient gets 3 points. If the patient answers yes to 3a, then the second part of the question becomes: What keeps you awake? At this point in time, one can decide how to score the answer to 3a. However, please remember patients may have no trouble falling asleep, but they may be awakened from sleep. In this case, even though the patient may have no difficulty falling asleep, one still has to ask whether or not they awaken from sleep. The patient should be given the benefit of the doubt, and be given the lower score on question 3a or 3b. Again, please remember that both questions 3a and 3b are three-part questions, in that you ask (1) Do you have trouble falling asleep, and if the answer is yes, then (2) What keeps you awake, and after that answer is obtained, then (3) How many nights a week? The same procedure applies for question 3b.

QUESTION 4

Does weather have any effect on your pain? The answer to this question should be straightforward. Please notice that there is a distinction between an effect of both wet and cold weather, as opposed to wet or cold weather, and there is a distinction between constantly affecting the pain, or occasionally affecting the pain. Some real organic pains, such as arachnoiditis, are not affected by the weather, but any negative bias produced by an answer to this question is removed by answers to subsequent questions.

QUESTION 5

How would you describe the type of pain that you have? This requires thorough questioning of the description of the pain by the interviewer. The best way to proceed would be (1) Is the pain constant or intermittent? (see Question 6) (2) How would you physically describe the pain? If the patient starts by describing it in terms of excruciating, etc., interrupt and ask if perhaps you could offer some suggestion, such as burning, sharp, shooting, etc. This will help lend some structure to the answer to the question, since it is very difficult for patients to describe their pain. After you have asked the question in open-ended form, using the potential answers on the test. If they still use subjective, inprecise terms, i.e., horrible pain, severe and crippling pain, etc., score 4 points.

QUESTION 6

See #5 above. If there are two pains or more, give the patient the benefit of the doubt, and score the lower of the two scores, for each type of pain. That is, if a patient has a constant burning pain in the leg with occasional dull aching pains in the back, the patient should get 0 points on question 6, because one of his pains is constant.

QUESTION 7

The answer to movement or position affecting the pain should be clear. Again, there are some organic conditions that are totally unrelieved by changes in position, but these are usually the result of previous surgeries. Note the distinction between answer a and answer b.

QUESTION 8

What medications have you used in the last month? The examiner is referred to the self-scoring version of the Screening Test, where the various medications are listed by group.

QUESTION 9

What hobbies do you have? If the hobby is non-active, arbitrarily assign 2 points to the answer and go on to the next question. Non-active hobbies include reading, watching television, sewing, knitting, etc. If they try a hobby they used to enjoy but spend less time at it, score 1 point.

QUESTION 10

Deals with sexual activity. The only exception to the various answers listed above would pertain to people who abstain from sexual activity, either due to their religious vows, or due to some difficulty with their marital situation, death or illness of a partner, or due to personality disorders which prevent them from acquiring a consistent-partner. In this case, one should arbitrarily assign a value of 2 as the point score for this question, since it would be quite difficult to assess the psychological status, but one suspects that there is pathology.

QUESTION 11

Are you still working and doing your household chores? The answer to this should be straightforward.

QUESTION 12

The financial question deals with a variety of complex issues. What I found as the most accurate way of scoring this question would be determining income from four sources: (1) Workmen's Compensation, (2) private disability insurance, (3) Social Security disability insurance, (4) Other sources of private income, such as investments, rental property income, etc. Then, I would qualify the sources of income, asking if the money the patient receives from various sources is tax-free or taxable. After his current income is determined, then I would review the patient's income at the time of the injury, and obtain both the gross income, as well as the after-tax (take home) income. If the patient has stopped working one year or more before the date of the interview, then I would also ask the patient what would they now be earning if they were still working, taking into account Union raises, normal promotions, etc. Again, I would ask both the pre-tax and post-tax (take-home) income. I would discount overtime pay and only judge base pay as the basis of income, since Workmen's Compensation claims are also calculated not on overtime pay, but on the salary. Into this financial calculation, I would also add the wife's income. Before and after total income is evaluated, then one can decide where the patient should fall in terms of the answer to his financial question.

QUESTION 13

The question about lawsuits should be straightforward.

QUESTION 14

This question should be asked in an open-ended fashion, just the way that it is illustrated on the Screening Test. If the patient says get better or be the way I used to be, this should be counted as "getting rid of the pain." They do not have to specifically mention pain *per se,* but if they indicate that they want some improvement in their physical status, they should be given the benefit of the doubt, and this should be considered as "getting rid of the pain."

QUESTION 15

Have you every been depressed or thought of suicide? This question pertains to their prepain adjustment, as well as their postpain adjustment. It is very important to make this distinction. I think the question should be asked in the following fashion: "Before you had the pain, were you ever depressed, had you ever thought of suicide, or had you ever attempted suicide?" After that answer is obtained, then I would ask the question again, as it pertains to after the pain. If they were depressed before the pain, but there was no personal loss creating depression, or they don't know why they were depressed, score 3.

REFERENCES

Atkinson, J. H., Ingram, R., Kremer, E., Saccuzzo, D. (1986). MMPI subgroup: And affective disorders in chronic pain patients. *Journal of Nervous and Mental Disease, Vol. 174,* No. 7, pp. 408-413.

Black, R. G. (1982). *The clinical management of chronic pain.* (pp. 211-224). In N. Hendler, D. Long, & T. Wise (Eds.), *Diagnosis and treatment of chronic pain.* Littleton, MA: John Wright-PSG, Inc.

Carroll, E. J., Martin, F. I. R., & Davies, B. (1968). Resistance to suppression by dexamethasone of plasma II-OHCS in severe depressive illness. *British Medical Journal, 3*:285-287.

Dworkin, R., Richlin, D., Handlin, D., & Brand, L., (1986). Predicting treatment response in depressed and nondepressed chronic pain patients. *Pain, 24*(3):343-353.

Engel, G. (1959). Psychogenic pain in the pain prone patient. *American Journal of Medicine, 26*:899-918.

Ford, C. V. (1984). *Somatizing disorders.* In H. Roback (Ed.), *Helping patients and their families cope with medical problems.* San Francisco: Jossey-Bass Publishers.

Ford, C. V. (1986). Somatizing disorders. *Psychosomatics, 27(5)*:327-337.

France, R., & Krishnan, K. R. R., (1985). The dexamethasone suppression and a biological marker of depression and chronic pain. *Pain, 21(1)*:49-55.

Gamsa, A., Braha, R., & Catchlove, R. (1985). The use of structure group therapy sessions in the treatment of chronic pain patients. *Pain, 22(1)*:91-96.

Haley, W., Turner, J., & Romano J. (1985). Depression in chronic pain patients: Relation to pain, activity, and sex differences. *Pain, 24(3)*:343-353.

Hall, R. C., Hall, A. K., & Gardnar, E. R. (1979). In *Comparison of tricyclic antidepressants and analgesics, The management of chronic postoperative surgical pain.* Read before the Annual Meeting of the Academy of Psychosomatic Medicine, San Francisco.

Hendler, N., Derogatis, L., Avella, J., & Long, D. (1977). *EMG biofeedback in patients with chronic pain.* In *Diseases of the nervous system. Vol. 38*, pp. 505-509.

Hendler, N., & Fernandez, P. (1980) Alternative treatments for patients with chronic pain. *Psychiatric Annals,10(12)*:25-33.

Hendler, N., Viernstein, M., Shallanberger, C., & Long, D. (1981). Group psychotherapy with chronic pain patients. *Psychosomatics, 22(4)*:332-340.

Hendler, N. (1981). *Diagnosis and nonsurgical management of chronic pain.* (pp. 80-92). New York: Raven Press.

Hendler, N. (1981). *Diagnosis and nonsurgical management of chronic pain.* (pp. 64-100). New York: Raven Press.

Hendler, N. (1981). *Diagnosis and nonsurgical management of chronic pain.* (pp. 12-15). New York: Raven Press.

Hendler, N. (1982). The anatomy and psychopharmacology of chronic pain. *Journal of Clinical Psychiatry, 43*:15-20.

Hendler, N. (1982). *The four stages of pain.* (pp. 1-8). In N. Hendler, D. Long, & T. Wise (Eds.), *Diagnosis and treatment of chronic pain.* Littleton, MA: John Wright - PSG, Inc.

Hendler, N. (1984). Depression caused by chronic pain. *Clinical Journal of Psychiatry, 43(3)*, Sect. 2:30-36.

Hendler, N. (1984). *Chronic pain.* (pp. 79-106). In H. Roback (Ed.), *Helping patients and their families cope with medical problems.* San Francisco: Jossey-Bass Publishers.

Hendler, N., Mollett, A., Viernstein, M., Schroeder, D., Rybock, J., Campbell, J., Levin, S., & Long, D. (1985). A comparison between the MMPI and the "Hendler back pain test" for validating the complaint of chronic back pain in men. *The Journal of Neurological & Orthopaedic Medicine & Surgery, 6(4)*:333-337.

Hendler, N., Mollett, A., Viernstein, M., Schroeder, D., Rybock, J., Campbell, J., Levin, S., & Long, (1985). A comparison between the MMPI and the "Mensana clinic back pain test" for validating the complaint of chronic back pain in women. *Pain, 23(3)*:243-252.

Hendler, N., Filtzer, D., Talo, S., Panzetta, M., & Long D. (1987). Hysterical scoliosis treated with amobarbital narcosynthesis. *The Clinical Journal of Pain, 2(3)*:179-182.

Hendler, N., Mollett, A., Talo, S., & Levin, S. (1988). A comparison between the Minnesota multiphasic personality inventory and the "Mensana clinic back pain test" for validating the complaint of chronic back pain. *Journal of Occupational Medicine, 30(2)*:98-102.

Hendler, N., & Talo, S. (1989). *Chronic pain patient versus the malingering patient.* (pp. 14-22). In Kathleen Foley & Richard Payne (Eds.), *Current therapy of pain.* Toronto: B.C. Decker.

Hendler, N., & Talo, S. (1989). *Role of the pain clinic.* (pp. 23-32). In Kathleen Foley & Richard Payne (Eds.), *Current therapy of pain.* Toronto: B.C. Decker.

Hendler, N. (1989). *Validating the complaint of pain: The Mensana clinic approach.* (pp. 385-397), In Peter McL. Black (Ed.), *Clinical Neurosurgery,* Vol. 35.

Jacobsen, E. (1964). *Anxiety and tension control.* (pp. 108-111). Philadelphia: J.B. Lippincott and Co.

Krishnan, K. R. R., France, R. D., Pelton, S., McCann, U. D., Davidson, J., & Urban, B. J. (1985). Chronic pain and depression, I. Classification of depression and chronic lower back pain patients. *Pain, 22(3)*:279-287.

Large, R. (1985). Prediction of treatment response in pain patients: The illness self concept repertory grid and EMG biofeedback. *Pain, 21(3)*:279-287.

Maruta, E., Swanson, D., & Swanson, W. (1976). Pain as a psychiatric symptom: Comparison between low back pain and depression. *Psychosomatics, 17*:123-127.

Payne, B., & Norfleet, M. (1986). Chronic pain and the family: A review. *Pain, 26(1)*:1-22.

Pilowsky, I., & Bassett, D. L. (1982). Pain and depression, *British Journal of Psychiatry, 141*:30-36.

Reich, J., Rosenblatt, R., & Tupin, J. (1983). DSM-III: A new nomenclature for classifying patients with chronic pain. *Pain, 16(2)*:201-206.

Rowat, K. M., & Knafl, K. A. (1985). Living with chronic pain: The spouse's perspective. *Pain, 23(3)*:259-271.

Rutrick, D. (1981). Psychotherapy with chronic intractable benign pain patients. *Pain, Suppl. 1(331)*:S271.

Scott, D. L. (1974). *Modern hospital hypnosis.* Chicago: Yearbook Medical Publishers.

Slater, E.(1965). Diagnosis of "hysteria." *British Medical Journal, 1*:1395-1399.

Stephens, J., & Kamp, M. (1962). On some aspects of hysteria: A clinical study. *Journal of Nervous and Mental Disease, 134*:305-315.

Teitelbaum. (1965). *Hypnosis induction techniques.* (pp. 24-29). Springfield, IL: Charles C. Thomas.

Turk, D., & Flor, H. (1984). Ideological theories and treatments for chronic back pain, II: Psychological models and interventions. *Pain, 19(3)*:209-233.

Walters, A. (1973). *Psychiatric considerations of pain.* (pp. 1,516-1,645). In J. Youmans (Ed.), *Neurological surgery* (1st ed., Vol. 3). Philadelphia: Saunders, W.B.

Webb, W., Jr. (1983). Chronic pain. *Psychosomatics, 24(2)*:1053-1063.

Chapter 7

THE NON-PHARMACOLOGICAL MANAGEMENT OF CHRONIC PAIN VIA THE INTERDISCIPLINARY APPROACH

Margaret S. Texidor, Ph.D.

Professor Texidor describes the non-pharmacologic management of chronic pain goals and objectives using the interdisciplinary approach. In doing so, she describes the distinction between the loose multidisciplinary concept of care to the integration of team goals and members within the interdisciplinary model. Dr. Texidor explores with the reader, the goals of counseling for effective and adaptive management within the patient's/client's cognitive, emotional, social, and behavioral world. The reader comes to understand that effective use of coping techniques require active participation by the client, as well as an ownership in his or her pain problem. Skills needed for creation and application of self-care are also discussed. This chapter is significant for its discussion of techniques for both recovery and prevention of relapse, as well as an understanding of the role environmental support plays in maintenance of both health and illness behavior.

Chapter 7

THE NON-PHARMACOLOGICAL MANAGEMENT OF CHRONIC PAIN VIA THE INTERDISCIPLINARY APPROACH

Margaret S. Texidor, Ph.D.

With anticipation that a variety of professional disciplines will have occasion to read this chapter, it is both appropriate and necessary that several terms be defined here at the outset. In reference to the consumer of health care services, the usual terms for that individual consist of "patient", "client", and sometimes "consumer"; for the purpose of this chapter, the term client will be used. The primary definition of chronic pain used here is the one expressed by Bonica (1990), who has stated that chronic pain is "that pain which persists a month beyond the usual course of an acute disease or a reasonable time for an injury to heal or that is associated with chronic pathologic process that causes continuous pain or the pain recurs at intervals for months or years." He also adds that this type of pain "may be caused by psychopathology or environmental factors, and that it never has a biologic function but is a malefic form that often imposes severe emotional, physical, economic, and social stresses on the patient and on the family, and is one of the most costly health problems for society." In an earlier edition of his book, Bonica (1990) wrote, "In most of these cases, apprehension, fear, worry, and anxiety—all mental effects of the pain—seem to have as much to do with the physical deterioration of the patient as does the pain itself. . .I believed was the effect and not the cause of prolonged pain." Moreover, he suggests that his conviction, over the subsequent 35 years, has indeed been strengthened.

THE INTERDISCIPLINARY APPROACH

The interdisciplinary approach to patient management may be the most constructive and efficient means to produce a viable result with respect to the treatment of chronic pain (Schulz & Texidor, in press). Fordyce (1981) and Melvin (1980) suggest that a clear distinction exists between an interdisciplinary approach and a multidisciplinary one. The multidisciplinary model provides treatment to a client by providing intervention accomplished by several treating disciplines. However, this treatment is rendered by each professional without the requirement of input from the others. Although this model has been found to be successful in providing consultation and managing pain, as well as developing research findings about chronic pain (Fields, 1981), there is no overlapping style in this model, no distinct need for any one discipline to synchronize therapy with any of the others. In essence, there is no need for synergism or consonance in the provision of treatment.

With interdisciplinary case management, however, it has been suggested that the work "can only be accomplished by a firmly interactive effort" on the part of all disciplines involved (Fordyce, 1981). Only when the therapeutic effort is managed by simultaneous service furnished by an interactive professional team can the desired outcome be reached. As Fordyce (1981) asserts, "The essence of the matter is that each of the participating professions needs the others to accomplish what, collectively, they have agreed are their objectives." This model provides basis for integration of the work of several professional disciplines through synchronization in the entire treatment process. Cleland and King (1972) suggest that the true systems model attempts to reach a common goal by team members working with team-defined segments leading to the final team goal. Although they will do so from the particular perspective of his or her own professional discipline, the objectives are specified around and about a single agreed upon goal; in this case, the resolution of the combination of problems and issues which the chronic pain client is experiencing represents the goal.

Furthermore, it is extremely important that the professionals develop these goals together with the client, because the client needs to be assisted, as a part of this teamwork, to develop a clear perception about his or her participation as a functional member of the team, a virtual partner in the work. In this instance, the client assists with the actual establishment of the goals of the treatment in order that he or she will be more likely to own both the goals and the work of accomplishing them. The aim here is that ultimately the client will be more likely to invest in the work of problem resolution in concert with the professionals whose consultation he or she has sought. This process provides a client-centered type of therapy that is founded, fostered, and supported by the interdisciplinary model of health care delivery.

With the use of the interdisciplinary model for treating chronic health situations, professionals actually delegate responsibility back to the client, and often also to the spouse and/or significant other or family members while providing guidance in the process. The responsibility for outcome becomes a shared one. As such, the client and his or her external influencing systems are permitted, in fact encouraged, to become an active part of the team, holding clear responsibility within the work. Goals are set which are not only acceptable to the client, but are also realistic within the lifescope of that client. Thus, it is the client who actually permits, accepts, and conducts the personal work of changing (Texidor, in press). The professionals function in a consultant role in their interactions with the client; they guide, facilitate, and support the client to grow, adapt, and become.

Such an interdisciplinary team is usually comprised of professionals from one or more specialties in medicine, one or more mental health disciplines (mental health counseling, psychology, social work), nursing, nutritional management, physical therapy, occupational therapy, and in some cases, vocational rehabilitation. Occasionally, sub-specialists from these disciplines may participate, for example, an oncologic nurse specialist or a psychometrist. The make-up of the team is often based upon services generally available at a given health care facility, or by choice of the individual who directs such a pain program. Often a nurse may serve as the team coordinator and facilitator. And, of course, the client and the "significant other" are also team members. The team concept should be explained to the client on or before the first visit, with reinforcement of his or her participation done by all team professionals during first interviews. This concept should be reiterated on a regular basis during any phone contacts and during all ensuing interactions between professionals and client.

Regardless of the professions represented on such a team, among such teams that work with people experiencing chronic pain, there seems to be a well defined set of three major goals for this work (Long, 1980; Brena, Chapman, & Decker, 1980). The essential theme, one which can be consistently seen within the literature on this topic, encompasses the concept of the internal personal environment; it includes mind-body connectedness, self-responsibility, self-care, self-help, day-by-day, indeed moment-by-moment choice in active decision making, in order to bring about change. This solidly refutes the Cartesian concept of separation of body from mind (Bonica, 1990; Rossi, 1986; Texidor, 1984). The second construct is one of external environment of the individual which addresses the ideas of interpersonal relationship and dynamics therein (Long, 1980; Flor, Turk, & Rudy, 1987; Sanders, 1988; Weiner, 1988) and the actual physical environmental factors which may have bearing on the client's problem. There is a third construct, consistently addressed in the literature, that of client education which is needed to support the other two (Long, 1980; Flor, Turk, & Rudy, 1987; Pellitier, 1979; Texidor 1984).

The basis for interdisciplinary treatment of chronic conditions, in summary, holds to the facts that: (1) the whole person is composed of multiple and various systems (Lazarus, 1978) (e.g. anatomical, physiological, cognitive, emotional, social-cultural, and spiritual systems) which interact (Simons & Simons, 1989); (2) this person is quite different from the simple sum of his or her systems (Pellitier, 1979; Cleland & King, 1972); and (3) the environment plays an important role. In providing treatment, it is essential to address not only these separate systems, but also the product of the interactions among them (Texidor, Hawk, Thomas, Friedman, & Weiner, 1987). The essence of interdisciplinary work is the synergistic nature of it; and, synchronization is a key factor necessary to produce an overall "most effective" therapeutic outcome. With these constructs in mind, the purpose of this chapter is to explore the goals, objectives, and processes associated with nonpharmacological management of chronic pain.

GOALS

Chronic pain is commonly defined as pain which has been experienced for a six-month duration or longer. However, as noted previously, Bonica (1990), defines it more succinctly as that pain which "persists a month beyond the usual course of an acute disease or reasonable time for an injury to heal, or pain that recurs at intervals for months or years." With this definition, he argues that the six-month definition is inappropriate because acute diseases or injuries heal usually in two to six weeks, and if pain still exists after that time, it must be considered chronic in nature. The term "chronic pain syndrome" as defined by Black as persistent pain caused by operant or psychologic mechanisms is inappropriate since there are many chronic pain syndromes; these are reviewed in detail by Bonica (1990). He also argues that the term "chronic benign pain" is equally inappropriate as chronic pain is never benign (Bonica, 1990).

Flor and Turk (1989) state that "the extent and nature of physiological pathology that is necessary or sufficient to result in the PERCEPTION of pain" is not yet agreed upon, either. There is doubt whether this will ever be known for any given individual, although it may be estimatable at some time in the future. These collaborators suggest that presently, it is probably more appropriate to refer to abnormal psychophysiological patterns as either antecedents or consequences of chronic pain that maintain or exacerbate the pain symptom, rather than to view them as causative factors. There are a number of pain syndromes that have been suggested as having a psychophysiological component (Flor & Turk, 1989; Margoles, 1989; Mallek, Neff, & Nakamoto, 1984). These include, but by no means are limited to, headaches (migraine and tension), temporomandibular disorders (TMD), and chronic neck, shoulder, and low back pain (CLBP). These have been seen as having vascular and musculoskeletal etiology, respectively. These syndromes are extremely prevalent in this society, and are of interest to researchers because there is often no readily apparent organic pathology evident which supports the presence of pain itself or the amplitude of it. Such anomalies have been observed clinically since the late 1940s (Wolff, 1950). As Tollison has reviewed the magnitude of the problem of pain within this text, the emphasis here will not be to re-explore this area. However, it is perhaps meaningful to express the current extent of CLBP alone. CLBP has been determined to exist in the experience of some 20 million people in this country (Sarker, 1982; Bonica, 1990) costing billions of dollars annually. Margoles (1989), Fields (1987), and Simons (in press, 1984) discuss multiple factors which support the perpetuation of chronicity associated with some types of CLBP. These perpetuators may include mechanical, structural, physiological, psychological, metabolic, biochemical, and/or hormonal, all as single entities or, more often, in combination with one another. This could be viewed as though a "domino effect" occurs with this problem. Regarding TMD, Mallek, et al. (1984) suggest that there are two forms of this disorder; these are orthofunction and dysfunction. They state that there is little agreement as to the etiology of the functional disturbance, and address the roles of nutrition and stress response as associated factors. Eggleston (1980) discusses stressor agents classified as nutritional, environmental, or structural, and their impact on TMD. He states that functional disorders are physiopathological such that the pathology exists with no presidposing organic problem. As Bonica (1990) suggests with regard to chronic pain, "In most cases, apprehension, fear, worry, anxiety—all mental effects of the pain—seem to have much to do with the physical deterioration of the patients as does the pain itself. . .the effect and not the cause of prolonged pain."

No matter what factors with which the pain experience consists or is associated, and regardless of etiology, the mind and body are connected and therefore are impacted together by the experience (Rossi, 1986; Texidor, 1984). Accordingly, one major goal in managing pain in a nonpharmacological manner is to produce effective adaptive management of the cognitive, emotional, and behavioral components of the individual regarding the role of perception and the experience of pain. These relate to both the internal environment of the individual, and to his or her internal responses to this environment. It would also follow that when the cognitive, emotional, and behavioral aspects are disturbed by perception stimulated change in the internal environment relative to the pain experience, there is concurrent change with regard to the external environment of the individual, rather like the effect of a pebble thrown into a lake. The observable ripple effect ensues which disturbs the remainder of the lake surface. Furthermore, this ripple effect may flow in both internal-external directions as well. Hence, a second major goal for pain management in the nonpharmacological sense is to effect adaptive modification regarding an individual's interaction with external factors such as environmental conditions and communication with others.

It is equally as important to address social support issues associated with the management of pain. These relate to the external environment of the individual and his or her responses to it. With the interplay between the internal and external environments, there is: (1) need for client comprehension of this fact if the management of this interplay is viewed as potentially productive with a given client and (2) there is consequently, a need to work with these integrated internal/external systems toward healthy adaptation.

Gorski and Miller (1982) discuss chronic illness as a "disease in which there is gradual onset of progressively more severe symptoms." They suggest that with chronic illness, there is lag time from physical health to obvious debilitation, which is a process of lengthy duration. We have previously discussed that chronic pain is defined as pain of about six or more months duration. This then represents such lag time. Gorski and Miller (1982) discuss chronic disease as providing an entire lifestyle change with concurrent associated broad spectrum changes in the physical, cognitive-emotional, behavioral, and social arenas of living. They suggest that these changes "become habitual and deeply ingrained in the personality. Even if the physical symptoms are treated, the person has become psychologically, behaviorally, and socially dependent upon the continuation of the symptoms of the disease." Therefore, as it takes a considerably long time to adapt to physical illness and to modify all other components to that adaptation, it also takes time to move to wellness producing all the adaptations associated with this dynamic change to recovery. "As there are benefits and disadvantages to illness, so are there gains and losses to recovery. When the physical aspect of disease is treated without treating the other aspects, the untreated levels produce an alternate disease or induce relapse to the previous disease state" (Gorski & Miller, 1982). Simply put, an individual develops a relationship with their illness and learns to incorporate it into their lifestyle. These new habits, behavioral, emotional, cognitive, social, and physical, allow the disease to be tolerated to some extent. Once an individual gets used to the feelings and physical limitations of the disease, he or she tolerates living with illness, even though he or she may not appreciate it. These changes support the fullest possible functioning with the illness, despite it or in light of its presence.

Therefore, recovery, including relapse prevention, must address all aspects of the chronic illness adaptation, not just the physical aspects. "Physical recovery alone is only partial" (Gorski & Miller, 1982) and represents, perhaps, only a temporary recovery. The combination of multiple perpetuating factors and the concept of recovery without relapse are the bases for the requirement of the interdisciplinary approach.

SPECIFIC AIMS

Taking these two major goals into account, there are several specific aims which are germane to working with persons experiencing chronic pain. Of critical importance are the general aims of supporting and facilitating patient adaptation to the concept of "dealing with pain", while simultaneously learning how to temper the usual and natural urge to fight against the pain. This "fighting" usually intensifies anger, anxiety, or guilt responses and is therefore supportive to maintenance of pain. The second and equally as important objective is to foster gradual adaptation regarding the impact and management of the emotions of fear, guilt, and anger associated with both the experience of pain and other general (and probably associated) living experiences. Thirdly, fostering client perception, motivation, and ability regarding active participation in pain reduction associated with pain severity, body area involved, and duration where possible are valuable to the reduction of pain; they support the evolution of both active participation and sense of control. These areas requiring adaptation are often termed those of "problem ownership" and "coping skills development."

Frequently, as we are socialized in our society, we come to understand that there are professionals to whom we go when our physical ailments "need fixing." It is within this context that our own individual role and responsibilities associated with being healthy, in this instance pain-free, are often diminished or, in fact, may never have been cultivated at all. With the maturation of perceived self-control or self-management regarding pain, despite the fact that pain continues to exist, comes a much enhanced self-concept through expanded senses of awareness and self-mastery. In support of such growth, it is also apropos to foster gradual adaptive body use regardless of presence of pain once the severity, area, and duration become even slightly perceived as manageable by the client, given that the anatomical and physical parameters will tolerate such use without incurring extended damage or disruption.

Concurrently, the facilitation of a sense of moving on with living, despite the fact of pain as an existing entity, is another major objective. In order to maintain an upward-bound attitude and ambience, supporting continued progress with associated enhanced self-concept and self-mastery development despite living with pain is a critical issue.

BASIC PROCESSES

There are a number of basic processes which may be applicable once an appropriate evaluation has been completed. With respect to the internal environment, the first is known as managing the pain-anxiety cycle. It is appropriate that individuals experiencing chronic pain become aware of the possible contributions they may inadvertently make to their pain by the automatic invocation of their stress response to any given stimuli or perception, and the ensuing associated physiologic reactivity. Clients need to understand that this physiologic response is but a built in mechanism for protection and survival, and that it is somewhat controllable through a combination of awareness and employment of intentional interventive strategies. Important tasks of treatment, therefore, are the development of knowledge about the cycle and provision of assistive experience regarding interventive strategies which may be applied with the sensing (body symptoms), feeling (emotions), thinking (cognitions), and behavioral components connected with the cycle. Likewise, it is fitting that the client become aware of and skilled with these options for intervention. Some of this work may incorporate assistance with development of numerous options that can be individualized to the specific client lifestyle and lifescope.

Regardless of what options are developed, the next phase is a most critical one. The development of actual skill with use of each option or strategy is necessary. Here, theory is well and good; however, without actual successful application of it, skill with application and integration at the behavioral level will not occur. Ultimately, the goal here is for the client to not only actively select but also to employ the options, appropriately matched to stressor or stress response in an effective, assertive, and consistent manner. Thus, elements of this portion of a pain management program include, but are not limited to, the tasks outlined in Table 1.

A number of self-regulatory methods exist which may be specifically employed to produce a reduction of sympathetic arousal. These include, but are not limited to, the use of relaxing recall, creative imagery, progressive muscle relaxation, certain breathing techniques, and biofeedback. In addition, body use (the use of exercise) may be effected in order to decrease the product (energy) of arousal in an advantageous way.

A variety of pain reduction self-management strategies may be employed at three levels of functioning to reduce sympathetic arousal. These can be taught-learned to create successful intervention (Rossi, 1986; Borysenko, 1987), thereby enhancing self-concept, while simultaneously reducing stress responsiveness within an individual. These levels of intervention are: (1) cognitive or thought management, (2) emotional management, and (3) behavioral management, which importantly includes nutritional intake management.

Cognitive strategies consist of techniques such as refocusing, the purposeful use of humor and/or music, cognitive restructuring such that one interprets pain as a helpful message (e.g., a friend for early awareness and as a prompt for purposeful and assertive adaptation to the application

Table 1.

A. **Development** of physiological status assessment and awareness skills.

B. **Identification** of and work with one's own physiologic response to stressors.

C. **Identification** and management of those stressors which can be modified, of both internal and external nature.

D. **Development** of strategies to assist one to be less stress responsive.

E. **Assertive** employment of these strategies to effectively manage the stress response.

F. **Development** of support systems to decrease perceived presence of stress.

G. **Reduction** of internal responses to co-dependent interactions with others through self-awareness and assertive change in the internal response patterns associated with communication styles.

H. **Development** of symptom recognition as a tool. This includes cue awareness such as symbolic internal dialogue (self-talk) or interactive word usage cues, body posture or position cues, recognition of pain-associated feelings and thought content cues.

I. **Development** of the perception of the presence of pain and the use of it as a helpful message upon which to make pro-active choices about self-care on one's own behalf (e.g. reframing the meaning of pain from fear/anger/fight to useful and usable information).

J. **Development** of skill with early symptom recognition, rather than paying attention only at extreme pain level periods (e.g. after-the-fact awareness).

K. **Choice** and use of strategies early-on to prevent pain accrual, de-intensify or attenuate the physiologic product of the thought response, the emotional response, and/or the behavioral response.

of self-care methods). Other cognitive strategies which may be learned and instituted include such techniques as thought interruption, thought substitution, living in the present (which is often called here/now thinking), and rehearsal. Additionally, strategies such as assertive collection of additional information, validation of current information, modification or alteration of internal dialogue, and the use of reflective/explorative conversation may prove extremely helpful. The interpretation of pain as a collaborator used to invoke self-management can be a focal point for adaptive growth.

Further, the concerted use of problem solving models to foster and support self-care and choice are significant in enhancing self-concept and perceived self-mastery. It is appropriate to engender the generalization of the use of these strategies to other similar situations as well. All may be couched in reflection on producing change for living in the present and for contributing to the creation of successful outcomes now for the future.

The use of transactional analysis (Berne, 1964) as a framework to comprehend and work with inner dialogue (self-talk) (Meichenbaum, 1977) (e.g., thinking through self-imposed "shoulds/oughts" and responses to them) can be of considerable assistance with both internal interactions and those which take place with other individuals in the life of the client. Values clarification and work associated with adapting thoughts about personal values and attitudes can assist with building and maintaining the upward-bound ambience. For example, exploring with the client how he or she can be okay by existing in the present while letting go of the past and decreasing future thinking may open new and viable perspectives. Then the more important task of how to do so is facilitated to the surface and can then be explored also. These constructive adaptations fully support movement on to the creation of a proactive perspective, a view of being a participant in living rather than being just a responder to what life presents.

With respect to emotional management strategies, a first and major step, which is difficult for some, centers around the identification of feelings. This is especially true for males, and moreso for those who have been active in the business world. These types of men and women are thinkers who are less likely to deal with feelings as a part of day-to-day awareness, either their own or those of others. However, once this level of identification has occurred, the definition of past emotional responses to certain types of perceptual and/or interactive situations may be brought about. With this step achieved, the assertive creation of new responses to old stimuli may be undertaken. Other strategies may include preparation for emotional impact, the development of multiple meanings of an idea while fostering multiple consequent feelings. In addition, the purposeful creation of emotions/emotional responses for application with future events incorporating the actual exploration and rehearsal of these response options, frequently given as between session "homework", can be very helpful.

Behavioral strategies which can be useful involve at least those behaviors constructive to a healthy lifestyle. They, too, must be explored as options for choice by the client rather than as requirements by the counselor. In this way the adult decision maker is allowed, in fact, encouraged to emerge. These behavioral options encompass behaviors such as body posturing, body positioning, and purposeful energy use. After initial evaluations have been completed by a physical therapist, and an occupational therapist, a plan for body ability maintenance may be incorporated into the behavioral strategies options. This plan should include both gradual and progressive body use enhancement and adaptive body use methods.

The nutritionist, supported by all other members of the team, may opt to work with specific behaviors such as nutritional intake strategies (Travell & Simons, 1983), glucose levels/calories/energy, and the management of specific nutrients. Special attention should focus on intake of vitamins that contribute to neurologic transmission and health such as B vitamins, folacin, and vitamins C, and D. Of equal importance in managing chronic pain syndromes are adequate intake of electrolytes needed for muscle use such as potassium and calcium. Minerals needed for health, such as magnesium, phosphorous, iron, copper, zinc, and manganese, should also be addressed during behavioral approaches to nutrition associated with chronic pain management. Other aspects of nutrition, such as nutrients needed for adequate energy use, like oxygen transport, and supportive to healthy maintenance of hemoglobin and hematocrit levels, should be addressed in the behavioral component as well. Further, and of critical importance to the management of some types of chronic pain problems, is body weight management, as this may effect anatomical posture and body use associated with cardiovascular-pulmonary tolerance of exercise. Other body use issues that are important to address within the behavioral realm are range of motion, flexibility, and strengthening. These may be critical in clients who over several years of having chronic pain have become essentially muscularly debilitated from inactivity and associated fear. These optimally will be dealt with by at least the nutritionist, the physical therapist, and the counselor, and will be supported by all other team members from the vantage point of each individual discipline involved. Massage, realignment, and thermal applications may be helpful; however these should be employed when indications for benefit are clear, as these are not patient-active solutions, but rather may be used as means to a secondary gain of attention which may in turn reinforce pain behavior.

With regard to the external environment and associated factors, it is important to consider both the client's relationship with the environment itself, and his or her relationship with other people, encompassing both social and cultural issues. All of the following methods may, or may not, include the conjoint work of the identified pain client and their significant other. However, greater progress is often seen when the significant other does participate, especially with regard to communications/interactions. With a basis for understanding what the client is working toward or with, the significant other person may be developed to become an active support system for client achievement and success with new skills and the application of them. Central to relationship issues are communications and behavioral interactive skills development. Education about and applications of transactional analysis constructs in communications (Berne, 1964) may be a most effective vehicle, providing a framework for interactions management. The application of "checking out" implied/perceived intent and/or meanings with others, and the creation of effective confrontation behaviors can be productive as well. The overall aim is the development of the adaptive "adult" methods for constructive, health-oriented interactions.

The role of decision making for taking charge of self is critical and central to communications management. The concept of $1 + 1 + 1$ math for healthy relationships (James, 1979) may readily assist the less verbal-oriented communicator with regard to the concept of communication in relationships. Awareness of strategies that both self and others use to attain goals in a relationship can be examined (Dyer, 1978). Roles others may take to be supportive regarding pain management need to be explored and addressed.

Overall, the creation and application of skills focused for assertive self-care through awareness and active choice is the underlying theme with regard to nonpharmacologic management of chronic pain. The end product of nonpharmacologic management when successful is a person who has adjusted to having some level of his or her pain, who can be and is proactive on their own behalf, with a sense of ability, accomplishment, and self-mastery regardless of the continued existence of the pain. Because of the numerous aspects of the individual involved, the interdisciplinary approach is probably the most appropriate and effective means to this end.

SUMMARY

The purpose of this chapter has been to present a discussion of the goals, objectives, and some of the viable processes available for the management of chronic pain. In addition, these have been presented within the context of and with rationale for the use of the interdisciplinary approach. With regard to the latter, synchronization of treatment rendered by a team of professionals is a key factor. Likewise, participation as part of this team by the client and family (or significant other) is of major importance. With regard to the former, the physical, emotional, cognitive, behavioral, social, cultural, and spiritual aspects of the person with chronic pain must all be tapped into in order to maximize results of treatment. Thus, the client's internal and external environments, and products of the interaction of these need to be taken into account with regard to assessment, planning, and rendering treatment. Chronic pain develops with possible maladaptation regarding all aspects of an individual; and this takes place over a considerable period of time. Effective management of chronic pain , therefore, implies recovery over a course of time; and recovery implies relapse prevention for the remainder of an individual's life.

REFERENCES

Berne, E. (1964). *Games people play.* New York: Grove Press, Inc.

Borysenko, J. (1987). *Minding the body, mending the mind.* Reading, MA: Addison-Wesley Publishing Company.

Brena, S. F., Chapman, S. L., & Decker, R. (1980). Chronic pain as a learned experience: Emory university pain control center. *National Institute of Drug Abuse Research Monograph Series, 36,* 76-83.

Bonica, J. (1990). *The management of pain, Vol. I.* Philadelphia: Lea & Febiger.

Cleland, D. L. & King, W. R. (1972). *Management: A systems approach.* New York: McGraw-Hill Book Company.

Dyer, W. (1978). *Pulling your own strings.* New York: Avon Books

Eggleston, D. W. (1980). The interrelationship of stress and degenerative diseases. *The Journal of Prosthetic Dentistry, 44(5),* 541-544.

Fields, H. (1987). *Pain.* New York: McGraw-Hill Book Company.

Fields, H. (1981). Pain II: New approaches to management. *Annals of Neurology 9,* 101-106.

Flor, H. & Turk, D. C. (1989). Psychophysiology of chronic pain: Do chronic pain patients exhibit symptom specific psychophysiological responses? *Psychology Bulletin, 105(2),* 215-259.

Flor, H. & Turk, D. C. & Rudy, T.E. (1987). Pain and families, I & II. *Pain, 30(1) and 31(2),* 3-27, and 29-45.

Fordyce, W. (1981). On interdisciplinary peers. *Archives of Physical Medicine, 62:* 51-53.

Gorski, T. T. & Miller, M. (1982). *Counseling for relapse prevention.* Independence, MO: Herald House-Independence Press.

James, M. (1979). *Marriage is for loving.* Reading, MA: Addison-Wesley Publishing Company.

Lazarus, A. (1978). What is multi-modal therapy? A brief overview. *Elementary School Guidance and Counseling, 13(1)*, 6-11.

Long, D. M. (1950). A comprehensive model for the study and therapy of pain: Johns Hopkins pain research and treatment program. *National Institute of Drug Abuse Research Monograph Series, 36*, 66-75.

Mallek, H., Neff, P., & Nakamoto, T. (1984). Interactions of nutrition and temporomandibular joint dysfunction. *Ear, Nose and Throat Journal, 63:* 499-504.

Margoles, M. S. (1989). Comprehensive evaluation and treatment of the patient with myofascial pain syndrome. *Journal of Neurologic and Orthopedic Medicine and Surgery, 10*, 344-346.

Melvin J. (1980). Interdisciplinary and multidisciplinary activities and ACRM. *Archives of Physical Medicine, 61*, 379-380.

Meichenbaum, D. (1977). *Cognitive-behavior modification.* New York: Plenum Press.

Pellitier, K. R. (1979). *Holistic medicine.* New York: Dell Publishing Company.

Rossi, E. L. (1986). *The psychobiology of mind-body healing.* New York: W. W. Norton and Company.

Sanders, R. (1988). Somatic communications: Interpersonal theory and therapy of psychosomatic disorders. In *Medical psychotherapy* (pp. 95-111). Toronto: Hans Huber Publishers.

Sarker, S. (1982). Pain centers: An alternative for management of chronic pain. *Health Care Management Review, 7(4)*, 77-84.

Schulz, I. & Texidor, M. S. (in press). The interdisciplinary approach: An exercise in futility or a song of praise. *Medical Psychotherapy.*

Simons, D. G. (1984). Myofascial pain syndromes and their treatment. In J. V. Basmajian and R. L. Kirby (Eds.), *Medical rehabilitation,* Appendix I. Baltimore: Williams & Wilkins Publishers.

Simons, D. G. (in press). *Myofascial pain and dysfunction: The trigger point manual. Vol. 2.* Baltimore: Williams & Wilkins.

Simons, D. G. & Simons, L. S. (1989). Chronic myofascial pain syndrome. In C. D. Tollison (Ed.) *Handbook of chronic pain management,* p. 523. Baltimore: Williams & Wilkins.

Texidor, M. (1984). Knowledge, attitudes, and behaviors: The effects of a seminar in wellness, holistic assessment, and collaborative approach on school social workers. *Dissertation Abstracts International, 42*, 1416A.

Texidor, M. S., Hawk, R., Thomas, P., Friedman, B., & Weiner, R. (1987). *Holistic counseling.* Alexandria, VA: The Holistic Counseling Special Interest Network of The American Mental Health Counselors Association.

Texidor, M. (in press). Chronic pain management: The interdisciplinary approach and cost-effectiveness. In K. Anchor (Ed.) *The handbook of medical psychotherapy: Cost-effective strategies in mental health.* Toronto, Canada: Hogrefe & Huber Publishers.

Travell, J. & Simons, D. G. (1983). *Myofascial pain and dysfunction: The trigger point manual*. Baltimore: Williams & Wilkins Publishers.

Weiner, R. S. (1988). Credentialing practices: Resistance to innovation. *Medical Psychotherapy*, 1:191-202.

Wolff, H. G. (1950). *Headache and other pain*. New York: Oxford University Press.

Chapter 8

PHARMACO-THERAPEUTIC MANAGEMENT OF SELECTED PAIN PHENOMENA

Robert B. Supernaw, Pharm. D.
Arthur F. Harralson, Pharm. D.

Doctors Supernaw and Harralson provide the reader with a classification and rationale for use of medication in the management of painful conditions. Building upon a taxonomy of distinction between acute pain states and that of chronic benign pain, as well as pain associated with cancer, this chapter describes the indications and potential complications for pharmacologic therapy. The philosophy of the authors is that the drug regimen should be equal to the task of alleviating pain. This philosophy of agressive dosing, termed "descending the ladder" is portrayed in graphic form. Tables presented will benefit the reader for clinical selection.

Chapter 8

PHARMACO-THERAPEUTIC MANAGEMENT OF SELECTED PAIN PHENOMENA

Robert B. Supernaw, Pharm. D.
Arthur F. Harralson, Pharm. D.

As is the case with almost any medical problem, the best pharmacotherapeutic approach to acute and chronic pain management is no drug therapy at all. However, the option of not using drugs in managing many pain syndromes is not viable. When the clinician has determined that the pain condition is significant and beyond the scope of being treated solely with physical medicine (e.g., ice packs, massage, physical therapy), drug therapy is indicated.

In order to determine the best pharmacotherapeutic response to pain, the nature and severity of the pain must be assessed. Whether the pain is acute or chronic must be taken into account as well as whether the pain is malignant, benign organic, psychogenic, vascular, or depression-related. Additionally, the pain should be graded as mild, moderate, severe, or excruciating before an appropriate drug regimen and drug delivery system are formulated.

ACUTE PAIN

When a patient presents in acute distress, often the clinician's attention is first drawn to the comfort of the patient, and alleviating the pain is attempted even before the cause of the distress is considered. For this reason, the clinician must make a quick and accurate assessment of the relative degree of the pain. In acute pain, the same classification system is used as for chronic pain (i.e., mild, moderate, severe, and excruciating).

Mild Acute Pain

Since, by definition, acute pain is limited in its duration, it need not be aggressively treated. Often, it need not be treated at all. If a decision is made to treat the mild acute pain, first consideration should be given to aspirin. For the aspirin-allergic patient, acetaminophen is an excellent alternative, although it has no anti-inflammatory activity.

Aspirin may be given in oral tablet form, 650 mg (two 325 mg tablets) every four hours. As a salicylate, aspirin represents the class of drugs most commonly prescribed for pain management. It is rapidly absorbed, primarily in the duodenum. Although it is an acid, it is a weak acid (pKa = 3.5) for which absorption is enhanced in an alkaline GI system. Therefore, buffered aspirin does have a shorter absorption time, but this difference is considered insignificant. All salicylates are metabolized in the liver. Salicylates are widely distributed and highly albumin-bound. For this reason, caution is urged when treating the anticoagulated patient taking an oral anticoagulant that is also highly protein bound (up to 97% bound). Aspirin may displace an oral anticoagulant, and if as little as 3% of the anticoagulant is displaced, a 100% increase in the unbound drug level will result in significant bleeding complications. Salicylates also inhibit platelet adhesion which places the anticoagulation patient at an even greater risk.

Aspirin has excellent analgesic activity. It is effective for post-operative pain, musculoskeletal pain, headache, fever-related pain, and some visceral pain. It is particularly effective in pain that is secondary to an inflammatory process. In the dose of 650 mg, aspirin is used as the standard yardstick against which all other analgesics are measured.

An alternative to aspirin for the acute pain patient is acetaminophen. It is considered to be approximately equipotent to aspirin in its analgesic activity, and it has the same indications for pain as does aspirin with one important exception. Acetaminophen does not have anti-inflammatory properties; therefore, it is of limited value in pain where inflammation may play a role. A word of caution with acetaminophen is warranted. Because significant conjugation of acetaminophen takes place in the liver, excessive doses of acetaminophen may overtax the body's ability to keep-up with the conjugation process, and the levels of a hepatotoxic metabolite increase, frequently resulting in extensive liver damage or even death.

Moderate Acute Pain

Aspirin is also the primary choice for moderate acute pain; however, if aspirin is not appropriate and the clinician is not prepared to leap to a narcotic analgesic, then a rapid onset nonsteroidal anti-inflammatory analgesic may be indicated. If a rapid onset of action is not a consideration to be taken into account, then, of course, an oral nonsteroidal anti-inflammatory drug (NSAID) may be used. These will be considered later in this chapter. However, if onset of action is a significant consideration, a parenteral dosage form of an NSAID is appropriate. Ketorolac tromethamine (Toradol, Syntex) is the only injectable NSAID available at this time. Given as an IM injection, ketorolac tromethamine exhibits effective analgesic activity in about 30 minutes. It is given in a dose of 30-60 mg IM followed by 15-30 mg IM every 6 hours, not to exceed 150 mg for the first day and 120 mg per day, thereafter. Ketorolac tromethamine has the advantages of rapid onset of action, little or no narcotic or central analgesic activity resulting in no respiratory depression, little potential for abuse, and few GI side effects.

As a post-operative analgesic, Ketorolac appears to be equipotent to standard narcotic agents (O'Hara, 1987; Yee, 1986). Given in a dose of 30 mg, it appears to be at least as effective as 12 mg morphine or 100 mg meperidine, when each is given intramuscularly. It also appears to continue its analgesic activity for a slightly greater duration of time when compared to the usual narcotic analgesics; however, this increased duration may not prove to be a significant advantage.

If the clinician feels that an oral medication is appropriate and also feels that a narcotic is indicated for an acute moderate pain presentation, the combination of aspirin or acetaminophen with codeine is an appropriate choice. In a study of 100 patients, codeine sulfate 65 mg and aspirin 650 mg was judged by the patients to be superior in its pain-alleviating activity when compared with (i) oxycodone 9.75 mg and aspirin 650 mg, (ii) pentazocine hydrochloride 25 mg and aspirin 650 mg, (iii) propoxyphene napsylate 100 mg and aspirin 650 mg, (iv) promazine hydrochloride 25 mg and aspirin 650 mg, (v) pentobarbital sodium 32 mg and aspirin 650 mg, (vi) caffeine 65 mg and aspirin 650 mg, (vii) ethoheptazine citrate 75 mg and aspirin 650 mg, (viii) aspirin 650 mg alone, and (ix) placebo (Moertel, 1974). When codeine is added to aspirin or acetaminophen, the side effects of the opiates present themselves. The most bothersome of these side effects are the gastrointestinal effects. It is common for patients taking these combinations to complain about constipation, gastric distress, as well as nausea. Sedation may also occur; so patients should be warned about taking precautions in driving or operating machinery. Patients should also be cautioned about the additive CNS depressant activity when alcohol is consumed.

Severe Acute Pain

For acute pain episodes that are considered severe, more potent and rapid-onset pharmacotherapy is necessary. There are three rather obvious criteria that would indicate aggressive treatment of pain with a narcotic agent, such as morphine. First, if the clinician has previously tried non-narcotics in reasonable doses and has achieved less than effective results; second, if the pain is considered to be significantly more debilitating than moderate pain; and third, if the patient has a history of pain relief when narcotics are used; and rapid relief is required, then a parenteral narcotic is appropriate.

Of the parenteral narcotics available, clearly, morphine sulfate is the standard. While it should be remembered that unless the patient is in acute distress, oral dosage forms are preferred, the clinician should not hesitate to administer morphine sulfate injection in acute severe pain situations. Unlike other drug regimens where the practitioner starts-off at a relatively low dose and gradually ascends to higher doses or adds other drugs until the condition is managed (e.g., hypertension, hyperlipidemia), the drug regimen immediately should be equal to the task of alleviating the pain. This philosophy of aggressive dosing, termed descending the ladder, is graphically illustrated in Figure 1. It has gained acceptance, at least partially, because too often fears of addiction and respiratory depression have led to too timid dosing of narcotics (Marks, 1973). Simply stated, a dose that is felt to be adequate should be administered, and the subsequent doses are slightly tapered-down until the pain threshold is discovered. Then, the dose is adjusted just slightly upward to alleviate the pain on an around-the-clock basis without overdosing. This system should lead to lower maintenance doses because the patient is rapidly brought into the realm of comfort rather than gradually.

A usual initial dose of parenteral morphine sulfate (i.e., IM or SC) for an adult is 10-20 mg. If an effective oral dose of morphine is known, then one-sixth of that dose should be administered parenterally. If the pain is excruciating, then a greater dose is appropriate in order to begin to descend the ladder. After the initial dose, the patient will need repeated doses every 4-6 hours. With parenteral morphine, the patient should begin to feel relief within a few minutes. If morphine is going to be continued, it should be changed to an oral dosage form as there is no real advantage to continuation of the parenteral form (Twycross, 1974). For long-term maintenance, consideration should be given to long-acting morphine sulfate (MS Cotin, Purdue Frederick). The long-acting dosage form appears to provide 12-hour relief at a dosage of approximately 75% of regular oral dosage forms (Cundiff, 1989).

As with all aggressive treatment regimens, the clinician will be most diligent in monitoring side effects, especially since the opiates have CNS depressant activity. Sedation should be carefully evaluated. Significant sedation will present itself at narcotic levels above the pain threshold. The ideal dose will be achieved if sedation is not significant and pain control is maintained. Sedation later in therapy may be an indication of accumulation toxicity effect. If this is the case, it may be difficult to cut-back the

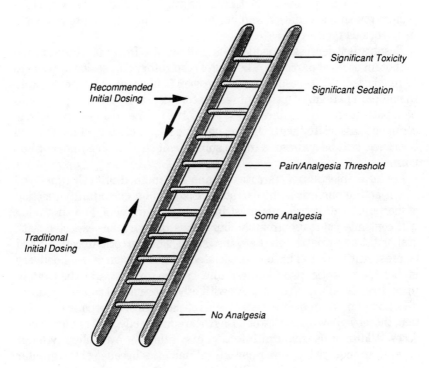

Figure 1. Analgesic Dosing Ladder

dose late in therapy without causing the pain to recur. Short of reinitiation of the dosing regimen, the more use of amphetamines or methylphenidate may be attempted. While the use of one drug to cover-up the adverse effects of another is considered irrational polypharmacy, for patients in acute distress, intractable pain, or for those who are terminally ill, the use of these CNS stimulants may be indicated as long as the sedation is simple sedation and not mental confusion, symptomatic of a more serious toxicity.

Respiratory depression is also a fear of many clinicians who administer potent doses of narcotics. The fear of respiratory depression appears to be misplaced. While respiratory depression is fairly easy to demonstrate in non-pain patients, significant respiratory depression is not common in pain patients receiving narcotics (Walsh, 1981). The adverse drug effects commonly associated with chronic narcotic use, including addiction and tolerance, will be addressed in the subsequent section on severe chronic pain.

Epidural injection of narcotics is another method of both rapid and longer-acting narcotic administration. Epidural (or extradural) injection of morphine will result in almost immediate pain relief, and that relief will continue for approximately four times the duration expected with oral or IM administration (Leavans, 1982). The narcotic injection must be preservative-free. The logic associated with this form of drug delivery is that the narcotic, usually morphine, can be given nearer the CNS to work directly on the receptors. As with other parenteral routes, epidural injection of morphine eliminates the first-pass effect of hepatic degradation, thereby allowing for lower doses to be equally effective to higher oral doses. Additionally, epidural injection may allow for even slightly lower doses than required for other parenteral narcotics because of the greater systemic absorption of IM or SC administered doses. Therefore, it has been shown to have significant advantages for the obstetric pain patient; however, to date, little other benefit has been achieved with the use of epidural injection for other pain patients, and adverse effect profiles for these administrations appear to be no better than those for conventional injections (McQuay, 1989). Significant itching has also accompanied epidural injections of narcotics. These seem to be alleviated with the combined use of hydroxyzine (Vistaril Pfizer; Atarax Roerig) with the narcotic.

CHRONIC PAIN

Chronic pain may be thought of as a completely different medical problem than its acute phase. Chronic pain has elements of acute pain, but it is generally more psychologically innervated, debilitating the personhood as well as the physical nature of the body being treated. For this reason, the patient suffering chronic pain should be treated just as aggressively as the patient suffering acute distress.

Mild Chronic Pain

As with mild acute pain, the treatment standard has for years remained aspirin and acetaminophen. The relative differences between these drugs have been discussed previously. Both of these drugs are well tolerated when used on a chronic basis, and larger dosing schedules rarely cause problems. The toxicity associated with excessive doses of acetaminophen, causing liver damage, have been associated with doses of 5 gm or more per day for two to three weeks (Seeff, 1986).The precautions have been discussed, but special mention should be made of the positive antiplatelet effects secondary to chronic aspirin use. Even in extremely low daily aspirin doses, the antiplatelet adhesion effects of aspirin appear to diminish the incidence of thromboembolic morbidity and mortality. Many non-pain patients are now taking aspirin as a prophylactic measure against vascular disease and stroke.

Moderate Chronic Pain

The second step in chronic pain care is to increase the dosage of the initial analgesic choice. This step is usually effective in most moderate pain complaints. If it is not effective, then a drug regimen change to a nonsteroidal anti-inflammatory drug may be indicated. These agents are summarized in Table I. As with acetaminophen, there is some concern of hepatotoxicity with the NSAIDs (Lewis, 1984). NSAIDs are not necessarily more potent than aspirin; however, they are worth trying if the chronic pain is not responsive to aspirin therapy. No one agent listed in Table I appears to be superior to any other. Selection is made on the basis of clinician preference. These drugs are widely prescribed and have a well deserved reputation for safety and efficacy. In addition to their intrinsic anti-inflammatory activity, they are very good analgesics. Currently, ibuprofen is available over-the-counter. In the future, other NSAIDs will surely follow; however, in 1989, naproxen (Naprosyn, Syntex) was the 13th most widely prescribed drug in the U.S. in terms of new and refill prescriptions. It is clear that being a prescription only medication has not adversely affected the use of NSAIDs.

Using naproxen as the prototype, the NSAID is administered at a 500 mg initial dose followed twice daily, approximately 12 hours apart, with doses of 250 mg. Naproxen and sulindac sulfide are dosed twice daily, as is the sustained-release formulation of indomethacin. Other NSAID are dosed three to four times daily. Only piroxicam, with an extremely long half-life, can be single daily dosed. The NSAIDs are excellent as anti-inflammatories and analgesics, and they are particularly effective in

Table I. Nonsteroidal Anti-inflammatory Drugs Used for Pain Management

Generic & Trade Name	Usual Dosage	Max. Daily Dose	Half-Life (Hrs)
Fenoprofen (Nalfon)	300mg–400mg tid-qid	3200 mg	3
Flurbiprofen (Ansaid)	50mg–100mg tid-qid	300 mg	3 to 4
Ibuprofen (Motrin)	300mg–800mg tid-qid	3200 mg	1.8 to 2
Ketoprofen (Orudis)	50mg–75mg tid-qid	300 mg	3 (ave)
Naproxen sodium (Anaprox)	250–550mg bid	1000 mg	13
Indomethacin (Indocin)	25mg–50mg tid	200 mg	4.5 (ave)
Indomethacin SR (Indocin SR)	75mg bid	150 mg	4.5 to 6
Sulindac sulfide (Clinoril)	150mg bid	400 mg	16.4
Tolmetin (Tolectin)	200mg–400mg tid-qid	2000 mg	5
Meclofenamate (Meclomen)	50mg–100mg	400 mg	2
Piroxicam (Feldene)	20mg daily	20 mg	50 (ave)
Diclofenac sodium (Voltaren)	50mg–75mg tid-qid	200 mg	1.2 to 2

menstrual pain and cramping. Most new NSAIDs are rapidly and well absorbed, but food seems to decrease absorption. Patients should be instructed to take these drugs on an empty stomach to maximize their efficacy. Because of the potential hepatic complications, there is no reason why acetaminophen should be continued when an NSAID such as naproxen in begun.

An alternative step in moving to a level above the level of simple aspirin or acetaminophen pharmacotherapy is maintaining the initial drug selections and adding codeine. This is best accomplished using products such as ASA with codeine (Empirin #3, Burroughs Wellcome) or acetaminophen with codeine (Tylenol #3, McNeil) as single fixed-dose agents. The addition of the codeine greatly enhances the analgesic activity and is extremely effective in most chronic moderate pain.The precautions regarding the CNS depressant activity of codeine have been discussed, and the clinician would be well advised to discuss these precautions with the patient who is using codeine in pain control. Additionally, in chronic pain management, if codeine is to be employed, care should be exercised with a patient on any other CNS depressant (e.g., tranquilizers, antipsychotics).

Codeine has an onset of action at approximately 30-45 minutes with a duration of analgesic activity of four to six hours when given orally. Constipation is frequently seen in patients on chronic codeine therapy, but it can be overcome with occasional use of mild laxatives. As has been discussed, drowsiness may also limit the use of codeine at the workplace. Nevertheless, ASA and acetaminophen with codeine have each gained wide acceptance as excellent analgesics for chronic moderate pain control.

Severe Chronic Pain

If the pain condition is not alleviated with the use of aspirin, nonsteroidal anti-inflammatory drugs, or with aspirin or acetaminophen combined with codeine, more potent narcotic agents are indicated. Over the years, several narcotics have been widely used in the management of severe pain that is chronic in nature. Pain cocktails and morphine sulfate are have been widely used narcotics.

The original pain cocktail is Brompton's Mixture, dating back to the 1800s. It was formulated using morphine, cocaine, alcohol, and chloroform. It is now thought that the cocaine was used to numb the throat, and the chloroform was used to give the mixture a bitter taste, a requirement for all British medicines in those times. Because these two ingredients are not appropriate (and chloroform is not permitted in medications in the U.S.), contemporary pain cocktails, usually labelled as "Hospice Mixture," contain just morphine sulfate in solution. Some pain clinics allow their pain cocktails to include any other patient-specific medications that

Table II. Characteristics of PCA Devices Available in the U.S.ᵃ

Device Name	Functions	Bolus	Prefilled Syringe	Security System	Lockout Interval Range
Abbott Lifecare Infusor 1821	PCA	volume	yes; 30 mL	key	5–99 min
Abbott Lifecare Infusor 4100	PCA/continuous PCA/continuous	mg	yes; 30 mL	key	5–99 min
Bard Ambulatory PCA	PCA continuous PCA/continuous	mg or volume	no; 100 or 250 mL reservior	yes	3–240 min
Baxter PCA System*	PCA	fixed volume	use with Baxter Infusor; not prefilled	optional pole mount	6 min fixed
Becton Dickinson PCA Infusor	PCA continuous PCA/continuous	mg	yes; IMS prefilled 30 mL	key	5–99

Device	Mode	Dosing	Reservoir	Lock	Time range
Graseby PCA System	PCA continuous PCA/continuous	mg	no; B.D. disp 60 mL	key	3–40 min
Harvard PCA Pump 6464-001	PCA/continuous PCA/continuous	volume	yes; 50 mL	key	3–60 min
MiniMed PCA Device-404-S	PCA continuous PCA/continuous	volume	no; 3 mL disp syringe	case locks	0–799 min
Pancretec Provider–5000	PCA continuous PCA/continuous	mg or volume	no; use with 50–3000 mL iv bag	key	1 min–200 h
Pharmacia Deltec-Model 5200 PXC	PCA continuous PCA/continuous	mg	no; use with medication cassette	key	5–199 min
Stratofuse PCA PSM-9000	PCA continuous PCA/continuous	volume	yes; IMS prefilled 30 mL	key	5–60 min

* Includes Baxter Infusor (5 mL/h) and patient-control module.

a Reprinted with permission of publisher: *DICP, The Annals of Pharmacotherapy*, 23:901, 1989.

are physically compatible with the hydroalcoholic mixture. Frequently, antidepressant medications will be added, but these are not required to justify the label of pain cocktail. The addition of other agents has been shown to have not demonstratable advantage over morphine sulfate solution alone.

When a narcotic is indicated in chronic pain care, morphine sulfate is the narcotic of choice. There are no advantages of parenteral administration of morphine in chronic pain care, except in the few cases where the patient cannot take or cannot tolerate oral medications. The initial oral dose of morphine sulfate is variable, based upon the clinician's assessment of the severity and nature of the chronic pain. Doses of from 10 mg to 90 mg may be required. Tablet strengths customarily available are 10 mg, 15 mg, and 30 mg. There are no established upper limits to the dose to be given to the patient suffering from severe chronic pain. Many clinicians feel that any dose that helps the patient in maintaining a relatively comfortable state, without causing mental confusion or significant respiratory depression is justified. Oral morphine will have to be redosed every four hours to achieve continued pain relief.

Some clinicians have felt that when chronic pain is not manifesting itself, the patient should not be taking medication. Therefore, these practitioners feel that chronic pain medication should be administered on an as needed (PRN) basis. It has now been demonstrated that around-the-clock administration of pain medication provides superior analgesia. Not allowing the pain symptoms to recur causes less mental and physical trauma and can actually lead to less medication used with better pain control. Pain memory, when the patient begins to feel pain and anticipate continued pain distress, can be eliminated when the pain control pharmacotherapy is regularly scheduled.

In chronic narcotic use, there persists a fear of tolerance and addiction. Clearly, these fears are overemphasized. In studies, addiction has been shown to be of minor concern in the patient with chronic pain. In one study, nearly 12,000 pain patients receiving narcotics were followed, and of these only four patients became addicted (Porter, 1980). Tolerance to the narcotics is also of little concern. Patients do not seem to require ever-increasing doses of narcotics unless they are stricken with a progressively pain-intensifying illness.

Another system that has recently gained popularity is patient-controlled analgesia (PCA). A PCA device, about the size of a pack of playing cards, is programmed to deliver regular doses of a narcotic directly into the patient (usually IM), and the microprocessor is adjusted to a set dose around-the-clock. Additionally, the PCA device allows the patient to administer bolus injections of medication when the pain level increases. The device will not allow the patient to overdose, as limits are programmed into the portable device. The more sophisticated models can give the practitioner a print-out of doses administered including bolus doses administered by the patient. Studies have shown that PCA devices are very effective in controlling pain with minimal side effects (White, 1988). A list of several commercially available PCA devices is presented in Table II. Most of these devices are simple microprocessors with small battery-driven motors that activate screw-driven plungers that inject predetermined amounts of medication into the muscle. Some clinicians prefer to add a steroid, such as dexamethasone, 0.02 mg per ml, to the narcotic to limit needle trauma and inflammation. Also, the implant site should be rotated about every four days. With PCA devices, the patient has a renewed sense of being in control of his pain, an exhilarating and liberated feeling for most chronic pain suffers.

Chronic Pain that is Opioid-insensitive

By definition, chronic pain that is opioid-insensitive does not respond to narcotic analgesics. Usually, this pain is either aberrant or organic with nerve compression or nerve destruction (McQuay, 1989). Nerve destruction is common in tumor-related disease, post-herpetic neuralgia, and trigeminal neuralgia. Some patients provide the greatest clinical challenge presenting with pain of both opioid-sensitive and opioid-insensitive pain at different sites. With nerve-related chronic pain that is opioid-insensitive, unconventional drug therapy is indicated. Trials with tricyclic antidepressants; anticonvulsants, such as carbamazepine (Tegretol, Geigy); steroids; or even a phenothiazine, such as hydroxyzine are appropriate choices. Often, just when the clinician is prepared to surrender, the patient responds to an unconventional analgesic.

Tricyclic antidepressants are rather curious analgesics. Clearly, antidepressant medications are effective in the treatment of endogenous depression. Since one of the symptoms of depression is chronic pain, usually vague in description, antidepressants exert an analgesic effect indirectly by combating the depressive illness. It is also postulated that tricyclics also have an intrinsic analgesic activity which assists in chronic pain management. This activity is secondary to tricyclics' ability to effectively block the reuptake of serotonin. Additionally, tricyclics may also have a potentiating effect on narcotics, thereby facilitating chronic pain management. The analgesic activity of the tricyclics is most likely a combination of all three of these phenomena. Studies have demonstrated their effectiveness in the management of chronic pain in hundreds of patients (Tollison, 1988). The analgesic activity of tricyclics occurs within five to seven days, rather than the 10-14 days required for antidepressant effects.

Chronic Malignant Pain

The World Health Organization (WHO) has taken a leadership role in the formulation of a pharmacotherapeutic algorithm for the management of cancer pain (WHO, 1986). This three-step algorithm provides a simple and logical approach to appropriate management and should lead to a lower incidence of undertreatment.

Step One

Patients whose cancer pain is either mild or moderate are to be treated with a non-narcotic analgesic. Aspirin, acetaminophen, or an NSAID is recommended. Additionally, any specific analgesic adjuvant may also be employed, if the specific indication exists. This step is similar to that recommended for mild or moderate nonmalignant pain.

Step Two

Any cancer patient who is without pain relief with the first step, or who presents with moderate to severe pain is to be given an oral narcotic analgesic as well as any specific adjuvant analgesic, if an indication exists. Additionally, the WHO recommendation is for around-the-clock dosing of the opioid to limit the ability of the pain to present itself. Subsequent doses are, therefore, given before the previous dose wears off.

Step Three

Patients who are nonresponsive to the second step, or who present with severe cancer pain should be given a potent opioid narcotic reserved for severe pain. Also, adjuvant analgesics may be given along with other nonopioids, if required. These doses should be given around-the-clock, rather than on a PRN basis. For step three cancer pain, WHO suggests that alternate routes of administration be attempted if the oral route proves ineffective or cannot be utilized.

Minor Chronic Muscle Pain

Muscle pain that is minor but bothersome may be treated topically, if traditional oral analgesic and anti-inflammatory agents prove ineffective. These topical analgesic agents are classified as counterirritants, and the exhibit analgesic action by dilation of the vasculature and increasing the blood flow to the affected muscle. The FDA advisory panel on nonprescription topical analgesics has labelled the following product ingredients as relatively more potent counterirritants as well as safe and effective: allyl isothiocyanate, stronger ammonia water, methyl salicylate, and turpentine oil, capsaicin, capsicum, capsicum oleoresin. Many patients achieve substantial muscle pain relief with the appropriate use of these counterirritants, but patients should be warned to discontinue use of these products if excessive irritation develops.

SUMMARY

Many pain patients are undertreated because of unwarranted fears on the parts of clinicians regarding adverse drug reactions including respiratory depression, tolerance, and addiction. These effects would be extremely problematic; however, they do not seem to occur often enough to warrant timidity in the pain management approach. Pain is an excessively debilitating medical and psychologic problem that warrants aggressive initial treatment and diligent continued care.

REFERENCES

Crabbe, Sarah J. (1990). Ketorolac: A non-narcotic analgesic. *Hospital Therapy,* 755-764.

Cundiff, D., McCarthy, K., Saverese, J. J., et al. (1989). Evaluation of a cancer pain model for the testing of long-acting analgesics: The effect of MS Cotin in a double-blind, randomized crossover design. *Cancer, 63:* 2355-2359.

Giles, G. W. A., Kenny, G. N. C., Bullingham, R. E. S., et al. (1987). The morphine sparing effect of ketorolac tromethamine. *Anesthesia, 42:* 727-731.

Leavans, M. E., Hill, C. S., Cech, C. A., et al. (1982). Intrathecal and intraventricular morphine for pain in cancer patients: Initial study. *Journal of Neurosurgery, 56:* 241.

Lewis, J. H. (1984). Hepatic toxicity of nonsteroidal anti-inflammatory drugs. *Clinical Pharmacy, 3:* 128.

Marks, R. M. and Sachar, E. J. (1973). Undertreatment of medical inpatients with narcotic analgesics. *Annals of Internal Medicine, 78:* 173.

McQuay, H. J. (1989). Opioids in chronic pain. *British Journal of Anaesthesiology, 63:* 213-226.

Moertel, C. G., Ahmann, D. L., Taylor, W. F., et al. (1974). Relief of pain by oral medications. *Journal of the American Medical Association, 229:* 55.

O'Hara, D. A., Fragen, R. J., Kinzer, M., et al. (1987). Ketorolac tromethamine as compared with morphine sulfate for treatment of post-operative pain. *Clinical Pharmacology & Therapeutics, 41:* 556-561.

Porter, J., et al. (1980). Addiction rare in patients treated with narcotics. *New England Journal of Medicine, 302:* 123.

Seeff, L. B., et al. (1986). Acetaminophen hepatotoxicity in alcoholics - A therapeutic misadventure. *Annals of Internal Medicine, 104:* 399.

Tollison, C. D. and Kriegel, M. L. (1988). Selected tricyclic antidepressants in the management of chronic benign pain. *Southern Medical Journal, 81(5):* 562-564.

Twycross, R. G. (1974). Clinical experiences with diamorphine in advanced malignant disease. *International Journal of Clinical Pharmacology, 9:* 184.

Walsh, T. D., Baxter, R., Bowerman, K., et al. (1981). High-dose morphine and respiratory function in chronic cancer pain. *Pain, S1:* 39.

White, P. F. (1988). Use of patient-controlled analgesia for management of acute pain. *Journal of the American Medical Association, 259:* 243-247.

World Health Organization (1986). *Cancer pain relief.* Geneva, Switzerland: WHO.

Yee, J. R., Koshiver, J. E., Allbon, C. et al. (1986). Comparison of intramuscular ketorolac tromethamine and morphine sulfate for analgesia of pain after major surgery. *Clinical Pharmacology & Therapeutics, 6:* 253-261.

Yee, J. R., Stanski, D., Cherry, C. (1986). A comparison of analgesic efficacy of intramuscular ketorolac tromethamine and meperidine in post-operative pain. *Clinical Pharmacology & Therapeutics, 39:* 237.

Chapter 9
UNDERSTANDING AND TREATING LOW BACK PAIN

William Harsha, M. S., M. D., J. D.

Doctor Harsha, a prominent orthopedic surgeon, describes how back pain has been better understood and treated using the total approach to patient impairment and disability. In understanding the complaints of back pain, an understanding of pathophysiology, level of subjective suffering, and time since onset, are described as important variables for consideration.

The reader will also benefit from the discussion on methods for taking an organized history. Doctor Harsha describes staging treatment and provides insight of the relative benefit for back surgery based on his years of clinical experience.

A deposition on this topic is included in the Appendix section entitled, "Depositions."

Chapter 9
UNDERSTANDING AND TREATING LOW BACK PAIN

William Harsha, M. S., M. D., J. D.

Understanding low back pain complaints has been a problem for physicians through the years. Misunderstanding what pain complaints mean to the patient, along with failure to treat or over-treat, based solely on presence or absence of objective physical findings, has often led to confusion by the physician and dissatisfaction by the patient.

As physicians, we are given sophisticated objective scientific diagnostic tools and sophisticated treatment plans to help our patients. In the mid-1900s, this often has led to de-humanization of the patient. During the last decade, however, diagnosis and treatment using the total patient approach to impairments, disability or lack of wellness has been widely accepted by physicians. It has become apparent that objective demonstration of the impairment by diagnostic techniques available explains a small percentage, perhaps 30 per cent of the patient's complaint. The balance has to rest with understanding and evaluation of what is commonly called "subjective" complaint.

Failure by examining physicians, treating physicians, and administrative triers of fact, to recognize this dichotomy frequently does the patient a disservice and regularly compounds the patient's impairment. Techniques to relate subjective complaints to the pathophysiology in the patient — in this instance, in the low back — need to be carefully addressed by the physician who is examining or treating low back pain patients.

A great deal is known about the epidemiology of low back pain complaints. This knowledge is based on how the combination of interested persons view the low back patient. That combination includes the patient's subjective input, the physician's input — albeit frequently formed only on narrow objectivity, but more frequently by current enlightened times based on the whole man evaluation concept — and the input by interested third party evaluators.

Ten per cent of all adults, 30 to 40 years of age, (the population of the highest initial incidence) will experience their first significant episode of low back pain and of these, 25 per cent will have recurring low back problems. Overall, 75 per cent or more of adult persons in the United States will experience significant back pain at some time in their lives. In initial treatment, 60 per cent of those affected with low back pain will see first a family practitioner; 25 per cent will see a specialist in back pain; 15 per cent will be seen initially by a chiropractor. Five per cent will require hospitalization for their first episode of low back pain, and of those, one to two per cent will require some type of surgical procedure. Most authors have classified persons involved in trucking, warehousing, construction work, and heavy manufacturing work as "high risk of injury." Truck drivers who spend long hours in 18-wheeler transports cross country driving and those required to load and unload top the risk of injury list. Manual material handlers also are high on this list. Nurses and nurses' aides involved in patient handling — lifting and moving — are in the group of frequent low back injury patients. Lifting injuries account, in one series, for 49 per cent of workers' compensation low back injuries. Twisting is associated in that series with 18 per cent of low back injuries. Bending is associated with 12 per cent. Reaching, arching back, pulling, and pushing substantially increase intradiscal pressure. This is particularly true if pulling, reaching or carrying objects out in front of the person is required.

In understanding the pathophysiology of low back pain, lumbar spine disorders should be viewed in a systematic way. We can divide low back pain disorders into two major diagnostic categories that do tend to overlap:

(1) those caused by irritation of peripheral nerves within the spinal canal or irritation as the nerves exit the spinal canal and

(2) those low back pain complaints resulting from incompetence of the soft tissues that connect one or two segments to another.

In the initial questioning of the patient, the physician can separate these groups frequently by asking the question, "Is the pain worse in the back or in the leg(s)?" It is important in the initial evaluation to know whether the patient is suffering from a problem of less than three months' duration, which is called "acute" in this paper, or from a problem of more than three months, which is called "chronic" in this paper.

Seventy-five per cent of all pain complaints of the low back that have an acute onset, with obvious injury or not, become comfortable with minimal impairment within two months. This includes also the recurrent low back pain problem that has attacks of pain. They frequently resolve with one or two months' conservative treatment, going a number of months without a flare-up, and then recur again. Chronic back pain, which may last for months or years, does frequently present itself and is far the most difficult of the two categories of pain experiences to treat.

Leg pain is usually the result of nerve root irritation or compromise and can be irritation, compromise, or stretching and may be acute or chronic. Acute single nerve root irritation produces a typical buttock, thigh, leg, or foot pain pattern that, though having both subjective and objective components to its presentation, is usually easily identified by the skilled examiner. If the same nerve root becomes the site of chronic irritation, the same pain pattern may be present, or it may become altered or diminished with the passage of time. This patient requires greater attention to the subjective components of the impairment. A careful, unhurried history by an experienced empathetic examiner is most productive for an accurate diagnosis in these areas.

Acute nerve root irritating or compromising complaints are caused by pathologies that directly apply to the nerve root. The acute protruded intervertebral disc is common, but certainly not the only pathological situation. Acute inflammatory hypertrophy of synovia about the posterior facets impinging on nerve root; acute compromises to the circulation to the nerve root; or acute inflammatory responses all can produce a single nerve root irritating response with a radicular pattern that is predictable. Pathological involvement of the lumbosacral plexus or the peripheral nerves going to the lower extremity certainly has to be evaluated at the same time.

It is true, however, that chronic nerve root irritation is usually the result of soft tissue reactive hypertrophy, such as bulge of an intervertebral disc, and at the same time, bulge or swelling of the facet capsule, with or without skeletal enlargement, such as osteophytes about the borders of the vertebral elements in the area of the nerve root tunnel. A wealth of other pathologies that are less common, such as metabolic bone disease with bone hypertrophy or reactive changes in the area of the nerve root, trauma with fracture, or residuals of old fracture with bony hypertrophies. Loss of intervertebral disc space height, allowing narrowing of the nerve root tunnel and impingements of nerve roots, may occur either in the lateral recess or in the nerve root tunnel itself. Both the intervertebral joint space and its intervertebral disc may degenerate in time causing back and/or leg pain. This seems to happen most frequently at the more mobile joints in the low back, lumbar 4-5 most often involved, L5-S1 next and L3-4/5 next.

A situation where the backache is the prime complaint and leg pain is less or absent, earmarking the pathophysiology can present a greater problem. Frequently there are radicular or neurological subjective symptoms, but rarely are there objective neurological deficits in this situation.

Another concept that needs to be studied at this stage of evaluation is the mechanical stability of the joint systems in the low back. Unstable joints systems and particularly, unstable facet systems, will be a source of low back pain in itself. It is to be understood that intervertebral disc spaces and the facet joint spaces are richly supplied by nerve fibers that have sensory nerve filaments in them and can be the source of noxious input interpreted by the brain as pain.

In the acute low back situation, acute soft tissue sprains, muscle ligament sprains, and sprains of supporting facet structures and intervertebral disc spaces occur. Most of these heal quickly. However, when they fail to heal completely, allowing increasing motion and its resulting degenerative change, symptomatic segmental instability develops. In the acute low back sprain patients, where muscles or ligaments or both, are partially disrupted or over-stretched, 90 per cent appear to recover and reconstitute their normal functional anatomy in the area of sprain, 10 per cent do not heal and leave anatomical abnormalities. Annulus fibrosis is the ligamentous support to intervertebral disc areas, and ligamentous structures about the facets, the anterior and posterior longitudinal ligaments and the intraspinous ligaments all have a rather poor blood supply and have a retarded or frequently incomplete healing ability.

Many authors have pointed out that it is impossible for the spine, after injury, to be at rest. There is a physiological balance between the overloading of the spine with persistent supportive tissue muscle ligament insult and the repair of that insult and the reconstruction of new connective tissue at the site of the injury. When this situation is in balance, stability of the segment is present. Here again, it is important to realize that these soft tissue insults and their status of healing are not visible by any diagnostic objective demonstration that the physician has available. Nonetheless, they represent a substantial number of patients who have been injured or have pathological changes in their low backs that are developmental or postural that have low back pain.

These spinal disruptions can be codified as they are seen in anatomical dissections. In that sense, Dr. Mooney pointed out that these dissections are not as neat as they appear but form a logical basis for a pathophysiological understanding of the problem. Referred pain in the buttock and thigh may be caused by mechanical irritation in lumbar facet joints. The presence of leg pain does not necessarily indicate a nerve root problem. If there are no signs of nerve root irritation, pain in the buttock or over the greater trochanter may well be the result of mechanical instability.

Intervertebral disc pathology can present as:

    a. Degenerative Changes. Probably due to either mechanical or chemical abnormalities. It would appear that there are three stages recognizable in such a degenerative change:
        (1) Dysfunction without a great deal of pathology visible.
        (2) Instability due to the changes in the disc itself.
        (3) When the disc ultimately becomes stable but degenerates nonetheless.

b. Traumatic Disc Changes. Annular or radial tears are usually associated with compound multiple small stresses.

c. Central Disc Disruption. Includes invasion by disc material of the vertebral body and its cancellous tissue.

d. Various degrees of disc bulging, prolapse, or extrusion occur.

e. Resorptive disc changes, which appear to be caused by multiple factors, both mechanical, chemical and immunological. The mechanical reaction to such change usually causes osteosclerosis in the adjacent areas of the vertebral bodies.

f. Reactive changes in addition to the changes already detailed. These include inflammation and/or immunological states. Additional nerve supply may invade such damaged tissues with increased amount of noxious stimulus.

g. Facet and ligamentous changes. The posterior facet joint is a diarthrodial joint covered by articular cartilage, lined by synovium and surrounded by capsule. The posterior capsule is formed by collagen fibers; the medial and anterior capsule is formed by lateral extensions of the ligamentum flavum and is thus 80 per cent elastin and 20 per cent collagen. The elastic nature of this part of the capsule may increase or reduce the strength of the posterior joint.

The relationship of his low back/leg complaint to systemic disease is important. The diabetic with neuropathy, the patient with acute onset of herpes zoster, the patient with osteopenia, the patient with potentially metastatic disease all present peculiar additions to the history-taking.

It is important to understand how the patient handles his back and his acts of daily living.

1. Is his posture balanced in respect to the low back?
2. Is he unusually lordotic?
3. Is his low back unusually flat?
4. Are there congenital deformities of the low back?
5. Is he in a fixed, bent forward posture at work?
6. Does he sit for hours at a time?
7. Does he work with his arms out in front of him unsupported with his arms over his head so the low back is arched?
8. Does he have one knee/hip bent as he sits or stands?
9. Does he work in a jarring or vibrating environment or use a vibrating tool?

Knowing what the patient does with his back on a day-to-day basis is important. An organized history from the patient — a fill-out form — is helpful.

This office uses a pain drawing similar to those used in many pain clinics, in addition to a patient history. The pain drawing is also useful as a follow-up of the patient as to how he perceives his low back pain impairment is progressing. In the pain drawing, the area of pain intensity and the character of that pain is the patient perception. This gives important insight as to how the patient views his pain.

The physical examination is a most important tool. It may be second in importance to adequate history and evaluation of subjective complaints. The consistency of those complaints, a good understanding of what the pain complaint means to the patient in all parameters of his present life situation are elements of this evaluation. In other words, understanding what the pain complaint means to the patient from a bio-psycho-social-spiritual point of view is a principal part of the diagnosis.

Evaluation of the patient so far as his posture and his body mechanics is important. His gait, stance, and abnormalities of these need to be noted and related to the impairment. Unlike other joints of the body, the joints of the low back are deep within soft tissues and are not amenable to palpation or not amenable to testing of ranges of motion by the examining hand in more than a subtle way; that is, a combination of ranges of many motions. It is rarely possible to notice swelling about the joints. Localized tenderness is helpful in the slightly built individual, but the more stocky one is misleading. The range of motion measurement of the low back is a total experience of the lumbar spine. I have never been satisfied that I can palpate or measure intersegmental ranges of motion.

Measurement of low back muscle strength is difficult. It is a total measurement because there is a multiplicity of interwoven and complex muscular responses to either stabilize or move the segments of the low back. Measurement of low back muscle strength automatically measures to a degree the strength and mobility of hip musculature.

You can obtain a great deal of information from watching a patient move about — getting in and out of his clothes, going from chair to examining table, and watching him walk in an examining gown. I am careful to explain to my patient that I am not trying to trap him, but that I want to see how he moves in his normal natural way. It is difficult to adequately examine a hostile or suspicious patient. Low back pain impaired patients are much more sophisticated than they were 10 to 15 years ago.

In examining patients while they are standing, a study of the patient's ability to bend forward and hyperextend, to side bend right and left, and to twist right and left is carried out. Ask the patient to do this on his own and then encourage him to the maximum — to the point of "real discomfort" — not to go past the point of pain. I have found that once a patient is hurt by the examining physician, it is extremely difficult to get him to further cooperate in that examination. It is not difficult to pick up limitations of motion in some parts of the back. The upper lumbar spine may well move more freely than the lower part, owing to muscle guarding. It is important to determine where this guarding is located. The relationship to what the patient says is tender to deep pressure is helpful, but not as important. Areas of tenderness in the low back are not as helpful in evaluation as they are in the mid- or upper back or neck. The location of myofascial trigger points by their sharply localized tenderness and the presence of snapping signs, such as described by Travell are important. There are several typical areas of myofascial trigger points about the low back — pelvic crest, buttock, greater trochanteric area — that are very helpful and also point to areas of therapeutic input. Range of motion of hips and knees is important to evaluate as part of a complete low back examination.

In the physical examination of the low back, the examiner is testing range of motion of intervertebral disc space and facets in the low back, sacroiliac joints, and hip joints. Testing for areas of soft tissue pathology in the low back can also be identified.

Neurological examination of the lower extremities is important, especially when there are positive neurological defects, atrophy of calf muscles, weakness of dorsal plantar flexors or inverters or everters of the foot, or weakness of toe extensors. Absent or diminished or asymmetrical ankle or knee reflexes and alterations of perception to pin prick about the thigh, calf, and foot are equally important and can quite accurately lead to a specific nerve root which is compromised.

Contralateral pain produced by straight leg raising is an important observation, practically always nerve root compromise on the opposite side, most often being extruded intervertebral disc. The sciatic stretch test, assessed by straight leg raising and other tests, is also a helpful adjunct. It is important to know that absence of so-called objective or hard neurological defects in the lower extremity does not rule out nerve root irritation as one part of back pain. It takes a fair amount of compromising of the nerve root to alter its function. Nerve root irritation can regularly be demonstrated by sciatic nerve stretch maneuvers when hard neurological defects are absent. The best neurological test in the lower extremity is the test that stresses the sciatic nerve, or occasionally the femoral nerve for nerve root irritation higher in the lumbar area. The patient's ability to outline the area of paresthesia or dysesthesia with his finger during the course of examination, and that outline following a specific dermatome, is strongly suggestive of that nerve root being irritated. It has been important to realize that there is a difference in nerve root compromise and in nerve root irritation. That difference is essentially the difference as recited in the first paragraph of this paper. Nerve root compromise represents perhaps 30 per cent of objective findings in leg pain or discomfort.

The consistency of the area of pain complaints of which the patient complains, or the dysesthesias of which he complains, including following dermatomal levels, represents 70 per cent of the subjective diagnostic information.

In trying to trap the malingerer, the use of confusion tests is of little value to me. I find that when I set myself in a posture to confuse and entrap a patient, I do this with an already pre-conceived bias and have not adequately assessed what the patient complaint means to the patient. It is a great fallacy and a great disservice to the patient to allow the physician's negative bias to control his opinion. If he feels the patient is faking from the outset, over-reacting, or acting inappropriately in response to various tests, when so many of these patients are very tense, anxious patients with a high emotional level, a false diagnosis is probable. Many hyper-reacting patients react more with a mass reflex response than a calculated, isolated act of deception. I recognize that it is naive to believe that there are no individuals who are skillful and coached in their ability to fake or malinger a complaint, just as I realize that it is a God-given attribute for a patient to be self-serving when he presents himself for a diagnosis, treatment, or disability evaluation. I do believe it is rare that a deliberate faker or malingerer is seen in the orthopedist's office. Taking a little more time with the suspect patient and understanding what his pain means to him and frankly confronting him as to the inconsistency of his tests and asking him to allow me to reassess the situation, has resolved that issue without fail. Again, I believe the patient is poorly served to be categorically segregated from the patient with real or so-called objective disease, based on his personality, his hyper-reactiveness, his state of anxiety, his "over-reacting" and particularly, when that reflects the bias of the examining physician. The physician who understand his patient as a whole; that is, what did objectively precipitate the pain, what is the ongoing impairment so far as being demonstrated objectively as well as subjectively, and what the psychological and social ramifications of the impairment mean to the patient. Putting these elements together, an effective treatment plan for the patient can be formed. This patient will probably do well. The patient who is treated solely on the basis of one parameter; that is, treated only if he has an objective finding and therapeutically ignored in respect to his subjective complaints and findings, will practically always do poorly. In evaluating and assessing low back pain, several factors are associated, such as certain occupations that involve heavy lifting and vibration, participation in certain sports, cigarette smoking, emotional stress, sedentary life styles, and lack of cardiovascular fitness.

The isokinetic strength measurement of back muscles has been studied as a risk indicator for low back problems. There are several studies suggesting that testing for isokinetic lifting strength is effective in identifying individuals at risk for industrial low back pain problems. The isometric endurance of the back muscles can be evaluated simply by measuring in seconds how long the patient, prone on a table, is able to keep the unsupported upper part of the body horizontal in air.

Maximal isokinetic strength can also be measured with testing machines set at various positions. Some machines are interfaced with computers to provide a readout of forces generated by the person tested. These data are then compared with a growing data base.

Pain is not a disability; only the reaction to pain may be disabling. A pain complaint is the most common reason a patient presents himself to a physician for diagnosis and treatment. To give the patient optimal care, the physician must not only find the cause of his pain and eliminate it, he must also help the patient understand his pain and the way that his body reacts to that pain complaint. Pain is both a necessary and troublesome part of the human sensory experience. Pain response is necessary to provide the body with a feedback mechanism that warns of external threat or internal illness. The pain response is troublesome when the physiological warning has been acknowledged but the pain persists and combines the psychological factors producing suffering. That suffering can be termed an appropriate stress response. The intensity of the patient's pain complaint will be directly related to the intensity of the stress of the pain as the patient perceives it. The pain is a necessary warning signal that something isn't right with the body-mind complex. This warning signal, however, is regularly a threat or a concern to the patient—a concern that brings the patient to his physician.

Health care professionals described two kinds of pain, acute and chronic. Acute pain is that pain complaint that appears suddenly and has a predictable length of time, and usually, a predictable cure. There is a noxious stimuli producing that acute pain which can be readily identified and removed. Acute pain is usually simple pain because complications seldom result from it. As a parallel, chronic pain can be called complicated pain because the longer duration of this type of pain often produces complications in the form of a wide range of emotions that represent the patient's unique reaction to this stress.

A patient's reactions to pain stress increase in number and intensity the longer the pain complaint persists. As complications continue reducing the individual's tolerance of pain, the patient's perception of pain increases as does the stress from it. The physician must remember that the patient's perception of pain is more important than how the physician perceives his pain. Doctors often suggest that while they may have observed a particular pain experience many times in the past in their practice, the patient often is experiencing this pain stress for the first time.

The body-mind response to a pain stress reaction may be mild or severe, but it always takes the same course, varying only a degree. It is change from familiar to a new and unfamiliar that parallels the anxiety attached to the pain stress response.

The typical patient's response to pain stress stimulus goes through several stages as follows:

1. denial
2. anger
3. depression

Denial is the attempt to correct a problem by pretending it doesn't exist. This is an immature, child-like approach that we all engage in. At this stage, the patient does not admit, either to himself or to others, that he feels frightened or threatened by the pain complaint. The patient, therefore, does nothing about it, ignoring it and wiping it from his conscious view. Even when the patient sees a physician, it is usual for him to minimize the importance of the pain complaint.

The value of denial is that it allows the patient a brief period in which to become familiar with the new situation of the pain complaint. The denial only becomes pathological as it continues and prevents a patient from progressing through the stress reaction to its completion.

If denial persists, a doctor may become confused because the repressed anxiety increases the intensity of the patient's pain, lowering pain tolerance. The patient complains loudly and in a very demanding way of pain, but shows very little personal distress. A doctor, out of confusion, can refer to a patient as neurotic, a malinger, or hysterical. What is really happening is that the patient is going through a normal stress reaction and has become fixated in the first stage of denial. At this stage, beneficial treatment from the physician is allowing, even insisting that the patient talk about his fears at as deep a level as the patient is capable. It is very difficult for many patients to understand and express their real feelings of anxiety and fear. It is at this stage that inappropriate administration of mind-altering chemicals that numb these feelings can, and do, prolong the denial phase.

Bargaining, compromising, argumentative, and even demanding behavior is another part of the denial process that occurs in the initial superficial response to stress. This is an attempt to undo what has happened. It reflects the magic thinking of the child's mind which people carry into adulthood that is frequently used at this phase. The child believes a thought is the same as an act. A patient at this stage will often use the phrases "if only" and "before it happened, I was able to do" because they are attempting to undo the pain stress. Doctor shopping is common at this stage. The patient tries to reinforce his perception that he truly knows himself.

The next stage of the pain stress reaction is anger or anger combined with depression. These are referred to as deeper or "gut" levels of defense. Anger is by definition a state of anxiety or tension and hostility when the expectation is frustrated or a goal is not achieved. When a patient experiences pain, the expectation is that the doctor can remove the pain. If the pain is not diminished to the patient's satisfaction, anger results.

Anger is a normal response to stress, be it pain, change, or loss. Unfortunately, most people were taught early in life to repress anger, especially toward authorities because the accompanying behavior was not socially acceptable. Doctors in our society are seen as authority figures. Anger has more energy than any other feeling. When it is repressed, energy builds up and eventually produces depression or other psychological responses such as muscle tension, headache, etc. Some of the anger may escape repression and be experienced indirectly as teasing or joking or as maladaptive behavior such as martyrdom.

Another common method of indirectly dealing with anger is referred to as the passive aggressive behavior in which a person does nothing or does the opposite of what is expected. Even some direct methods of expressing anger are destructive, such as blaming others, blaming yourself, seeking revenge, and vindictiveness. Revenge is a particularly destructive method of dealing with anger because it has two-fold effect. The patient suffers internally as he or she ruminates and then later causes suffering to others when he or she directs the force of his or her anger outwardly. Our legal system presents a vehicle through litigation to seek revenge in a socially acceptable way.

Depression, which is found as a loss of interest and frequently is described in part as lack of motivation on the patient's part, occurs when anger is repressed. This symptom lowers pain tolerance more effectively than any other factor increasing a patient's perception of pain. The doctor now may become confused and often angry because the patient's complaints of pain far outweigh his organic findings. If the doctor becomes too frustrated by this experience, he may attack or reject the patient or see the patient as neurotic or even as malingering. The doctor's attack causes the patient to respond with increased anger or other emotions of being hurt. This attitude of depression further lowers the tolerance of pain, an ever downhill spiral evolving. Thus the depression may deepen even to the point of suicide ideation.

A further breakdown of the doctor-patient relationship can occur when the patient sees his doctor as a "God-like" individual who can always produce what the patient wants. Along with this, the doctor's expectations of the patient are frequently frustrating because he expects the patient to recover when he, the doctor, treats him.

Appropriate management of pain stress reaction or any other illness is to allow the patient the opportunity to express anger and frustration over what he or she experiences. Encouraging the patient to vent his concerns, fears, and anger to an empathetic, understanding, nonjudgmental professional is a powerful therapeutic tool. The doctor needs to understand and accept his authority posture and encourage his patient to release such feelings. Patients who are allowed to talk about these feelings to an understanding listener can generally rid themselves of the distress in a few minutes and move on to the next stage in pain stress reaction without feelings of depression.

Pain stress reaction is diminished when a stage of acceptance by the patient is reached. At this point, the patient no longer denies what is happening, is not trying to undo the process, and is, for all practical purposes, ready to face the reality and not wallow in anger, frustration, self pity, guilt, or depression. He is able to cooperate fully with the physician by putting energy into whatever treatment is indicated rather than tying up the energy in the self-defeating emotions of fear, anger, etc. If pain complaint, in fact, cannot be eliminated and the person must learn to accept and cope with his pain complaint, he then can accept the situation and work on methods to raise his tolerance of pain. With the understanding of the chronic pain stress complaints, doctors can offer their patients an active, productive life and relieve the patient of self-defeating behavior patterns and/or avoid the use of mind-altering chemicals or other diminishing therapies. Pain is not a disability; only the reaction to pain may be disabling.

SURGERY IN LOW BACK PAIN PROBLEMS

The placing of the section on surgery at the last of the chapter is appropriate as surgical intervention in low back pain problems is unusual. Indications for surgical intervention must include consideration of all the factors mentioned before.

Urgent emergency indications are those where injury or disc protrusion have produced acute spinal cord or nerve root compression with function loss in extremities and loss of urinary and fecal continence. Vertrebral fracture with bone displaced into spinal canal and central intervertebral disc protrusions in lumbar spine (cauda equinae syndromes) are typical examples.

Urgent indications for surgery include ligament and more commonly, fractures of vertebral bodies or posterior elements that render the spine unstable and at risk of increasing impairment. Here a variety of spinal fusions using rigid internal fixation is appropriate.

The most common low back surgery is carried out for intervertebral disc protrusions in which nerve root irritation is intractable and/or in which progressive neurological defects are noted. There is a wide variety of opinion among back surgeons when disc surgery is indicated. A period of two weeks conservative treatment after onset of symptoms is a minimum requirement unless there are progressive neurological findings. Most surgeons are aware of research showing that the acute protruded intervertebral disc symptoms may improve with leg pain improving in time without surgery. If half of patients are operated and half are not, at the end of two to three years, most will have the same residual impairment, usually none.

Essential diagnostic testing prior to intervertebral disc surgery include MRI of CT scans showing the area or disc protrusion and its relationship to the nerve root. Myelography is still favored by some surgeons, but has been replaced by CT scanning and MRI studies. In spinal stenotic lesions, either central or lateral that interfere with nerve root function, bony decompression operations removing the offending bone may be very helpful in pain and functional impairment problems related to the stenotic lesions. These lesions may be congenital due to hypertrophic changes, or both.

Protruded intervertebral disc problems combined with spinal stenotic problems statistically show the best result with surgical intervention.

Adequate decompression for spinal stenosis may render the spine unstable and spinal fusion of the decompressed segment may be necessary.

Spinal fusion for the chronically painful low back syndrome has, by in large, fallen into disrepute, though some orthopedists advocate spinal fusion for the unremitting pain, due to traumatized or degenerative intervertebral discs (internal disc disruption). Use of discography to demonstrate the painful disc was a popular diagnostic test in years past and has again become popular to demonstrate this lesion. Conservative care directed to lessening overload to the disc and pain acceptance is a presurgical requisite and usually avoids surgery.

Spinal fusion for congenital or developmental spondylolythesis that present with intractable pain is a common indicator for spinal fusion as a treatment for low back pain.

The bottom line to the management of low back pain shows that fewer than three per cent of these pain problems are favorably affected by surgical intervention. The incidence of failed back syndromes is high and represent significant impairments.

Low back pain, dealt with by multifaceted methods of physical therapy (largely rehabilitative exercise, flexibility training and back school), combined with a wide range of social and psychological therapies is the most effective way to lessen pain complaint with return to maximum function is the ultimate goal.

For more information on Understanding and Treating Low Back Pain, see Appendix C.

REFERENCES

Biering-Sorenson, F. (1983). A prospective study of low back pain in the general population. I. Occurrence, recurrence and etiology. *Scan Journal of Rehab Med. 15*:71-79.

Dandy, W. E. (1929). Loose cartilage from intervertebral dissimulating tumor of the spinal cord. *Archives of Surgery, 19*:660.

Dandy, W. E. (1944). Newer aspects of ruptured intervertebral disc. *Annals of Surgery,* 119:4.

Evaluating of low back disorders in the primary care office. (1984, January). *Journal of Muscloskeletal Medicine.* (pp.16-26).

Kirkaldy-Willis, W. H. & Farfan, H.F. (1982). Instability of lumbar spine. *Clinical Orthopedics, 165*:110.

Kirkaldy-Willis, W. H., Wedge, J. H., Yong-Hing, K., et al. (1982). Lumbar spine lateral nerve entrapment. *Clinical Orthopedics, 169*:171.

Kirkaldy-Willis, W. H., Wedge, J. H., Yong-Hing, K., et al. (1978). Pathology and pathogenesis of lumbar spondylosis and stenosis. *Spine, 3*:319.

Mooney, V., & Robertson, J. (1976). The facet syndrome. *Clin Ortho. 115*:149-176.

Nachemson, A. (1976). The lumbar spine: An orthopedic challenge. *Journal of Spine, 1*:59-71.

Offierski, C., & MacNab, N. (1980). Hip spine syndrome. *Spine, 5*:316-321.

Ransford, A., Carins, D., & Mooney, V. (1976). The pain drawing as an aid to the psychological evaluation of patient's low back pain. *Spine, 1*:126-134.

ADDITIONAL READINGS

Sale, D. (1987). Influence of excercise and training on motor unit activation. *Exer Sports Sci Rev. 15*:95.

Gonyea, J. (1980). Role of exercise in inducing increases in skeletal muscle fiber number. *Journal Appl Physiol. 48*:421.

Hickey, D. S., et al. (1980). Relation between the structure of the annulus fibrosus and the function and failure of the intervertebral disc. *Spine. 5*:106.

Rosenberg, L., et al. (1982). *Structure of the intervertebral disc.* In A. White II & S. Gordon (Eds.), *American Academy of Orthopedic Surgeons; Symposium on Idiopathic Lowback Pain.* (pp. 339-356). St. Louis: CV Mosby Co.

Spiker, R., et al. (1984). Mechanical response of a simple finite element model of the intervertebral disc under complex loading. Journal Biomech. 17:103.

Nachemson, A. (1960). Lumbar intradiscal pressure. *ACTA Ortho Scand* 43 (suppl). 1-104.

Wilder, D. (1987, May). *The biomechanics of lumbar disc herniation and the effects of overload and instability.* Presented at the meeting of the American Back Society, Anaheim, California.

Kirkaldy-Willis, W. (1988). *Managing low back pain.* New York: Churchill Livingstone.

Farfan, H., et al. (1985). Mechanism of the lumbar spine. *Spine, 6*:249.

Gracovetsky, et al.: The abdominal mechanism. *Spine, (11) 4*:317.

Mooney, V., et al. (1976). The facet syndrome. Clin Orthop. 115:49.

Nachemson, A. (1981). The role of spinal fusion. *Spine, 6*:306.

Frymoyer, J. (1981). The role of spinal fusion. *Spine, 6*:284.

Hirsch, C. (1963). The reliability of lumbar disc surgery. *Clin Ortho. 29*:189.

Burton, V. (1981). Causes of failure of surgery on the lumbar spine. *Clin Orthop., 157*:191.

Wiltse, L., et al. (1976). Classification of spondylolysis and spondylolithesis. *Clin Orthop., 117*:23.

Simmons, D. (1985). Myofascial pain syndromes: Principles and diagnosis. *Manual Medicine., 1*:67.

Bosacco, S. (1986). Lumbar discography: Redefining its role. *Orthop., 9*:399.

O'Brien, J. (1983). The role of fusion for chronic low back pain. *Orthop Clin of North America., 14*:639.

Farfan, H., et al. (1981). The present status of spinal fusion in the treatment of intervertebral joint disorders. *Clin Orthop., 158*:198.

Heithoff, K., et al. (1985). Evaluation of the failed back surgery syndrome. *Orthop Clin of North America, 16*:417.

McKenzie, R. (1981). *The lumbar spine, mechanical diagnosis and treatment.* Waikenae, New Zealand: Spinal Publications Ltd..

Rothman, R. & Simeone, F.(1985). *The spine.* Philadelphia: WB Saunders Co..

Jayson, M. (Ed.). (1976). *The lumbar spine and back pain.* New York: Grune and Stratton, Inc.

Harsha, W. (1978, October). *Nerve root compression due to spinal and/or nerve tunnel stenosis.* Presented second annual meeting American Academy Neurological and Orthopedic Surgeons. Las Vegas.

Harsha, W. (1980, September). *Pain clinic approach to low back disability.* American Academy of Psycosomatic Medicine. Miami, Florida.

Harsha, W. (1984). *Multi-faced assessment of chronic back pain: Pain and stress coping skills.* Presented World Congress of Pain Meeting. Seattle.

Chapter 10

THE ROLE OF NEURAL BLOCKADE IN THE MANAGEMENT OF COMMON PAIN SYNDROMES

Steven D. Waldman, M.D.

Dr. Waldman provides the reader an excellent overview of the role of neural blockade in the management of pain. Neural blockade is described as both an aid for differential diagnoses as well as a palliative procedure. Dr. Waldman, in keeping with the emerging shift toward multidisciplinary care, argues that anesthetic blocking techniques must be integrated into a comprehensive treatment plan.

This chapter will be a real aid for today's practitioner. Specific techniques for relieving pain associated with specific syndromes will serve the clinician as a reference and practice guide. Each subsection is followed by a discussion of practical considerations as well as a discussion regarding potential for complication.

Chapter 10

THE ROLE OF NEURAL BLOCKADE IN THE MANAGEMENT OF COMMON PAIN SYNDROMES

Steven D. Waldman, M.D.

INTRODUCTION

Pain is the most common medical complaint of civilized man. The Nuprin Pain Report estimates that there are over 70 million Americans with pain severe enough to require medical care (Saper, 1987). The cost of pain to society in terms of medical bills, lower productivity, absenteeism, etc. is staggering. The purpose of this chapter is to provide the pain management specialist with an overview of the role of neural blockade in the management of common pain syndromes encountered in clinical practice. Practical suggestions to simplify the care of these sometimes difficult patients are also included.

Neural blockade with local anesthetic may be used as a diagnostic procedure to identify specific pain pathways and to aid in the differential diagnosis as to the origin and site of pain. Neural blockade with local anesthetics may also be used in a prognostic manner to predict the effects of destruction of a given nerve. In addition to helping determine the efficacy of destruction of a given nerve, prognostic neural blockade can allow the patient an opportunity to experience the numbness, loss of function, and other side effects that may attend the destruction of a nerve. Therapeutic neural blockade with a local anesthetic, combined with steroid, or rarely neurolytic agent, can be useful in relieving a variety of painful conditions. Neural blockade should not be viewed as a stand alone treatment for most pain syndromes, but should be intelligently intergrated into a comprehensive treatment plan.

SYMPATHETIC NERVE BLOCKS

SPHENOPALATINE GANGLION BLOCK

Indications

Blockade of the sphenopalatine ganglion with local anesthetic is useful in the management of acute migraine, acute cluster headache, and a variety of facial neuralgias including Sluder's, Vail's, and Gardner's syndrome (Waldman, 1990; Phero & Robbins, 1985; Diamond & Dalessio, 1982; Kitrelle, Grove & Seybold, 1985). This technique may also be useful in status migrainous and chronic cluster headache.

Anatomy

The sphenopalatine ganglion (pterygopalatine, nasal, or Meckel's ganglion) is located in the pterygopalatine fossa, posterior to the middle turbinate (Katz, 1985). It is covered by a 1 to 5 ml layer of connective tissue and mucous membrane. The ganglion is a 5 mm triangular structure comprising the largest group of neurons in the head, outside the brain. There are major branches from the sphenopalatine ganglion to the trigeminal nerve, carotid plexus, facial nerve, and the superior cervical ganglion.

Technique

Sphenopalatine ganglion block is accomplished by the application of local anesthetic to the mucous membrane overlying the ganglion (Waldman & Waldman, 1987)(see Fig. 1). The patient is placed in the supine position. The cervical spine is then extended and the anterior nares space is inspected for polyps, tumor, or foreign body. A small amount of 2% viscous lidocaine, 4% topical lidocaine, or 10% cocaine solution is then instilled into each nostril. The patient is asked to inhale briskly through the nose. This draws the local anesthetic into the posterior nasdal pharynx serving the double function of lubricating the nasal mucosa and providing topical anesthesia, allowing more easy passage of 3 1/2 inch cotton-tipped applicators. These applicators are saturated with the local anesthetic chosen and then advanced along the superior border of the middle turbinate until the tip comes in contact with the mucosa overlying the ganglion. 1.2 ml of local anesthetic is then placed along the cotton tipped applicator in each nostril. The applicator acts as a tampon allowing the local anesthetic to remain in contact with the mucosa overlying the ganglion and then diffuse through the mucosa to the ganglion. The applicators are removed after 20 minutes. The patient's pulse, blood pressure and respirations are monitored for untoward effects secondary to sphenopalatine ganglion block.

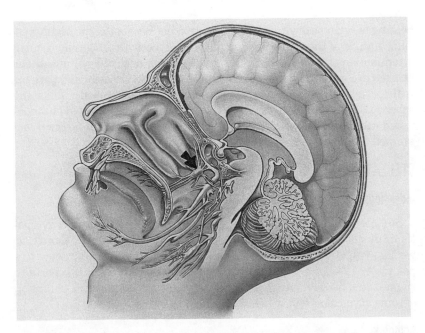

Fig. 1. Sphenopalatine ganglion. Courtesy of Astra Pharmaceutical Products, Inc., ©Anazak Productions.

Practical Considerations

Clinical experience has shown that this technique can be useful in aborting the acute attack of migraine or cluster headaches (Diamond & Dalessio, 1982; Kitrell, Grouse & Seybold, 1985). Its simplicity lends itself to use at the bedside, in the emergency room, or in the headache or pain clinic. Although some experienced in this technique feel that cocaine represents a superior local anesthetic for this indication, the various political issues surrounding the use of this controlled substance make the use of other local anesthetics such as lidocaine a more practical option. For the acute headache sufferer, this technique can be combined with oxygen inhalation via mask through the mouth while the cotton-tipped applicators are in place. Experience indicates that this technique will abort approximately 80% of acute migraine or cluster headaches. This technique is utilized on a daily basis for chronic headache and facial pain conditions with the end point being total pain relief. Our clinical experience suggests that pain relief will generally occur within five daily sphenopalatine ganglion blocks.

Complications

The major complication with this technique is epistaxis. This complication occurs more frequently during the winter months when forced-air heating may cause drying of the nasal mucosa. Because of the highly vascular nature of the nasal mucosa, local anesthetic toxicity may occur if attention is not paid to the total maximum mg dose of local anesthetic utilized to carry out sphenopalatine ganglion block. Occasionally patients will experience significant orthostatic hypotension following sphenopalatine ganglion block. For this reason the patient should be monitored carefully following the block and moved to a sitting position and allowed to ambulate only with assistance.

STELLATE GANGLION BLOCK

Indications

Stellate ganglion block is indicated in the treatment of reflex sympathetic dystrophy of the face, neck, upper extremity, and upper thorax, as well as sympathetically mediated pain of malignant origin and acute herpes zoster (Waldman & Waldman, 1987). There are clinical reports to suggest that stellate ganglion blocks may also be useful in the palliation of some atypical vascular headaches.

Anatomy

The stellate ganglion is located between the anterior lateral surface of the seventh cervical vertebral body and the neck of the first rib (Katz, 1985). The ganglion lies central to the vertebral artery and the transverse process and is separated by the longus colli muscle. The ganglion is medial to the common carotid artery and jugular vein and lateral to the trachea and esophagus.

Technique

The medial edge of the muscle is identified at the level of the cricothyroid notch (C6). The sternocleidomastoid muscle is then displaced laterally with two fingers. The pulsations of the carotid artery should then be identified. The skin medial to the carotid pulsation is prepped with alcohol and a 1 1/2 inch, 22-gauge needle is advanced until contact is made with the transverse process of C6. The needle is then withdrawn approximately 2 mm and careful aspiration is carried out, 7 ml of 0.5% preservative free bupivacaine is then injected. Careful monitoring of pulse, blood pressure, and respirations is indicated.

Practical Considerations

Daily stellate ganglion block with local anesthetic is beneficial for the above mentioned pain syndromes. Careful explanation to the patient regarding the special side effects of Honer's Syndrome from blockade of the stellate ganglion should be given prior to implementation of stellate ganglion block to avoid undue patient anxiety. Local anesthetic should never be injected if the transverse process of C6 cannot be identified with the needle, as doing so will lead to unacceptable high rate of potentially life-threatening complications.

Complications

Hematoma, hoarseness due to blockade of the laryngeal nerves, difficulty in swallowing, and pneumothorax can occur. Due to the proximity of the great vessels of the neck, intravascular injection, with almost immediate local anesthetic drug toxicity is a distinct possibility if careful aspiration and needle placement is not carried out. Epidural and subarachnoid anesthesia can occur if the needle is allowed to pass between the transverse process of C5 and C6 and impinge upon the cervical root.

CELIAC PLEXUS BLOCK

Indications

Celiac plexus block with local anesthetic is indicated as a diagnostic maneuver to determine if flank, retroperitoneal, or upper abdominal pain is sympathetically mediated via the celiac plexus (Portenoy & Waldman, 1990). This technique is also used in a prognostic manner to determine if celiac plexus block with neurolytic solution, such as alcohol or phenol, will provide relief of the pain of chronic pancreatitis or, more commonly, pain of upper abdominal and retroperitoneal malignancy, such as carcinoma of the pancreas, adrenal gland, etc. Daily celiac plexus block with local anesthetic is also used in the palliation of pain secondary to acute pancreatitis. Clinical reports suggest that early implementation of celiac plexus block with local anesthetic and/or steroid may markedly reduce the morbidity and mortality associated with acute pancreatitis.

Anatomy

The celiac plexus is situated in the prevertebral area at the level of T12-L1 vertebral body (Raj, 1985). It is composed of the ganglia of the right and left celiac, superior mesenteric, and aorticorenal ganglia and the dense network of sympathetic nerve fibers that connect them.

Technique

Diagnostic celiac plexus block with local anesthetic may be performed without radiographic guidance. However, it is the clinical impression of many pain management specialists that neurolytic celiac plexus block can be performed most safely utilizing CT guidance or, if CT guidance is unavailable, fluoroscopy. The use of radiographic guidance should improve not only the safety but the efficacy of the following technique.

The patient is well-hydrated with intravenous fluids and is placed prone on the CT scanning table. A scout film is obtained to identify the T12-L1 interspace. A CT scan is then taken through this area. The scan is reviewed for position of the aorta relative to the vertebral body, the position of intra-abdominal and retroperitoneal organs, and the distortion of normal anatomy due to tumor, previous surgery, or adenopathy. The level at which the scan was taken is then identified on the patient's skin and marked with a gentian violet marker. The skin is prepped with aneseptic solution. The skin and subcutaneous tissues at a point approximately 2 1/2 inches from the left of the midline is then anesthesized with 1% lidocaine utilizing a 22-gauge x 1 1/2 inch needle. A 13 cm x 22-gauge styleted Hinck needle is then placed through the anesthesized area and is advanced until the posterior wall of the aorta is encountered. The needle is then advanced into the aorta and the stylet is then removed. A free flow of arterial blood should then be present. A well-lubricated 5 cc glass syringe filled with preservative-free saline is then attached to the Hinck needle and the needle and syringe are then advanced through the anterior wall of the aorta (Feldstein, Waldman, & Allen, 1990) using the loss of resistance technique (Liebarman & Waldman, 1990). The glass syringe is removed and a small amount of 0.5% lidocaine in solution with water-soluable contrast media is then injected through the needle. A CT scan at this same level is again taken. The scan is reviewed for the placement of the needle and most importantly for the spread of contrast. Contrast should be seen in the pre-aortic area surrounding the aorta. None of the contrast should be retrocrural. After satisfactory placement and spread of contrast is confirmed, 12 to 15 cc of absolute alcohol or 6% aqueous phenol is then injected through the needle. The needle is flushed with a small amount of saline and then removed. The patient is observed carefully for hemodynamic changes including hypotension and tachycardia secondary to the resulting profound sympathetic blockade.

Practical Considerations

CT guided celiac plexus neurolysis utilizing the loss of resistance technique has been shown to be safe as well as efficacious for treatment for the above mentioned pain syndromes (Liebarman & Waldman, 1990). This technique may be performed in the lateral position for patients who are unable to lie prone because of intractable abdominal pain or because of colostomy, ileostomy appliances, and the like. This technique avoids the possibility of spread of neurolytic substance onto the lumbar plexus. Posterior retrocrural spread of local anesthetic and contrast injected prior to injection of the neurolytic substance will alert the clinician to the possibility of this complication and the needle can be repositioned. It is our clinical impression that the higher resolution and ease of identification of anatomic structures makes the use of the CT scanner far superior to the use of fluoroscopy for this technique (Liebarman & Waldman, 1990).

Complications

The most feared complication of celiac plexus neurolysis is the inadvertent injection of neurolytic substance onto the lumbar plexus, epidurally, subarachnoid, or intravascular. Inappropriate needle placement can result in damage to the kidneys. If the needle is placed too far anterior, injection into the pancreas or into the peritoneal cavity or liver can occur. As mentioned above, the incidences of these complications can be markedly reduced by the use of CT guidance.

When properly performed this technique results in profound sympathetic neural blockade. In the cancer patient who may have compromised cardiac reserve, this hypotension can be life-threatening. For this reason, the patient should be well-hydrated prior to the procedure and the blood pressure should be monitored closely following the procedure. The patient should be cautioned that orthostatic hypotension may persist for a period of days and patient should get up only with assistance until the orthostatic hypotension has been compensated for.

LUMBAR SYMPATHETIC NERVE BLOCK

Indications

Lumbar sympathetic nerve block with local anesthetic is indicated as a diagnostic maneuver to determine if lower extremity pain is sympathetically mediated via the lumbar sympathetic chain and for sympathetic dystrophy of the lower extremity. Prognostically, the lumbar sympathetic chain may be blocked with local anesthetic to determine if destruction of the lumbar sympathetic chain with neurolytic substances such as phenol and alcohol or surgical excision of a portion of the lumbar sympathetic chain will improve blood flow and/or relief of pain of the lower extremities. This technique is used therapeutically to treat acute peripheral vascular insufficiency, ischemia secondary to frostbite, acute herpes zoster of the lower extremities, and a variety of peripheral neuropathic pains of the lower extremities (Lobstrom & Cousins, 1988).

Anatomy

The lumbar sympathetic ganglion lies along the anterolateral surface of the lumbar vertebral bodies and antromedial to psoas muscle (Raj, 1985). The anterior vena cava lies just anterior to the right sympathetic chain and the aorta lies anterior and slightly medial to the sympathetic chain on the left.

The sympathetic innervation of the lower extremity arises from preganglionic fibers that take their origin from the cell bodies located in the

T10-L2 levels of the spinal cord. Nearly all postganglionic fibers to the lower extremity leave the sympathetic chain interval below L2. Anterior to the chain is the visceral peritoneum and the great vessels.

Technique

The technique of lumbar sympathetic block and neurolysis is quite similar to that described in the section above on celiac plexus neurolysis. Patient is placed in the prone position on the CT scanner table with a pillow underneath the abdomen to allow flexion of the thoraco-lumbar spine. This opens up the space between adjacent transverse processes. A scout film is taken and the L2 vertebral body is identified. The skin overlying the transverse process of L2 is marked with a gentian violet marker and then prepped with betadine. Utilizing a 1 1/2 inch x 22-gauge needle the skin and subcutaneous tissues are anesthetized with 1% Xylocaine. A 22-gauge x 13 cm styleted needle is then advanced through the previously anesthetized area until the tip rests against the vertebral body. The needle is then redirected in a trajectory to pass just lateral to the vertebral body. A well-lubricated glass syringe filled with preservative-free saline is then attached and loss of resistance technique is then utilized while the needle is advanced through the body of the psoas muscle. As soon as the needle tip passes through the fascia of the muscle a loss of resistance is encountered. This should place the needle adjacent to the sympathetic chain. A small amount of local anesthetic and water-soluable contrast media is then injected to assure appropriate spread of contrast material in the prevertebral region. Twelve cc of 0.5% preservative lidocaine or absolute alcohol are then injected via the needle. The needle is flushed with preservative-free saline and removed. The patient is then observed carefully for hypotension and tachycardia secondary to sympathetic blockade.

Practical Considerations

The use of CT guidance when performing lumbar sympathetic neurolysis can markedly decrease the risk of complications (see below). The patient should be warned that in all likelihood he or she will experience some backache following the procedure due to needle trauma to the muscles of posture. The patient should also be advised that following lumbar sympathetic block the affected lower extremity may feel hot and somewhat swollen relative to the non-affected extremity. This side effect is normal and will go away with time.

Complications

Complications (Lobstrom & Cousins, 1988) of lumbar sympathetic block are similar to that of celiac plexus neurolysis. Since the needle tip is more medial in its trajectory, damage to lumbar nerve roots as they exit the spinal column is a distinct possibility.

SOMATIC NERVE BLOCKS

OCCIPITAL NERVE BLOCK

Indications

Occipital nerve block with local anesthetic and steroid may be beneficial in the management of occipital neuralgia (Raj, 1989). Occipital neuralgia is characterized by suboccipital pain which is aching in nature. This pain radiates over the posterior lateral scalp. Superimposed electric shock-like pain may also be present. With prolonged attacks of occipital neuralgia the patient may also complain of deep retro orbital ache. Pressure over the greater and lesser occipital nerve on the affected side may recreate the patient's pain symptomatology. In some patients occipital neuralgia may trigger migraine headaches.

Anatomy

The greater occipital nerve perforates the semispinalis capitis and the trapezius muscles, approximately 3 cm lateral to the occipital protrubance, at the level of the linea nuchae. It is medial to the occipital artery, which can be palpated in some patients. The lesser occipital nerve is approximately 2 1/2 cm lateral to the greater occipital nerve, and is found directly above and behind the mastoid process.

Technique

Deep palpation of the musculature overlying the greater occipital nerve will generally recreate the patient's pain symptomatology and help localize this nerve's exit from the bony skull. If the occipital artery can be palpated, this will serve as an additional guide. The skin and hair overlying the greater occipital nerve is then prepped with alcohol and 2 to 10 ml of 0.5% bupivacaine and 80 mg of methylprednisolone is injected around the greater and lesser occipital nerve.

Practical Considerations

Occipital neuralgia is greatly over-diagnosed. Many patients carrying this diagnosis actually suffer from tension-type headaches. This may explain the less then optimal long-term results that many patients who undergo occipital nerve block experience. If the patient who carries a working diagnosis of occipital neuralgia does not respond to daily blocks of long-acting local anesthetic and depo-steroid preparations, a trial of cervical epidural steroids is indicated. Since the pain of posterior fossa tumor or tumor compromising the upper cervical nerve roots may mimic the pain of occipital neuralgia, these potentially life-threatening conditions must be ruled out prior to implementation of occipital nerve block. Currently, MRI scanning of the posterior fossa and upper cervical spine is the best way to rule out occult pathology in this anatomic region.

Complications

This block should be performed with care in patients who are anticoagulated. The needle should not be directed medially or inadvertent subarachnoid injection with resultant total spinal anesthesia may occur.

EPIDURAL NERVE BLOCKS

Indications

The use of epidural nerve blocks with local anesthetic and/or steroid are useful in the diagnosis and treatment of a variety of pain syndromes. The efficacy of this technique has been demonstrated for the relief of pain secondary to acute and chronic cervical, thoracic, and lumbar strain and radiculopathy, bilateral sympathetically mediated pain such as reflex sympathetic dystrophy, peripheral vascular insufficiency, or ischemic pain secondary to frostbite. Epidural neural blockade with local anesthetic and/or steroid is also useful in the management of acute herpes zoster and post herpetic neuralgia of the extremities or trunk.

Cervical epidural nerve block has also been shown to be efficacious in providing long-term relief in tension-type headache. Cronen and Waldman (1988) demonstrated this finding in a prospective study in a group of patients who had failed all treatment modalities, including the optiminal use of simple analgesics, nonsteroidal anti-inflammatory agents, anti-depressant compounds, and biofeedback. Cervical epidural nerve blocks are also useful in the palliation of pain secondary to cervicalgia and "whiplash" type injuries of the cervical spine. Clinical experience suggests that this technique is of value in patients with severe fibromyalgia of the cervical paraspinal musculature (Waldman, 1990).

Anatomy

The epidural space extends from the foramen magnum where the periosteal and spinal layers of dura fuse together to the sacrococcygeal membrane (Bridenbaugh & Greene, 1989) (see Fig. 2). The anterior portion of the spidural space is bounded by the posterior longitudinal ligament which covers the posterior aspect of the vertebral body and the intravertebral disc. Posteriorly, the spidural space is bounded by the anterior lateral surface of the vertebral lamina and the ligamentum flavum. Laterally, the epidural space is bounded by the pedicles of the vertebra and the intravertebral foramen. From a technical viewpoint the ligamentum flavum is the key landmark for identification of the epidural space. It is composed of dense fibroelastic tissue. It is thinnest in the cervical region. In the adult male the epidural space is narrowest in the cervical region, with an anterior/posterior diameter of 2-3 mm in the cervical region when the neck is flexed.

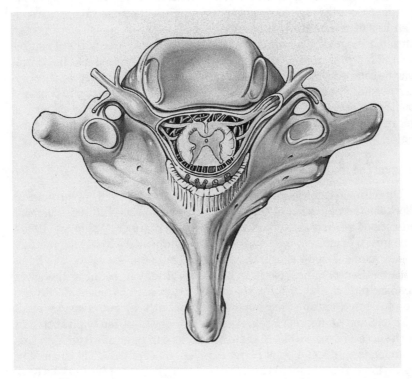

Fig. 2. The epidural space. Courtesy of Astra Pharmaceutical Products, Inc., ©Anazak Productions.

Technique

Epidural nerve block is most easily carried out with the patient in the sitting position with the cervical spine flexed and the forehead resting on a padded bedside table. The arms should rest comfortably in the patient's lap or at the patient's side. The skin overlying the appropriate vertebral interspace is prepped with antiseptic solution and a sterile fenestrated drape is then placed. Careful palpation of the spinous process and intervertebral space is carried out. The exact midline position is then identified. The skin and subcutaneous tissues are then anesthetized with 1% preservative-free lidocaine or 0.25% preservative-free bupivacaine. An

18-gauge or 20-gauge Hustead or Tuohy needle is then placed into the previously anesthetized area with a trajectory slightly cephalad and toward midline. The stylet is removed and a well-lubricated 5 cc glass syringe filled with preservative-free saline is then attached to the epidural needle. With constant pressure on the plunger of the syringe, the epidural needle is carefully advanced. The operator will sense the tip of the needle impinging on the dense ligamentum flavum. As the tip of the needle passes through ligamentum flavum into the epidural space a sudden loss of resistance will be experienced; 0.5 cc of air is then injected through the needle to confirm epidural placement. After careful aspiration, 0.5% preservative-free lidocaine or 0.25% preservative-free bupivacine combined with depotsteroid preparations is then injected through the needle. The epidural needle is removed and a 4x4 gauze pad is placed on the injection site and general pressure is applied. The patient is returned to the supine position and careful monitoring of blood pressure, pulse, and respirations is carried out until the patient is fully recovered.

Practical Considerations

Our clinical experience suggests that the use of steroid epidural nerve block for the palliation of the above mentioned pain syndromes is most efficacious when carried out in the following manner (Waldman, 1990): The initial epidural nerve block (ENB) is performed with 80 mg methylprednisolone (Depo-Medrol, Upjohn) and 7 ml of preservative-free bupivacaine (Sensorcaine, Astra) in the cervical region, 10 ml in the lower thoracic region, and 12 ml in the cervical region. Subsequent ENB were administered on an every-other-day basis with 40 mg of methylprednisolone and an appropriate amount of preservative-free bupivacaine in each successive nerve block. Up to six blocks can be administered in this manner, with the end point being complete relief of pain. The amount of methylprednisolone should be decreased in diabetics or patients who have received prior treatment with systemic gluccocorticoids. Epidural nerve block may be utilized early in the course of treatment for the above mentioned pain syndromes while waiting for other treatment modalities such as anti-depressants or physical therapy to become effective.

Complications

Since epidural interrupts both somatic and sympathetic nerve conduction, cardiovascular changes including hypotension and tachycardia may occur (Waldman, 1989). These cardiovascular changes can produce devastating complications if not promptly identified and treated. Respiratory compromise or failure may occur if blockade of the phrenic nerve or respiratory centers of the brain stem inadvertently occurs. For this reason epidural nerve blocks should be performed only by those trained in airway management and resuscitation. Appropriate monitoring of vital signs is imperative and resuscitation equipment must be readily available.

Minor untoward effects and complications of epidural nerve block include pain at the injection site, inadvertent dural puncture, and vaso-vagal syncope. Major complications include damage to neural structures, epidural hematoma, and epidural abscess. These major complications are rare, but can be life-threatening when they occur.

TRIGEMINAL NERVE BLOCK

Indications

Use of trigeminal nerve block with local anesthetic and steroids serves as an excellent adjunct to drug treatment of trigeminal neuralgia (Feldstein, 1989). The use of this technique allows rapid palliation of pain while oral medications are being titrated to effective levels (Phero & Robbins, 1985). This technique may also be of value in patients suffering from atypical facial pain. Other indications for trigeminal nerve block include pain in maxillary neoplasm, cluster headaches uncontrolled by sphenopalatine ganglion block, and acute herpes zoster in the area of trigeminal nerve not controlled by stellate ganglion block.

Anatomy

The trigeminal nerve is the largest of the cranial nerves, containing both sensory and motor fibers. The trigeminal nerve can be blocked utilizing an extra oral approach via the coronoid notch into the pterygo-palatine fossa (Feldstein, 1989). The fossa is a triangular space between the pterygoid process of the sphenoid bone and maxilla of the upper part infratemporal fossa.

Technique

Palpation of the coronoid notch is facilitated by having the patient open and close their mouth. The notch should be encountered approximately 4 cm anterior to the acoustic auditory meatus (see Fig. 3). The skin is anesthetized with antiseptic solution and a 1 1/2 inch 22-gauge needle is directed through the middle of the coronoid notch. The tip of the needle may encounter the lateral lamina of the pterygoid process. If blockade of the maxillary nerve is desired, the needle is withdrawn into the subcu-taneous tissue and is redirected with the tip 1 cm further anteriorly and 1 cm further superiorly from the first bony contact. Paresthesia may be elicited in the area of the maxillary nerve. If blockade of the mandibu-lar nerve is desired, the needle is withdrawn into the subcutaneous tissue and readjusted with the tip 0 cm posteriorly and 1 cm inferiorly.

Paresthesia in the distribution of the mandibular nerve may be elicited. After careful aspiration, 5 to 7 ml of 0.5% preservative-free bupivacaine in combination with 80 ml of methylprednisolone is injected. Subsequent daily nerve blocks are carried out in a similar manner, substituting 40 ml of methylprednisolone for the initial 80 ml dose.

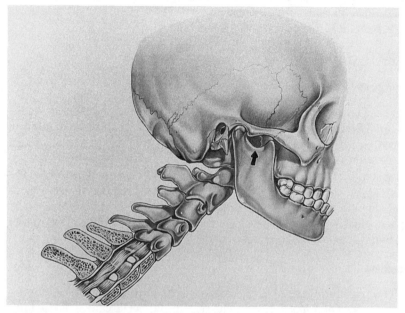

Fig. 3. The coronoid notch. Courtesy of Astra Pharmaceutical Products, Inc., ©Anazak Productions.

Practical Considerations

This technique represents an excellent emergency treatment for uncontrolled pain of trigeminal neuralgia. It can be utilized while carbamezepine (Tegretol), liorisal (Baclofen), phenytoin (Dilatin), or other medications are being titrated. With patients suffering from atypical facial pain secondary to temporomandibular joint dysfunction, this technique can be utilized to allow physical therapy and range of motion of the temporomandibular joint.

Complications

The major complication of trigeminal nerve block is inadvertent vascular injection. The pterygopalantine fossa is traversed with a large number of arteries and veins and for this reason careful and frequent aspiration should be carried out during injection of local anesthetic. Needle damage to this vasculature can result in significant hematoma formation. Although self-limited, it is recommended the patient be advised of this potential untoward effect so they will not be unduly alarmed should it occur.

MYOFASCIAL TRIGGER POINTS

Indications

Injection of myofascial trigger points with local anesthetic and/or steroid are indicated in the treatment of myofascial pain syndromes of the head and neck (Raj, 1989). These myofascial trigger points are discreet hypersensitive area's of muscle that in most instances result from previous trauma. Palpation of these trigger points can initiate pain, autonomic disturbance in a nonsegmental and referred distribution. Trigger points can occur essentially in any muscle of the head and neck. They are most frequently found in the trapezius, semispinalis capitis, spleenius capitis, occipitofrontalis, and the muscles of mastication and facial expression.

Technique

Localization of trigger points is accomplished by deep palpation and observation of the radiation of the patient's pain (Travell, 1976). The skin overlying the area is then prepped with alcohol, 0.25 ml of 1% preservative-free xylocaine or 0.5% preservative-free bupivacaine alone, or in combination with methylprednisolone, is injected into the trigger points.

Practical Considerations

Most patients with muscle contraction headache and atypical head and facial pain syndrome will have multiple myofascial trigger points. It has been our experience that a more central nerve block such as cervical epidural nerve block or trigeminal nerve block, may be more effective in treating and decreasing the number of these trigger points than actual injection into the multiple trigger points that may be present. Discreet trigger points that remain after epidural or trigeminal nerve blocks can then be injected quite easily. The patient should be informed that with trigger point injection when the local anesthetic wears off the patient may experience an exacerbation of pain symptomatology.

Complications

Due to the highly vascular nature of the head and face, intravascular injection is a possibility. Care should be taken to avoid inadvertent subarachnoid injection with resultant total spinal anesthetic when injecting trigger points near the midline of the neck and occipital region.

INTERCOSTAL NERVE BLOCKS

Indications

Intercostal nerve block with local anesthetic and/or corticosteroid can be performed at the bedside or in the outpatient setting. This procedure may palliate pain secondary to acute traumatic or pathologic rib fractures, chest wall metastasis, post thoracotomy pain, or right upper quadrant pain secondary to hepatic metastasis (Feldstein & Allen, 1980).

Intercostal nerve blocks may also reduce pain due to percutaneous drainage devices such as chest tubes or a nephrostomy tubes. Studies have demonstrated clinically significant improvement in pulmonary function in patients treated with this procedure (Feldstein, Waldman, & Allen, 1980).

Anatomy

The thoracic spinal nerves give off the white and gray rami communicantes of the sympathetic system which go to or come from the particular ganglion of the sympathetic chain. Distal to the rami communicantes, the nerve trunk divides into the dorsal and ventral branch. The dorsal branch innervates the skin and muscles of the back as well as the periosteum of the vertebra. The ventral branch follows the rib via the costal sulcus, into the dorsal thoracic region between the two lamina of the intercostal muscles into the lateral and ventral portion of the thorax. This intercostal nerve travels in tandem with the intercostal artery and vein (Raj, 1985).

Technique

Intercostal nerve block can be performed with the patient in the sitting, lateral decubitus, or prone position. The rib in the anatomic region to be blocked is identified by palpation and the skin in the posterior axillary line is prepped with aneseptic solution. A 22-gauge, 1 1/2 inch needle attached to a 5 ml syringe is advanced vertically until bony contact with the rib is made. The needle is withdrawn back into the subcutaneous tissues and the needle is then walked off the inferior margin of the rib, with care being taken not to advance the needle more than 0.5 cm. After careful aspiration, 3 to 5 ml of 0.5% or 0.75% preservative-free bupivacaine is injected. The needle is then removed. This technique may be repeated at each level subserving the pain, with care being taken to carefully monitor the total milligram dosage of local anesthetic injected.

Practical Considerations

Therapeutic intercostal nerve block is an excellent adjunct in the armormentarium of the pain management specialist to treat a variety of acute and chronic pain syndromes. Its simplicity lends itself to performance in the emergency room or at the bedside, providing appropriate resuscitation equipment and drugs are readily available. The highly vascular nature of the intercostal region makes careful monitoring of the total milligram dosage of local anesthetic mandatory. By utilizing long-acting protein bound local anesthetics such as 0.75% bupivacaine, this technique can be performed on a daily basis to provide long lasting pain relief for trauma and acute surgical incisions.

Complications

The major complication of intercostal nerve block is inadvertent and unrecognized pneumothorax. The incidence of this complication is approximately 0.5 to 1.0%. If the patient is being maintained on ventilatory support with positive pressure ventilation, tension pneumothorax can occur. As mentioned above, vascular uptake of local anesthetic with systemic toxicity is also a problem if careful dosage guidelines are not observed.

INTRAPLUERAL CATHETER

Indications

Recent studies have demonstrated that local anesthetic installation via intraplueral catheter is effective in the management of both acute and chronic pain (Reiestad & Stomstag, 1986). This simple technique may be performed on out-patients or at the bedside. Indications are essentially the same as for intercostal nerve block. In addition to these indications, several clinical reports have suggested that intraplueral catheter technique can be used to reduce pain below the diaphragm including pain secondary to pancreatic malignancy.

Technique

The patient is placed in the lateral decubitus position with the painful side upward. The 8th and 9th ribs at the posterior axillary line are identified and then prepped with antiseptic solution. Sterile drapes are placed and skin and subcutaneous tissues are anesthetized with 1% lidocaine. After adequate analgesia is obtained, a styleted Tuohy or Hustead needle is placed through the skin and into the subcutaneous tissue. A 5 ml syringe with 0.9% preservative-free saline is attached and the needle and syringe are walked over the superior margin of the rib to avoid damage to the neurovascular bundle. The intrapleural space is then identified utilizing either the hanging drop technique or the negative intrapleural pressure technique as described by Reistad et al. (1984). A catheter is then introduced through the needle and advanced approximately 10 cm through the intrapleural space, the Tuohy needle is then removed. 12 to 15 ml of local anesthetic is then injected to insure catheter integrity and to confirm adequate pain relief from the intrapleural catheter. If long-term use is anticipated, the catheter should be tunneled to avoid the risk of subcutaneous infection (Waldman, 1989).

Practical Considerations

This technique has proven quite useful in the acute pain management arena. Recent clinical reports have demonstrated that this technique can also be used on a long-term basis. This is accomplished by tunneling the intrapleural catheter to reduce the incidence of infection. As the pleural space is highly vascular careful attention to the total milligram dosage with local anesthetic used is indicated. In patients with significant pleural disease or pleural effusion this technique should be used with caution and the total dose of local anesthetic must decreased to avoid toxic blood levels.

Complications

The complications of this technique are similar to intercostal nerve block. In addition, if infection occurs empyema may result.

EPIDURAL BLOOD PATCH

Indications

Epidural blood patch is indicated for the treatment of post dural puncture headache following lumbar puncture, myeographic procedures, or inadvertent dural puncture occurring during attempted epidural anesthesia (Waldman, Feldstein, & Allen, 1987). This technique may also be utilized in the treatment of spontaneous low pressure headaches that may result from minor head or neck trauma.

Anatomy

The anatomy of the epidural space has been described above in the section on epidural nerve block. The epidural space is larger in the lumbar region relative to the cervical region and clinical experience indicates that a larger volume of autologous blood will be required to relieve post dural puncture headaches in the lumbar region relative to the cervical region.

Technique

The patient is hydrated with intravenous fluids and any co-existing nausea and vomiting is treated with antiemetics. After donning sterile surgical cap, gown, mask, and gloves, the anticubital fossa and skin overlying the area of dural puncture are prepped in a sterile manner with povidone-iodine solution. Identification of the epidural space is carried out and autologous blood is obtained in a sterile manner from the previously prepped anticubital vein. Seven to 10 ml of autologous blood is placed in the cervical region with 12 to 15 ml of autologous blood required for the lumbar region.

Practical Considerations

Many patients with post dural puncture headache have severe nausea and vomiting that may lead to significant dehydration. This results in worsening of the headache and makes venous access to obtain autologous blood quite difficult. The use of preprocedure hydration is therefore indicated. The most common reason for failure of epidural blood patch is the fact that the patient does not remain supine following the procedure. The patient and nursing staff must be instructed to closely adhere to the post epidural blood patch orders.

Complications

In addition to the complications attendant to identification of the epidural space, the most feared complication of epidural blood patch is that of infection. Although written about, the actual incidence of this potentially devastating complication (assuming that strict sterile technique is followed) is exceedingly rare. Occasionally a second and rarely a third epidural blood patch may be required to palliate the above mentioned pain syndrome.

SUMMARY

The use of neural blockade represents an excellent addition to the armamentarium of the physician caring for the patient in pain. Proper integration of these techniques into the comprehensive pharmacologic and behavioral treatment plan is essential if one is to maximize the efficacy of these techniques. An understanding of the anatomic, technical, and practical considerations of each specific type of nerve block should lead to a high degree of success and minimal complications.

REFERENCES

Bridenbaugh, P., & Greene, N. (1989). *Spinal neural blockade*. In M. Cousins & P. Bridenbaugh (Eds.), *Neural blockade* (p. 216). Philadelphia: Lippincott.

Cronen, M., & Waldman, S. (1988). Cervical steroid epidural nerve block in the palliation of pain secondary to intractable muscle contraction headache. *Headache, 28*:314-315.

Diamond, S., & Dalessio, D. (1982). *Cluster headache*. In *The practicing physician's approach to headache* (pp. 64-65). Baltimore: Williams and Wilkins.

Feldstein, G. (1989). *Percutaneous retrogasserian glycerol rhizotomy in the treatment of trigeminal neuralgia.* In G. Racz (Ed.), *Techniques of neurolysis* (p. 126). Boston: Kluwer Publishers.

Feldstein, G. (1989). *Percutaneous retrogasserian glycerol rhizotomy in the treatment of trigeminal neuralgia.* In G. Racz (Ed.), *Techniques of neurolysis* (pp. 125-132). Boston: Kluwer Publications.

Feldstein, G., Waldman, D., & Allen, M. (1987). Reversal of apparent tolerance to epidural morphine sulfate by epidural methylprednlsolone. *Anesth Analg. 67*:264-265.

Feldstein, G., Waldman, S., & Allen, M. (1985). Loss of resistance technique for transaortic celiac plexus block. *Anesth Analg. 65*:1092-1093.

Jakobson, S., Fridiksson, H., & Ivarsson, I. (1980). Effects of intercostal nerve blocks on pulmonary mechanics in healthy man. *ACTA Anaesthesiology Scand. 24*:482.

Katz, J. (1985). *Sphenopalatine ganglion.* In J. Katz (Ed.), *Atlas of regional anesthesia* (pp. 16-17). Norwalk: Appleton-Century-Crofts.

Katz, J. (1985). *Stellate ganglion.* In J. Katz (Ed.), *Atlas of regional anesthesia* (pp. 50-51). Nowalk: Appleton-Century-Crofts.

Kitrelle, J., Grouse, D., & Seybold, M. (1985). Cluster headache: Local anesthetic abortive agents. *Archives of Neurology 42*:496-498.

Kvalheim, L., & Reiestad, F. (1984). Interpleural catheter in the management of postoperative pain. *Anesthesiology, 61*:A231.

Liebarman, R., & Waldman, S. (1990). Celiac plexus neurolysis. *Radiology, 175*:874-876.

Lobstrom, J., & Cousins, M. (1988). *Sympathetic neural blockade.* In M. Cousins & P. Bridenbaugh (Eds.), *Neural blockade* (pp. 479-491). Philadelphia: Lippincott.

Lobstrom, J., & Cousins, M. (1988). *Sympathetic neural blockade.* In M. Cousins & P. Bridenbaugh (Eds.), *Neural blockade* (pp. 492-493). Philadelphia: Lippincott.

Lobstrom, J., & Cousins, M. (1988). *Sympathetic neural blockade.* In M. Cousins & P. Bridenbaugh (Eds.), *Neural blockade* (pp. 491-493). Philadelphia: Lippincott.

Phero, J., & Robbins, G. (1985). *Sphenopalatine ganglion block.* In P. Raj (Ed.), *Handbook of regional anesthesia* (pp. 24-26). New York: Churchill Livingstone.

Phero, J., & Robbins, G. (1985). *Trigeminal nerve block.* In P. Raj (Ed.), *Handbook of regional anesthesia* (pp. 18-21). New York: Churchill Livingstone.

Portenoy, R., & Waldman, S. (1990). Recent advances in cancer pain management. *IM Internal Medicine.* (In press).

Raj, P. (1985). *Chronic pain.* In P. Raj (Ed.), *Handbook of regional anesthesia* (pp. 113-115). New York: Churchill Livingston.

Raj, P. (1985). *Chronic pain.* In P. Raj (Ed.), *Handbook of regional anesthesia* (pp. 115-116). New York: Churchill Livingstone.

Raj, P. (1985). *Chronic pain*. In P. Raj (Ed.), *Handbook of regional anesthesia* (pp. 102-103). New York: Churchill Livingstone.

Raj, P. (1989). *Prognostic and therapeutic nerve blocks*. In M. Cousins & P. Bridenbaugh (Eds.), *Neural blockade* (pp. 899-900). Philadelphia: Lippincott.

Raj, P. (1989). *Prognostic and therapeutic nerve blocks*. In M. Cousins & P. Bridenbaugh (Eds.), *Neural blockade* (pp. 901-907). Philadelphia: Lippincott.

Reiestad, F., & Stomstag, K. (1986). Intrapleural catheter in the management of postoperative pain. *Regional Anesthesiology, 11*:89-91.

Saper, J. (1987). Highlights of the Nuprin pain report. *Topics in Pain Management. 2*:41-43.

Travell, J. (1976). *Myofascial trigger points*. In J. Bonica & D. Albe-Fessard (Eds.), *Advances in pain research and therapy* (pp. 919-926). New York: Raven Press.

Waldman, S. (1989). Complications of cervical epidural nerve blocks. *Regional Anesthesiology, 14*:149-151.

Waldman, S. (1989). Subcutaneous tunneled intrapleural catheter in the long term relief of right upper quadrant pain of malignant origin. *Journal of Pain Symptom Management, 4*:86-89.

Waldman, S. (1990). The role of neural blockade in the management of headache and facial pain. *Headache Digest*. (In press).

Waldman, S., & Waldman, K. (1987). Reflex sympathetic dystrophy of the face and neck. *Regional Anesthesiology, 12*:8-12.

Waldman, S., Feldstein, G., & Allen, M. (1987). Cervical epidural blood patch for treatment of cervical dural puncture headache. *Anesthesiology Review* 1987, pp. 23-25.

Chapter 11

HEADACHES:
Muscle Contraction, Migraine, and Cluster
R. Michael Gallagher, D. O.

Dr. Gallagher shares with the reader the many facets involved in the diagnosis and treatment of headache. A problem of epidemic proportion, headache intervention can be a frustrating experience for both the physician and the patient. A knowledgeable clinician will work with a headache patient toward improvement through initiation of both prophylactic treatment and abortive treatment. Treatment should follow a definite plan and this chapter will aid the clinician in understanding what elements make for a successful treatment plan.

Chapter 11

HEADACHES:

Muscle Contraction, Migraine, and Cluster
R. Michael Gallagher, D.O.

Headache is an exceedingly common patient complaint that has been described throughout recorded medical history. Approximately 42,000,000 persons in the United States alone suffer from chronic headaches (Diamond, & Diamond-Falk, 1982). The economic cost of this problem reaches staggering proportions. It is estimated by the National Headache Foundation that 157,000,000 work days are lost each year to illness related to the headache problem.

The vast majority of headaches, although painful and, in some cases, temporarily disabling, are not associated with serious illness or pathological conditions. However, chronic and recurring headaches can be distressing and interfere with normal daily life. Most of the chronic or recurring headaches fall into one of the primary headache disorders: muscle contraction, migraine, and cluster.

The exact mechanism of the primary headache disorders is not completely understood at this time. Traditionally, these headaches were divided into the vascular headaches, migraine and cluster, involving blood vessels, and the non vascular headaches, muscle contraction, involving the muscles of the scalp, face, and/or neck. Recently, however, this concept has been questioned by some investigators, and a more complex neuronal mechanism put forward (Moskowitz, 1984, Olsen, 1987). For practical purposes and ease of understanding, the traditional concept will be discussed in this chapter.

The medical management of the chronic headache patient can sometimes be a frustrating experience for both the physician and the patient. Help for the headache sufferer rests with the empathetic, knowledgeable clinician who is willing to work with the patient in a partnership directed toward improvement and not necessarily cure. Unfortunately, many suffering patients only seek medical attention during acute attacks and severe pain which is the most inopportune time for evaluation and diagnosis. The most productive time for evaluation is when the patient is headache free or not so incapacitated as to interfere with a complete history, physical examination, and development of a realistic, achievable treatment plan.

There are two elements of treatment that headache patients require: first, an attempt to prevent headaches from occurring (prophylactic treatment) and second, relief of such headaches that do occur (abortive or reversal treatment). The appropriateness of whether prophylactic treatment or only abortive treatment is needed depends on the frequency and severity of headaches and the responsiveness of the individual. When headaches are frequent or unresponsive to abortive treatment, prophylactic treatment is indicated. Abortive treatment is used in patients whose headaches are infrequent and for those headaches that break through in spite of prophylactic medication.

Whether prophylactic or abortive, treatment should follow a definite plan incorporating the physician and patient into a team proceeding to reduce the frequency and/or severity of headaches. The physician's impressions and physical findings should be completely explained to the patient and as detailed as necessary for complete understanding. The headache condition should be explained, emphasizing the fact that it is more than just a pain in the head and that it is controllable, not curable! Once a plan is developed, follow up and continuing care is the key to a successful result.

MUSCLE CONTRACTION HEADACHE

Muscle contraction headache or tension headache is the most common type of headache. It is characterized by intermittent or persisting pain, often described as squeezing pressure, an ache, a band like discomfort, or a weight on the head. The intensity is quite variable and usually non incapacitating. The headache can last from hours to days and, in some cases, persist for months. The precise mechanism for the pain of muscle contraction headache is not clearly understood, but it is believed that waste products of sustained muscle contraction provoke chemical stimulation of pain nerve endings.

The pain of muscle contraction headache is usually bilateral with some patients experiencing a "hat band" like sensation around the entire head while others experience pain in the temporal, occipital, forehead, or vertex. The location of symptoms can vary from attack to attack, and associated tightness of the neck and shoulders is common. Muscle contraction headaches are not preceded by prodromal symptoms characteristic of some migraine headaches, nor are they typically associated with nausea or vomiting.

Precipitating Factors

Muscle contraction headaches frequently occur during periods of stress or emotional upset. Many of these patients display evidence of anxiousness, and poor coping and adaptation skills. If headaches are frequent or near daily, depression may be involved and should be considered even in the absence of obvious signs such as mood changes, crying spells, or loss of appetite.

Organic processes are sometimes involved in the precipitation of muscle contraction headache. When the cause is organic rather than psychogenic, the pain is often resistant to usual treatment modalities. Organic causes can be numerous, but the more commonly encountered are degenerative joint disease of the cervical spine, trauma to the head or neck, temporomandibular joint dysfunction, and ankylosing spondylitis.

Treatment

Periodic muscle contraction headache is usually resolved following the cessation of stressful stimuli, the use of mild analgesics or muscle relaxants, manipulative therapy, or any combination of these. The above rarely is effective when muscle contraction headaches are chronic (daily or near daily), and the use of stronger medications risks habituation.

Simple analgesics, such as acetaminophen, aspirin, or ibuprofen, are often all that is needed to relieve the symptoms of acute muscle contraction headache. Other nonsteroidal anti inflammatory drugs such as naproxen (Anaprox), meclofenamate (Meclomen), or ketoprofen (Orudis) can be prescribed for more significant symptoms. For patients who do not find relief, aspirin in combination with the muscle relaxants orphenadrine (Norgesic) or carisorpodal (Soma Compound), or acetaminophen added to chlorzoxazone (Parafon Forte) may be of help. On occasion, and in some patients, muscle contraction headache can be extremely severe and require potentially addicting analgesic combination drugs containing butalbital or meprobamate. These drugs can give significant relief by providing analgesia and reducing anxiety often associated with pain. (see Table I) As with any potentially addicting drug, careful monitoring of amounts given and strictly prohibiting daily or near daily use is essential.

Prophylactic therapy may be needed for patients whose headaches are frequent, daily, or the result of organic abnormalities such as degenerative joint disease of the cervical spine, temporomandibular joint dysfunction, and ankylosing spondylitis. Pharmacological treatment can include the judicious use of sedatives or muscle relaxants, but most patients who respond do so only temporarily, and the risk of habituation is significant. The nonsteroidal anti inflammatory drugs and antidepressants are the most useful in preventing muscle contraction headache (Gallagher, & Freitag, 1987, Speed, 1982).

Table I. Muscle Contraction Headache Abortive Medications

Drug	Brand Name	Dose – Prn
naproxen sodium	Anaprox	275-550 mg. every 4-6 Hr.
meclofenamate sodium	Meclomen	50-100 mg. every 4-6 Hr.
ketoprofen	Orudis	50-75 mg. every 4-6 Hr.
orphenadrine/aspirin	Norgesic/Norgesic Forte	2 every 4 Hr./1 every 4 Hr.
carisoprodol/aspirin	Soma Compound	2 every 4 Hr.
chlorzoxazone	Parafon Forte	1 every 4-6 Hr.
butalbital/aspirin/caffeine	Fiorinal	1 every 4 Hr.
butalbital/acetaminophen/caffeine	Fioricet/Esgic	1 every 4 Hr.
butalbital/acetaminophen	Phrenilin	1 every 4 Hr.
butalbital/aspirin	Axotal	1 every 4 Hr.
meprobamate/aspirin	Equagesic/Micrainin	1 or 2 every 4 Hr.

Nonsteroidal anti inflammatory drugs can be useful in preventing headaches in chronic muscle contraction headache patients. (see Table II) Those with underlying organic disease such as temporomandibular joint dysfunction or degenerative joint disease of the cervical spine are particularly good candidates. These drugs interfere with the inflammatory process and have analgesic properties. Most patients who improve will do so in approximately two to three weeks. Patients who do not respond or who cannot tolerate a particular agent may be helped by a comparable agent from another class. Side effects include fluid retention, gastrointestinal distress, nausea, diarrhea, dizziness, and gastric and duodenal irritation. Renal function monitoring should be done as regular nonsteroidal anti inflammatory drug use can diminish renal function.

Table II. NSAID's in the Treatment of Muscle Contraction Headache

Class	Medication	Dosage
Oxicam	piroxicam (Feldene)	20 mg./day
Indole	indomethacin (Indocin)	25-50 mg. TID-QID
	(Indocin SR)	75 mg. BID
	sulindac (Clinoril)	150-200 mg. BID
Propronic acids	fenoprofen (Nalfon)	600 mg. BID-TID
	ibuprofen (Motrin, Rufin)	400-800 mg. TID-QID
	naproxen (Naprosyn)	250-375 mg. TID-QID
	ketoprofen (Orudis)	50-75 mg. TID-QID
Fenamates	meclofenamate (Meclomen)	50-100 mg. TID

Antidepressants in a single bedtime dose can be extremely effective in reducing and, in some cases, eliminating chronic muscle contraction headache. Their mode of action is believed to be through analgesic and antidepressant effects. Many patients who experience frequent muscle contraction headaches suffer with an underlying or reactive depression.

There are a multitude of antidepressants, and the appropriate selection of an agent is dependent upon the physician's familiarity with the drug and the needs of the patient. (see Table III) Their onset of action is gradual, and sometimes therapeutic response can take as long as four weeks. It is recommended that therapy begin with a low dose which can be gradually titrated to the individual patient. Side effects are variable with the agents, but more frequently include drowsiness, postural hypotension, weight gain, constipation, and dry mouth.

Table III. Antidepressants and the Treatment of Muscle Contraction Headache

Drug	Brand Name	Dosage
amitriptyline	Elavil	25-100 mg./day
desipramine	Norpramin, Pertofrane	25-100 mg./day
doxepin	Adapin, Sinequan	25-100 mg./day
fluoxetine	Prozac	20 mg. OD-20 mg. BID
imipramine	Tofranil	25-100 mg./day
nortriptyline	Aventyl, Pamelor	25-100 mg./day
protriptyline	Vivactil	5-10 mg. BID-TID
trazedone	Desyrel	50-150 mg./day

The beta blocker, propranolol HCl (Inderal), commonly used in migraine, is used by some physicians with success. It has been postulated that propranolol HCl has significant anxiolytic effects (Speed, 1982). The usual dosage is 60 160 mg/day. Beta blocking drugs are discussed elsewhere in this chapter.

Manipulative therapy can be of significant help alone or in combination with medication. Gentle soft tissue techniques to the scalp, cervical, or thoracic areas often release muscle tension and induce relaxation. High velocity low amplitude techniques to the cervical and upper thoracic areas often reduce pain associated with muscle contraction headache (Hoyt, Shaffer, Bard, et al., 1979).

Reduction of stress and muscle tension is probably the most beneficial treatment. However, before this can begin, the patient, with the assistance of the physician, must accept responsibility for the management of his or her own chronic headache problem. Stress reduction and relaxation techniques and programs are numerous; however, biofeedback seems to be the most effective and efficient method in the motivated and open minded patient. Biofeedback is described elsewhere in this chapter.

Consideration should be given to dynamic psychotherapy for those patients whose headaches are caused by significant emotional conflict or depression or whose headaches are unresponsive to treatment. Psychotherapy can range from supportive to long term and may involve the family physician, psychiatrist, or psychologist.

MIGRAINE HEADACHE

Migraine is a specific type of vascular headache characterized by recurrent attacks of severe pain and associated symptoms. It is considered by many to be the most problematic of headaches and is sometimes referred to as "sick headache". Migraine is not a disease in itself but is thought to be a familial affliction. The headaches frequently begin in childhood or adolescence, are usually manifest by age 30, and may diminish in frequency and intensity after age 50. Approximately 10 per cent of the population may be affected, with an adult male to female ratio of 1:3 (Vahlquist, 1955). In prepubescense, migraines occur equally in boys and girls (Bille, 1962).

Characteristically, migraine headaches are unilateral but can be bilateral or generalized. The attacks are periodic, occurring as often as four to six times per month to as infrequently as one or two per year. The headaches last 8 to 48 hours on average and usually cause partial or complete incapacitation. Onset of the pain can be gradual or rapid and is sometimes present on awakening.

The pain of migraine is throbbing or constant and is sometimes described as an extreme pressure sensation. A variety of associated symptoms can occur and may precede or outlast the pain. The majority of sufferers will experience gastrointestinal symptoms such as nausea, vomiting, anorexia, abdominal bloating, constipation, or diarrhea. Photophobia, phonophobia, alterations in fluid balance, pallor or coldness of extremities are common. Psychological disturbances such as depression, euphoria, or feelings of well being before attacks are frequently observed by family or friends of the sufferer.

There are countless types of migraine headache, but common, classic, and complicated are generally accepted as the most typical forms. Classic and common migraine are seen in the majority of sufferers.

The classic migraine headache is preceded by sharply defined neurological warning symptoms (aura) 20 to 40 minutes prior to the attack. Almost any type of symptoms can occur, but visual disturbances such as blind spots, zig-zag lines, or diplopia are experienced most frequently. These aural symptoms generally disappear as the headache becomes manifest, and on occasion, cease without progression to headache (acephalic migraine).

The common form of migraine affects approximately 85 per cent of all sufferers. It can be present upon awakening or begin with a dull ache or stiffness in the neck and slowly progress to full intensity. Nonspecific prodromal symptoms such as changes in mood, appetite, energy level, or sense of well being may precede the headache by hours to days. Writers, artists, and professionals who suffer with common migraine headache sometimes feel that their most productive work is accomplished just before an attack.

Complicated migraine headache is characterized by more severe neurological aural symptoms such as slurred speech, confusion, parasthesias, or paresis. These symptoms sometimes continue throughout the headache and occasionally remain after the pain has ceased. It is not uncommon for these patients to have been incorrectly diagnosed as having had a stroke or transient ischemic attack (TIA).

Precipitating Factors

Certain factors can play a significant role in the precipitation of migraine. These factors may vary from patient to patient, but often include dietary, environmental, psychological, and pharmacological factors. The elimination of these factors will not necessarily prevent headaches, but may decrease their frequency or intensity in some patients.

Dietary guidelines are frequently included in comprehensive treatment programs since headaches are affected by diet in 25 per cent of migraine sufferers (Selby, & Lance, 1960). Additives such as monosodium glutamate or a variety of components of food such as tyramine, nitrites, and phenylethylamine often are implicated. Tyramine, an amino acid which possesses sympathomimetic activity, can trigger migraine by inducing vascular changes. Even small amounts of Na nitrite (found in a variety of cured meats) and monosodium glutamate (found in oriental and many packaged foods) can precipitate attacks in susceptible individuals. (see Table IV") Alcoholic beverages (particularly wine) precipitate attacks in most patients due to the vasoactive properties of ethanol and tyramine found in many brands of liquor. Caffeine in excessive amounts can aggravate migraine, especially if consumption is suddenly reduced or delayed.

Table IV. Common Foods to Avoid in Migraine

Beans	Garlic	Peanut Butter
Caffeine	Hot Fresh Bread	Pickled Products
Chinese Food	Liver	Pizza
Citrus Fruits	Monosodium Glutamate	Pork
Chocolate	Nuts	Processed Fish
Fermented Foods	Olives	Processed/Cured Meats
Figs	Onions	Ripened Cheese

Other commonly reported triggering factors include too much or too little sleep, long exposure to sun or glare, flickering lights, fatigue, hormonal fluctuations as seen in menses and ovulation, exogenous estrogen supplements, and vasodilating medications. (see Table V)

Personality traits that are common in migraineurs include neatness, perfectionism, restlessness, creativity, or resistance to change. Migraine sufferers often accept responsibility freely and have difficulty in saying "no". These traits predispose the patient for increased stress and fatigue, which often increase the frequency of headache.

Table V. Migraine Precipitants

Excessive Sleep	Changes in Routine
Fatigue	Stong Odors
Stressful Events (Good or Bad)	Loud Noise
Excessive Sun and Glare Exposure	Exposure to Altitude
Hormonal Changes	Weather Changes

Treatment

Once the diagnosis of migraine is established, a comprehensive treatment plan to include both pharmacological and nondrug aspects can be recommended. General nonpharmacological measures include the elimination of triggering foods and beverages, sleep pattern adjustments and the adjusting of nonmigrainous medications which may promote headaches. Changes in occupational and personal lifestyles, regular exercise, and definite relaxation periods can be helpful.

Stress reduction can play an important role in helping to control migraine headaches. Precipitating stressful situations can be numerous and vary from prolonged environmental exposures in some patients to strenuous activity in others. With markedly stressed patients, it may be necessary to enlist the assistance of a psychiatrist, psychologist, or counselor. Biofeedback can be helpful in reducing the frequency or severity of migraine in some patients (Gallagher, & Warner, 1984). Biofeedback is a technique which utilizes electronic sensory monitoring of body processes to give an individual immediate feedback on changes in these processes such as muscle tension or blood flow. The individual learns to control thought processes and how to determine which thoughts produce beneficial results. Two beneficial results are reduction in muscle tension, which is associated with stress reduction, and warming of the hands, which is associated with diversion of blood flow from the head to the periphery. (see Fig. 1)

The timely administration of vasoconstrictive medication can reverse the vasodilation of cranial and scalp arteries and relieve migraine symptoms. Most attacks of migraine start with a dull headache or aural symptoms which gradually progress. When the pain begins to throb, localize, or become severe, a vasoconstrictor should be taken. The two commonly

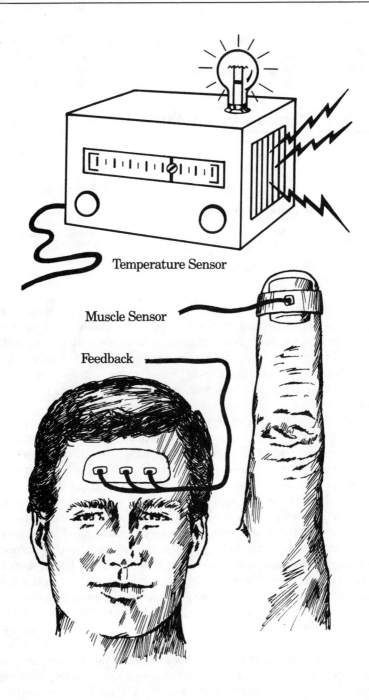

Fig. 1 Biofeedback

used vasoconstricting agents are ergotamine (Cafergot, DHE-45, Medi-haler, Wigraine, Ergostate, ErgoMar) and isometheptene (found in Midrin).

Ergotamine is the drug of choice and can be administered orally, rectally, sublingually, and parenterally. It is taken in repeated doses depending on brand and form and is generally restricted to no more than 6 mg/day or 12 mg/week. Frequent use of ergotamine can lead to ergot rebound headache, and for this reason should not be taken more frequently than every four to five days (Gallagher, 1983). Also, exceeding ergotamine dosage limitations may cause ergotism, a condition characterized by severe vasoconstriction with arteritis and possible gangrene of extremities. Side effects include nausea, vomiting, cramping, and parasthesias. It should not be taken in pregnancy, during febrile illness, or by those with peripheral vascular insufficiency, coronary artery disease, or hepatic impairment.

Isometheptene is found in Midrin capsules in combination with chloralphenazone and acetaminophen and is taken orally. It is preferred by many physicians as its limitations and side effects are less than those of medications containing ergotamine. Midrin use should not exceed five capsules in a 12-hour period. Side effects include fatigue and gastrointestinal disturbances. It should not be used in pregnancy or in those with peripheral vascular or coronary artery insufficiency, renal or hepatic dysfunction, glaucoma, hypertension, or in conjunction with monaminoxidose inhibitors (MAOI).

Simple analgesics or sedatives are sometimes helpful in the early stages of migraine headache because the headache often begins with dull pain and reactive muscle contraction. If the symptoms can be alleviated, the vasoactive process may sometimes be avoided. The judicious use of the more potent narcotic/non narcotic analgesics and antiemetics may be necessary in some patients whose headaches do not repond to initial therapy. Butalbital or codeine combinations are favored, but must not be permitted to be taken on a daily or near daily basis.

Occasionally, the migraine patient may experience a particularly long (over 36 hours) and debilitating headache which is referred to as "status migrainosis" (Couch, & Diamond, 1983). For such attacks, the administration of dihydroergotamine (DHE-45) intravenously or corticosteroids such as dexamethasone (Decadron) intramuscularly may be helpful (Callahan, & Raskin, 1986).

Daily prophylactic medication is considered for patients who experience frequent migraine attacks (three or more per month), whose headaches are unresponsive to usual abortive therapy, or whose headaches are associated with significant or prolonged neurological symptoms. The more commonly accepted medications are beta blocking agents, calcium channel antagonists, nonsteroidal anti inflammatory drugs, and antidepressants.

Beta blockers, such as propranolol (Inderal), are a relatively safe and effective migraine preventative. The mechanism of action is not completely understood, but is thought to involve the prevention of peripheral vasodilation through blockade of beta adrenergic receptors (Saper, 1983) and through anxiolytic properties (Speed, 1982, Kellner, Collins, Shulman, & Parthak, 1974). Propranolol is administered in divided doses of 80 240 mg per day or in a single long acting form at a daily dosage of 80 160 mg. Other beta blockers, such as nadolol (Corgard) 40 120 mg (Freitag, & Diamond, 1984), timolol (Blocadren) 5 30 mg (Gallagher, 1987), atenolol (Tenormin) 50 100 mg, (Stensrud, & Sjaastad, 1980), and metoprolol (Lopressor) 50 100 mg (Langohn, Gerber, Koletzki, et al., 1985), also prevent migraine in many patients. Side effects include fatigue, diarrhea, and depression as well as lowering of the heart rate and blood pressure.

The calcium channel antagonists are generally well tolerated and are proving to be helpful in many migraine sufferers. Verapamil (Calan, Isoptin) may be effective after two to eight weeks of therapy (Solomon, Diamond, & Freitag, 1987) and is the more frequently used of currently available agents. A total of 240 360 mg per day is administered in divided doses. The side effect profile is generally minimal and includes constipation and fluid retention. After continued use, its effectiveness diminishes in some patients. Other calcium channel antagonists, such as nimodipine (Nimotap), diltiazem (Cardizem), and nifedipin (Procardia), have been of help in the occasional patient.

The antidepressants, alone or in combination with beta blockers or calcium channel blockers, are often effective in reducing frequency and severity of migraine headache (Gallagher, & Freitag, 1987), and especially in those who experience frequent attacks. Their mode of action in migraine is not completely understood, but may involve an antidepressant effect or possibly an effect on neurotransmitter depletion. Drugs such as amitriptyline (Elavil), nortriptyline (Aventyl, Pamelor), doxepin (Adapin, Sinequan), or trazedone (Desyrel) are commonly used. (see Table VI)

The nonsteroidal anti inflammatory drugs have been of benefit to some patients in migraine prevention as well as symptomatic treatment. Their mode of action may involve both anti prostaglandin and antiplatelet aggregation effects (Kunkel, 1985). Naproxen (Naprosyn) (Ziegler, & Ellis, 1985) 750 1,000 mg/day, fenoprofen (Nalfon) (Diamond, Solomon, Freitag, et al, 1987) 1,800 2,400 mg/day, ketoprofen (Orudis) (Diamond, Freitag, Gallagher, et al., 1990) 150 225 mg/day may be used. Mefanamic acid (Ponstel) is sometimes used with success in migraine prevention in those headaches associated with menses. Commonly reported side effects include fluid retention, gastrointestinal distress, nausea, diarrhea, dizziness, and gastric and duodenal irritation. Renal function monitoring should be done as regular nonsteroidal anti inflammatory drug use can diminish renal function.

Table VI. Antidepressants in Migraine Prophylaxis

Drug	Brand Name	Dosage
amitriptyline	Elavil, Endep	50-150 mg./day
desipramine	Norpramin, Pertofrane	50-150 mg./day
doxepin	Adapin, Sinequan	50-150 mg./day
fluoxetine	Prozac	20-60 mg./day
nortriptyline	Aventyl, Pamelor	50-150 mg./day
protriptyline	Vivactil	10-40 mg./day
trazedone	Desyrel	50-200 mg./day

Migraineurs are unique individuals, and medication effectiveness and tolerance can vary from patient to patient. For this reason, medication changes and adjustments are often needed in the early stages of treatment. A significant number of other agents are available which may be effective. Some of these drugs include methysergide (Sansert), monoamine oxidase inhibitors such as phenelzine (Nardil) or isocarboxazid (Marplan), cyproheptidine (Periactin), clonidine (Catapres), dipyridamole (Persantine), ergonovine (Ergotrate) or small amounts of ergotamine as found in Bellergal S.

CLUSTER HEADACHE

Cluster headache is a devastatingly severe type of recurrent vascular headache. It is also sometimes referred to as histamine cephalgia, Horton's syndrome, or migrainous neuralgia. Its clinical constellation of symptoms with the characteristic patient behavioral tendencies during attacks should make it easily recognized and differentiated from a migraine or muscle contraction headache. Of the recurrent headache syndromes, it is probably the most distressing and brutal to the afflicted.

The headache is characterized by severe unilateral pain, often described as a burning, boring, or stabbing sensation in the area of the eye, temple, or forehead with radiation to the jaw, ear, or neck. During attacks, sufferers often pace or become extremely active, similar to patients experiencing renal colic. Frequently associated is ipsalateral lacrimation, eye injection, rhinorrhea, congestion, facial droop or sweating. The pain usually builds quickly over several minutes and lasts approximately 30-90 minutes.

Cluster headache attacks can occur numerous times daily, sometimes with regularity at the same hour each day. Early morning awakening with headache two to three hours after retiring is common. In its typical form, episodic cluster, the headaches cluster or group for periods of weeks to months and mysteriously disappear for months to years; thus the name "cluster headache". In its chronic form, which affects approximately 10-15% of sufferers (Ekbom, Olivarius, 1971, Kunkel, & Dohn, 1974), the headaches continue to occur indefinitely, affording the patient few headache free days.

The typical onset of cluster headaches is in the third or fourth decade of life, although it has been reported from as early as one year to the late 60s (Heyck, 1981). Unlike migraine, it is more prevalent in males with an estimated male to female ratio of 5:1. The etiology is not clearly understood; however, it is thought that complex vasomotor, hypothalamic, or neurohormonal disturbances are involved (Moskowitz, 1984, Saper, 1983, Kudrow, 1983).

Cluster patients frequently display a typical leonine face with ruddy complexion, thickened, coarse or pitted skin, and often with prominent furrows and creases (Graham, 1976). Sufferers tend to be conservative, responsible, resourceful, hard driving, conscientious, tense, and may abuse alcohol and cigarettes (Anonymous, 1980). The tremendous incapacitating pain and other symptoms can cause desperation, and it is not uncommon for these patients to consider suicide or to inflict injury upon themselves. In their quest to find relief, the afflicted often seek help from dentists, ophthalmologists, otorhinolaryngologists, orthopedists, chiropractors, accupuncturists, nutritionists, and so on.

Unlike migraine, diet does not seem to precipitate cluster, although an occasional patient will report that chocolate can be a factor. The one exception, however, is the consumption of alcohol during cluster periods.

The cluster attack will usually occur within 30 minutes of intake in 70 per cent of exposures (Horton, MacLean, & Craig, 1939). During remission periods while patients are not on preventative medication, alcohol appears to have no provoking effect.

The typical cluster headache is markedly different from other commonly encountered headache syndromes. (see Table VII) Although migraine and cluster share a few similar characteristics, their differentiation should not be difficult.

Treatment

There are few nonpharmacological measures that are helpful to cluster sufferers. However, the complete abstinence from alcohol during cluster periods is imperative. Alcohol undisputedly precipitates cluster attacks and will interfere with prophylactic therapy. The reduction of cigarette smoking and caffeine (Gallagher, & Freitag, 1987) and avoidance of day

Table VII. Headache Differential

	Migraine	Cluster	Muscle Contraction
Sex (M:F)	1:3	5:1	1:1
Onset (Avg)	4-30	20-40	any age
Location	usually unilateral	unilateral	bilateral, occipital frontal
Pain Character	variable, throbbing	lancinating, brutal	dull, tight pressure
Prodrome	visual aura vague aura	none	none
Duration	hours to days	30-90 minutes	hours to days
Family History	frequently present	none	sometimes present
Accompanying Symptoms	gastrointestinal, neurologic	Horner's syndrome, rhinorrhea, lacrimation	sore neck

time napping (Stensrud, & Sjaastad, 1980) may be of benefit to some patients.

The preferred approach to the treatment of cluster headache patients is prophylactic. The tremendous pain and relatively short but frequent attacks makes symptomatic treatment less practical and often ineffective. Appropriate pharmacological prophylactic regimens can reduce the frequency and severity of attacks in most patients.

When treating cluster patients, the benefits of therapy should be weighed against the hazards of taking medication. Patients should be monitored closely as some of the pharmacological agents prescribed in treatment can potentially cause problems. Ergotamine preparations, methysergide, calcium channel blockers, corticosteroids, and lithium are commonly used. Other agents such as cyproheptidine (Periactin), indomethacin (Indocin), chlorpromazine (Thorazine), antidepressants, and ergonovine (Ergotrate) have been used with limited success.

Ergotamine tartrate (Bellergal S, Cafergot, Wigraine) is a blood vessel constrictor. It is administered orally in divided doses throughout the day and will often limit the severity and frequency of attacks. The daily dose should be kept as low as possible (1-2 mg/day), and additional ergotamine for breakthrough headaches should not be permitted. Individual tolerance and sensitivity varies greatly, and patients should be followed closely for untoward reactions and complications. Side effects include nausea, vomiting, muscle cramps, peripheral vascular problems, intermittent claudication, arterial spasm, and chest pain. In addition, ergotamine should not be used routinely in the presence of febrile illness, coronary artery disease, marked hypertension, collagen vascular disease, renal or hepatic insufficiency, and in pregnancy.

Methysergide (Sansert), an ergot derivative, is considered by many to be the drug of choice in the treatment of cluster headache patients. Its mechanism of action is unclear, but it is thought to inhibit serotonin (Friedman, 1978). It is administered orally in divided doses not to exceed 8 mg/day. Upon initiation of therapy, some patients experience transient mental confusion, nausea, vomiting, muscle cramps or aches, and insomnia. If these symptoms persist for more than three days or the patient develops evidence of peripheral vasoconstriction, claudication, or angina, the medication should be stopped. Methysergide is contraindicated in the presence of peripheral vascular or cardiovascular disease, hypertension, active ulcer disease, cardiac vascular disease, hepatic or renal dysfunction, or pregnancy.

A rare but serious complication of methysergide therapy is an inflammatory fibrosis that can affect heart valves, lungs, pleura, or the retroperitoneal space. This condition is usually reversible with discontinuation of the drug (Gillman, Goodman, & Gillman, 1980). For this reason, a one- to two-month medication free period is mandatory after each four- to six-month period of use. During treatment, patients should be examined frequently and laboratory tests such as blood chemistries and urinalysis should be monitored periodically.

Corticosteroids, alone or in combination with ergot or methysergide, are frequently effective for difficult patients. Their mechanism of action is not completely understood but is thought to involve suppression of hormonal mechanisms. This treatment is more suited for the episodic type of cluster as its long-term use in chronic cluster could be hazardous. However, because of the extreme distress and suffering of some chronic cluster patients, its use can provide temporary relief while other drugs are being introduced.

Prednisone (Deltasone) or triamcinolone (Artistocort) are commonly prescribed, although others are effective. The steroids are given in divided doses that must be titrated to the individual. The average daily starting dose is 60 mg of prednisone or 16 mg of triamcinolone. The medication is then tapered over two to four weeks with adherence to usual steroid precautions. Side effects include fluid retention, weight gain, gastrointestinal disturbances, lethargy, and Cushing's syndrome. Contraindications are hypertension, diabetes, peptic ulcer disease, infection, active immunization, or pregnancy.

Calcium channel blocking drugs are a relatively new class of drugs that have been helpful to many patients, especially those suffering with the chronic form. It is believed that they alter smooth muscle tone of cerebral arteries by interfering with calcium ion function (Gallagher, & Freitag, 1987). Verapamil (Calan, Isoptin) is generally well-tolerated and more frequently utilized. It is taken in divided doses with an average daily dosage of 360 mg/day. The most frequently experienced side effects include constipation and fluid retention. Verapamil is contraindicated in hypotension, cardiac conduction disease, and significant renal or hepatic disease. Other calcium channel blockers sometimes used are nifedipine (Procardia) 40 80 mg/day and nimodipine (Nimotapp) 30 60 mg/day.

Lithium Carbonate (Eskalith, Lithobid) is reported to be effective in reducing frequency and severity of attacks in the treatment of patients suffering with the chronic form of cluster headache. Its mechanism of action has been debated but may involve its effect on cyclic changes in serotonin and histamine (Gallagher, & Freitag, 1987) or electrical conductivity in the central nervous system (Diamond, & Dalessio, 1978). It is administered orally in divided doses with a daily dosage of 600-1,200 mg. Serum lithium level monitoring is necessary in order to avoid toxicity. Effective therapeutic ranges vary greatly but generally should not exceed 1.2 meq/liter. Nonsteroidal antiinflammatory drugs and thiazide derivatives should be used with caution as these agents may potentiate risks of toxicity. Side effects include fatigue, tremor, sleepiness, diarrhea, decreased thyroid function, goiter, and fluid retention. Lithium is contraindicated in the presence of significant renal or cardiovascular disease.

Abortive therapy for cluster patients is of limited effectiveness because of the relatively brief headaches and the time necessary for medication absorption. However, in patients who experience longer headaches and in those who are not sufficiently controlled by preventative medication, abortive therapy may be needed. This is generally limited to ergotamine, analgesic/sedatives and oxygen inhalation.

Ergotamine preparations can be administered early in a cluster attack, sublingually (Ergomar, Ergostat), intramuscularly (DHE) or by inhalation (Medihaler). This may give relief to some, while simply delaying the completion of the headache in others. The usual ergotamine limitations must be observed which limits the amount that can be taken and the number of headaches that can be treated.

Analgesics and sedatives are of limited help, but often aid certain patients psychologically and reduce the anxiety associated with cluster attacks. Unmonitored use of these medicaments should be avoided, as potential habituation or toxicity can develop.

The inhalation of oxygen during cluster attacks is a relatively safe and effective treatment. In the majority of sufferers, oxygen will abort attacks within 12 minutes (Kudrow, 1981). Oxygen is administered at a rate of 7 liters per minute by facial mask at the onset of an attack and continued for up to 15 minutes. The main drawback to the use of the oxygen is the cumbersome equipment which makes it difficult to transport for patients whose attacks are unpredictable.

MIXED HEADACHE SYNDROME

Most headache patients experience one or possibly two distinct headache types with pain free periods between attacks. However, there is a group of patients who experience intermittent migraine attacks superimposed on a daily or near daily less intense headache similar to that of muscle contraction. This pattern is characteristic of the mixed headache syndrome. The mixed headache syndrome is one of the most difficult to manage of the chronic headache disorders.

The typical mixed headache patient will, in many cases, have a long history of evaluations and failed therapeutic attempts. Their constant fear of the daily or near daily headaches worsening will sometimes lead to self treatment and excessive medication use. The frequent use of prescription or over-the-counter analgesics (Kudrow, 1982), especially those containing caffeine or ergotamine, (Wainscott, Volans, & Wilkinson, 1974), can cause rebound headaches which perpetuate the problem and often renders other treatments ineffective. Psychogenic factors such as chronic stress, anxiety, "burn-out", or depression are usually present and further contribute to the ongoing problem.

The patient doctor relationship is critical in the management of mixed headache patients. A definitive, comprehensive treatment plan which addresses each element of the patient's problem must be developed and supervised by a single physician. The patient must be educated as to the nature of his or her headaches and how each aspect of treatment is expected to contribute to the control of the headaches. Once a plan is begun, continuity of care with regular follow-up visits is vital.

The treatment of the mixed headache syndrome will usually require prophylactic medications in addition to nonpharmacological measures such as diet, exercise, stress reduction, biofeedback, social adjustments, and counseling. Since these patients, in effect, experience co existing muscle contraction and migraine headaches, each individual component will require its own appropriate therapy. The management of muscle contraction and migraine headache has been described earlier in this chapter. Patients who do not respond to outpatient therapy or who are unable to withdraw from frequent analgesic or ergotamine use may benefit from hospitalizaiton at dedicated in patient headache units (Diamond, Freitag, & Maliszewski, 1986).

REFERENCES

Anonymous (1980). Matching therapy to headache type. *Patient Care,* 14:102.

Bille, B. (1962). Migraine in school children. *ACTA Paediatrica Scandinavica, 51 (suppl. 136)*:1.

Callahan, M., & Raskin, N. (1986). A controlled study of DHE-45 in the treatment of acute migraine headache. *Headache, 26*:168.

Couch, J., & Diamond, S. (1983). Status migrainosis: Causative therapeutic aspects. *Headache, 23*:94-101.

Diamond, S., & Dalessio, D. (1980). *Practicing physician's approach to headache* (2nd ed.). Baltimore: Williams & Wilkins.

Diamond, S., & Diamond-Falk, J. (1982). *Advice from the diamond headache clinic.* New York: International University Press.

Diamond, S., Freitag, F., Gallagher, R., et al. (1990). Ketoprofen in the prophylaxis of migraine. *Headache Quarterly, 1:* 75-77.

Diamond, S, Freitag, F., Maliszewski, M. (1986). Inpatient treatment of headache: Long-term results. *Headache, 26*:189-197.

Diamond, S., Solomon, G., Freitag, F., et al. (1987). Fenoprofen in prophylaxis of migraine, a double blind placebo study. *Headache, 27*:246-249.

Ekbom, K., & Olivarius, B. (1971). Chronic migrainous neuralgia: Diagnosis and therapeutic agents. *Headache, 11*:97-101.

Friedman, A. (1978). Migraine. *Medical Clinics of North America, 62:* 490.

Freitag, F., & Diamond, S. (1984). Nadalol and placebo: Comparative study in the prophylactic treatment of migraine. *Journal of the American Medical Association, 84:*343.

Gallagher, R. (1983). Ergotamine withdrawl causing "rebound headache." *Journal of the American Osteopathic Association, 82:*677-678.

Gallagher, R. (1987). Timolol maleate, a beta-blocker, in the treatment of common migraine headache. *Headache, 27:*84-85.

Gallagher, R. & , Freitag, F. (1987). Cluster headache: Diagnosis and treatment. *Journal of Osteopathic Medicine, 1:*10-18.

Gallagher, R., & Freitag, F. (1987). Muscle contraction headache: Diagnosis and treatment. *Journal of Osteopathic Medicine, 1(6):*8-17.

Gallagher, R., & Warner, J. (1984). Patient motivation in the treatment of migraine: A non-medical study. *Headache, 24:*269.

Gillman, A., Goodman, L., & Gillman, A. (1980). *Pharmacologic basis of therapeutics* (6th ed.). New York: MacMillan.

Graham, J. (1976). Cluster headache. In O. Appenzeller (Ed.) *Pathogenesis, treatment of headache.* New York: Spectrum.

Heyck, H. (1981). Headache and facial pain. *Chicago, Yearbook of Medical Publishers, 119.*

Horton, B., MacLean, A., & Craig, W. (1939). A new syndrome of vascular headache: Results in treatment with histamine, preliminary report. *Mayo Clinic Proceedings, 14:*257-260.

Hoyt, W., Shaffer, F., Bard, D., et al. (1979). Osteopathic manipulation. *Journal of the American Osteopathic Association, 78:*322-325.

Kellner, R., Collins, A., Shulman, R., & Parthak, D. (1974). The short-term antianxiety effects of propranolol. *Journal of Clinical Pharmacology, 5:*301-340.

Kudrow, L. (1983). Cluster headache. *Neurologic Clinics, 1:*370.

Kudrow, L. (1982). Paradoxical effects of frequent analgesic use. In M. Critchely (Ed.) *Advances in Neurology,* Vol. 33. New York: Raven Press.

Kudrow, L. (1981). Response of cluster headache to oxygen inhalation. *Headache, 21:*1-4.

Kunkel, R. (1985). Pharmacologic management of migraine. *Cleveland Clinic Quarterly, 52:*95-101.

Kunkel, R. & Dohn, D. (1974). Surgical treatment of chronic migrainous neuralgia. *Cleveland Clinic Quarterly, 41:*189-192.

Langohn, W., Gerber, E., Koletzki, E., et al. (1985). Clomipramine and metropolol in migraine prophylaxis: A double blind crossover study. *Headache, 25:*107-113.

Moskowitz, M. (1984). The neurobiology of vascular head pain. *Annals of Neurology, 16:*157-168.

Olsen, J. (1987). The ischemic hypothesis of migraine. *Archives of Neurology, 44*:321-322.

Saper, J. (1983). *Headache disorders: Current concepts and treatment strategies.* Boston: John Wright-PSG, Inc., 76-77.

Selby, G., & Lance, J. (1960). Observations in 500 cases of migraine and allied vascular headache. *Journal of Neurology, Neurosurgery, and Psychiatry, 23*:23.

Solomon, G., Diamond, S. & , Freitag, F. (1987). Verapamil in migraine prophylaxis: Comparison of dosages. *Clinical Pharmacology and Therapeutics, 41*:202.

Speed, W. (1982). How to ease the pain of muscle contraction headache. *Modern Medicine, 50*:127-140.

Stensrud, P., & Sjaastad, O. (1980). Comparative trial of tenormin (atenolol) and inderal (propranolol) in migraine. *Headache, 20*:204.

Vahlquist, B. (1955). Migraine in children. *International Archives of Allergy and Applied Immunology, 7*:348.

Wainscott, G., Volans, G., & Wilkinson, M. (1974). Ergotamine-induced headaches. *British Medical Journal, 2*:274.

Ziegler, D, & Ellis, D. (1985). Naproxen in prophylaxis of migraine. *Archives of Neurology, 42*:582.

Chapter 12

OROFACIAL PAIN AND TEMPOROMANDIBULAR DISORDERS

Differential Diagnosis

Charles McNeill, D.D.S.

By some accounts, 40 per cent of all cases of chronic pain seen in a pain clinic are due to craniofacial and neck pain. Dr. McNeill sheds light on the many factors relating to head and neck pain. This chapter will help describe the role of the dentist as a team member. The term temporomandibular disorder covers a number of musculoskeletal problems which lend themselves to evaluation and treatment by the dentist.

Characteristic symptoms of TMD include pain, limitation of mandibular range of motion, and resultant functional problems. Factors relating to predisposition and perpetuation of TMD are reviewed. The importance of a physical examination, review of records, and history leads the dentist to a differential diagnosis and is crucial for successful treatment. The role of imaging and testing is reviewed and the tables presented further highlight recommendations for management.

Chapter 12

OROFACIAL PAIN AND TEMPOROMANDIBULAR DISORDERS
Differential Diagnosis
Charles McNeill, D.D.S.

In dentistry, as in medicine, the diagnosis and management of chronic pain conditions are among the most perplexing problems confronting the clinician. Chronic pain is one of the most prevalent chronic illnesses costing society billions of dollars annually in lost work, health care services, and disability compensations (Bonica, 1984). Chronic pain syndromes are most frequent in the area of the head and neck (Crook, et al., 1984; Sternbach, 1986). It has been reported that craniofacial and neck pain may account for approximately 40 per cent of all cases of chronic pain seen in pain clinics (Donaldson & Kroening, 1979). A recent Harris poll found more adults working full-time miss work from headache than any other site of pain (Harris, et al., 1986). Headache is one of the most common symptoms reported by patients suffering from temporomandibular disorders (TMD) (Magnusson & Carlsson; 1978, 1980; Wanmann & Agerberg, 1986).

Bell subdivides head and neck pain into (1) headache, (2) orofacial pains, and (3) cervical pains (Bell, 1989). Disorders of the teeth, periodontium, and other intra oral structures constitute the major source of acute orofacial pain seen by dentists. Temporomandibular disorders are recognized as the most common chronic orofacial pain conditions confronting dentists and other health care providers (Bell, 1990). The responsibility of the dental profession in the management of head and neck pain symptoms is the confirmation or exclusion of certain orofacial pains, specifically pain conditions in teeth, associated supporting structures, intra oral structures, jaws, and temporomandibular disorders (TMD).

TEMPOROMANDIBULAR DISORDERS

Temporomandibular disorders (TMD) is a collective term embracing a number of clinical problems, often overlapping, that involve the masticatory musculature and temporomandibular (TM) joints (McNeill, 1990a), and are considered a subclassification of musculoskeletal disorders (Bell, 1989). They are characterized by pain in the preauricular area, TM joint, or muscles of mastication; limitation or deviation in the mandibular range of motion; and, TM joint sounds during mandibular function. In addition to this triad of pain, limited function, and joint sounds, nonpainful masticatory muscle hypertrophy and abnormal occlusal wear associated with oral parafunction, such as bruxism (grinding), are considered related problems (McNeill, 1990b).

Epidemiologic studies report that about 75 per cent of the population have at least one sign of dysfunction (joint noise, tenderness, etc.) and about 33 per cent have at least one symptom (face pain, joint pain, etc.) of temporomandibular disorders (Solberg, 1983; Rugh & Solberg, 1985; Schiffman & Fricton, 1988). The prevalence of at least one oral parafunctional habit is about 60 per cent; however, self report of oral habits occurring daily is less than 25 per cent (Ingervall et al., 1980; Schiffman et al., 1990). Signs and symptoms of TMD generally increase in frequency and severity from the second through the fourth decade of life (Dworkin et al., 1990). The majority of 3,428 patients with TMD in a recent study were between the age of 15 and 45 years with a mean age of 32.9 years (Howard, 1990). Although small sex differences have been found in some epidemiological studies (Agerberg & Carlsson, 1972; Helkimo, 1974a, 1974b), recent clinical tabulations report a ratios ranging from 6 to-1 to 9-to 1 of females to males seeking care for TMD (McNeill, 1985; Howard, 1990). Temporomandibular disorders are often self limiting or fluctuate over time as suggested by the declining prevalence with age. Unfortunately, there is limited knowledge regarding the natural history or course of TMD (Rasmussen, 1981a, 1981b; Nickerson & Boering, 1989). Prevalence figures may overstate the clinical significance of this problem because many studies include individuals with mild transient signs and symptoms that may not require treatment. In fact, of the large percentage of the population who have signs and/or symptoms, it is estimated that only about 5 per cent are in need of treatment (Rugh & Solberg, 1985; Schiffman et al., 1990).

Contributing etiologic factors include behavioral, psychosocial, and physical factors. Some factors prove to be only risk factors, others are causal in nature, while others result from, or are purely coincidental to, the problem. These factors are classified as predisposing, initiating (precipitating), and perpetuating to emphasize their role in the progression of TMD (McNeill, 1983a). Predisposing factors involve pathophysiologic, psychologic, or structural processes that alter the masticatory system sufficiently to increase the risk of developing TMD. Initiating factors that lead to the onset of symptoms are primarily related to trauma or adverse loading of the masticatory system. Overt trauma producing injury to the head, neck, or jaw can result from an impact injury, a flexion extension injury, an injury while eating, yawning, singing, or from prolonged mouth opening or extensive stretching as may occur during long dental appointments. A second form of trauma results from sustained and repetitious, adverse loading of the masticatory system that occurs during occlusal parafunction. Parafunction may result in adverse loading of the temporomandibular joint, muscles, as well as the teeth, causing excess tooth wear, sensitivity, and mobility. The intensity and frequency of parafunctional jaw activity (bruxism) may be exacerbated by stress and anxiety, sleep disorders, and medications (phenothiazines), alcohol, and other substances (Rugh & Harlan, 1988). Studies of oral parafunctional habits have demonstrated a positive association with TMD (Ingervall et al., 1980; Nilner & Lassing, 1983; Nilner, 1983; Mealiea & McGlynn, 1987; Schiffman et al., 1990). Perpetuating factors including parafunction sustain the patient's disorder, and thus, complicate their management. They are primarily factors that are related to the behavioral, social, emotional, and cognitive difficulties of the patient (Rugh, 1987).

DIFFERENTIAL DIAGNOSIS

Temporomandibular disorders constitute the major source of chronic orofacial pain, but there are other causes that must be considered. To establish order to the process of classifying craniofacial pain, a system using operational diagnostic criteria was developed by The World Federation of Neurology and The International Headache Society. The diagnostic classification system provides a logical and complete diagnostic classification for headache disorders, cranial neuralgias, and facial pain (Cephalgia, Vol. 8, Suppl. 7, 1988) (see Table I).

The American Academy of Craniomandibular Disorders has collaborated with these organizations in order to include TMD in the diagnostic classification (McNeill, 1990b). As listed in the diagnostic classification, orofacial pain can be associated with vascular disorders, trauma, infection, metabolic disorders, or substance abuse or withdrawal. Orofacial pain may also be associated with intracranial disorders and extracranial structures, or be related to cranial neuralgias, nerve trunk pain or deafferentation pain.

However, it is important to realize that psychiatric or psychological disorders may also cause, contribute to, or result from orofacial pain syndromes (Rugh, 1983). Therefore, it is critical for clinicians who manage orofacial pain conditions to have an extensive knowledge of all disorders that may be responsible for the symptoms regardless of disciplinary boundaries (see Table II).

The multitude of disease entities which present with similar pain patterns in the head and neck region mandate that dentists consider diseases unrelated to the masticatory system in their differential diagnosis.

Table I. International Headache Society Classification for Headache Disorders, Cranial Neuralgias and Facial Pain

1. Migraine
2. Tension type Headache
3. Cluster Headache & Chronic Paroxysmal Hemicrania
4. Miscellaneous Headaches, Unassociated with Structural Lesion
5. Headache Associated with Head Trauma
6. Headache Associated with Vascular Disorders
7. Headache Associated with Non vascular Intracranial Disorders
8. Headache Associated with Substances or Their Withdrawal
9. Headache Associated with Non cephalic Infection
10. Headache Associated with Metabolic Disorder
11. Headache or Facial Pain Associated with Disorder of Cranium, Neck, Eyes, Ears, Nose, Sinuses, Teeth, Mouth, or Other Facial or Cranial Structures
12. Cranial Neuralgias, Nerve Trunk Pain, and Deafferentation Pain
13. Headache Not Classifiable

Cephalgia, Vol. 8, Suppl. 7, 1988 Norwegian University Press, Publications Expediting Inc., or P. 0. Box 2459 Tolyen, 0609 Oslo 6, Norway

Likewise, physicians evaluating craniofacial pain must also consider TMD in their differential diagnosis. All clinicians must be aware that there can be a confusing overlap of signs and symptoms in spite of widely varying etiology. The process of differential diagnosis is critical because an incorrect or omitted diagnosis is one of the most frequent causes of treatment failure.

Intracranial and Extracranial Structures

Disorders of the intracranial structures, such as neoplasm, aneurysm, abscess, hemorrhage, or hematoma, and edema should be considered first in the differential diagnosis because they can be life threatening and may require immediate attention. The characteristics of serious intracranial disorders include new or abrupt onset of pain or progressively more severe pain, interruption of sleep by pain, and pain precipitated by exertion or positional change, (i.e., coughing, sneezing). Also, weight loss, ataxia, weakness, fever with pain, and neurologic signs or symptoms, such as seizure, paralysis, or vertigo and neurologic deficits are characteristic of intracranial disorders (Fricton et al., 1988). Besides masticatory structures, other extracranial structures should also be suspected as the source of pain. This includes disorders of the dental pulp, periodontium, mucosa, tongue, salivary glands, Lymph tissues, sinuses,

Table II. Differential Diagnosis of Orofacial Pain

Somatic Pain
  Intracranial Structures
    Neoplasm, Aneurysm, Abscess, Hemorrhage, Hematoma, Edema
  Extracranial Structures
    Temporomandibular Disorders and Other Orofacial Structures
    and/or Disorders

  Vascular Disorders
    Migraine, Migraine Variants, Cluster Headache, and Paroxysmal
    Hemicrania, Vascular Arteritis, Carodidynia

Neurogenous Pain
  Paroxysmal Neuralgias
    Trigeminal, Glossopharyngeal, Facial, Nervus intermedius,
    Superior Laryngeal Neuralgias

  Deafferentation Pain Syndromes
    Peripheral Neuritis, Postherpetic Neuralgia, Post traumatic and
    Postsurgical Neuralgia, Reflex Sympathetic Dystrophy

Psychogenic Pain
Somatoform Disorders
    Conversion Disorders, Psychogenic Pain Disorders, Hypochondria-
    sis, Somatization Disorders, Atypical Somatoform Disorders

Other Psychiatric Disorders and Symptoms
    Factitious Disorder with Physical Symptoms, Somatic Delusions

Nonpsychiatric Disorders
    Malingering, Chemical Dependency

---

eyes, ears, nose, and throat. When doubt exists about a specific diagnosis, consultation with an appropriate specialist is essential.

Neurologic Disorders

Neurologic disorders can be divided into two main categories of painful conditions, namely, paroxysmal and continuous pain conditions. The paroxysmal neuralgias associated with orofacial pain include trigeminal neuralgia, glossopharyngeal neuralgia, facial neuralgia, nervous intermedius neuralgia, and superior laryngeal neuralgia (Friction & Kroening, 1988). Occipital neuralgia is not listed here because the characteristic pain is located in the back of the cranium above the nuchal line rather than in the orofacial region. The common paroxysmal pain attack follows a distinct unilateral course and is described as electric like, stabbing or shooting pain. Attacks occur intermittently lasting for seconds to minutes with remission periods of days, months, or even years. Stimulation of a trigger zone within the distribution of the nerve affected sets off a volley of pain attacks. Trigeminal neuralgia (tick douloureux) commonly involves the maxillary and/or mandibular division causing pain in the area of their distribution (Loeser, 1977). Glossopharyngeal neuralgia is less common than trigeminal neuralgia. Cutaneous trigger zones are less common, but if present, are localized around the ear. Ordinary function such as coughing, chewing, swallowing, and talking may trigger pain. The pain is generally located in the ear, tonsillar area, throat, and pharynx (Stevens, 1987). Facial neuralgia (atypical facial neuralgia, atypical odontalgia) is described as persistent facial, jaw, gingival, or tooth pain not associated with physical signs or a demonstrable organic cause. Nervus intermedius (geniculate) neuralgia is rare and is described as a lancinating "hot poker" in the ear. The trigger area is usually in the external auditory canal. Superior laryngeal neuralgia is also a rare disorder characterized by severe pain in the lateral aspect of the throat, submandibular region, and underneath the ear, precipitated by swallowing, shouting, or turning the head (Cephalgia, 1988).

The continuous neurologic (neuropathic) pain disorders associated with orofacial pain are primarily considered deafferentation pain syndromes and include peripheral neuritis, postherpetic neuralgia, post traumatic or postsurgical neuralgia, and reflex sympathetic dystrophy. The pain is usually described as a persistent, ongoing, unremitting burning sensation. Patients frequently report abnormal sensations (dysesthesias) which are exacerbated by movement or touch. Neuropathic pain can occur as a result of inflammation, compression, distortion, demyelination, infarction, or paralysis of a nerve trunk. Referred pains and other central excitatory effects do not occur (Bell, 1989). One common neuropathic pain condition, postherpetic neuralgia ("shingles"), is usually a constant, intense, unilateral burning pain with hyperesthesia that occurs within days of an infection of a peripheral nerve or dorsal root ganglion with herpes zoster virus (Loeser, 1986). Post traumatic and postsurgical (anesthesia dolorosa) neuralgias are usually described as a continuous tingling, numbness, twitching, or prickly sensation. This deafferentation pain results from damage to the nerve by trauma or surgery. Since a disruption of the normal pathway which connects the neural elements of the dental pulp with the central nervous system occurs routinely with pulp extirpation during endodontic procedures and dental extraction, deafferentation pain is an important pain syndrome to consider in the differential diagnosis of orofacial pain.

Reflex sympathetic dystrophy (RSD) refers to a specific group of painful disorders initiated by an injury to peripheral tissues and sustained by neural mechanisms that include sympathetic efferent activity. The existence of this condition has been unequivocally demonstrated by the clinical observation that regional blockade of the sympathetic system produces immediate and complete relief of pain (Fields, 1987). The term causalgia has been used in the past for RSD initiated by trauma of a major peripheral nerve. Reflex sympathetic dystrophy is characterized by progressive autonomic dysfunction, i.e., changes in cutaneous temperature, color, texture, and perspiration followed by trophic changes in the skin, muscle, and bone (Kroening & Fricton, 1988).

Vascular Disorders

Vascular disorders associated with orofacial pain include migraine headache, migraine variants, cluster headaches, cranial arteritis, and carodidynia. The usual description of vascular pain is a throbbing, pulsation, or beating pain. Migraine headaches can be subdivided into migraine with aura (classic) and migraine without aura (common migraine) headache. Migraine with aura headaches characteristically are one-sided and have a prodromal vasoconstriction phase with visual aberrations. This is followed by vasodilation of the affected arteries resulting in throbbing (pulsating) pain lasting 4 to 72 hours with frequently accompanying nausea and/or vomiting and phono and photophobia (Edmeads, 1987). Migraine without aura headaches are similar to classic migraine, but proceeds into a headache without prodromata. At least five attacks are required as a diagnostic criterion to separate it from episode tension type headache. The site of pain in migrainous headaches is most frequently in the orbital, frontal, or temporal regions, but facial migrainous headaches also occur. The term "mixed muscular vascular combination headache" is being eliminated in favor of both migraine and tension-type headache being individually coded for patients with coexisting conditions (*Cephalgia,* 1988). Migraine with aura variants include ophthalmoplegic, retinal, basilar, and hemiplegic migraines. Ophthalmoplegic and hemiplegic migraines are severe variations of classic migraine. The symptoms are accompanied by ocular motor nerve palsy and/or partial or complete paralysis of motor function. Retinal migraine is described as repeated attacks of monocular scotoma or blindness lasting less than an hour.

Cluster headache, also known as Horton's headache or histaminic neuralgia, and chronic paroxysmal hemicrania, are similar to migrainous pain but much more intense and of shorter duration than migraine. The pain is usually reported as unilateral, excruciating, throbbing pain behind the eyes that occur in clusters of days to weeks with periods of remission of months to years. The headaches can be provoked by alcohol, histamine, or nitroglycerine. Cluster headache frequently presents characteristic autonomic effects, i.e., nasal congestion, lacrimation, conjunctive injection, edema of the eyelids and face on the affected side, which are commonly referred to as Horner's syndrome (Raskin & Appenzeller, 1980). Cluster headaches are 10 to 50 times less common than migraine and are found at least five to six times more frequently in men than women (Campbell, 1987). Chronic paroxysmal hemicrania is similar to cluster headache except they are shorter lasting, more frequent, occur mostly in females, and there is absolute effectiveness of indomethacin.

Headaches associated with other vascular disorders that can be related to orofacial pain include cranial arteritis and carodidynia. Cranial arteritis (temporal arteritis) is a giantcell inflammatory disease of the carotid artery system (vasculitis) and is rarely seen in people under 50 years of age. The problem can easily be misdiagnosed as muscular and/or TM joint disorders when the temporal artery is involved. The danger in delayed diagnosis is when there is involvement with the ophthalmic artery with the possibility of subsequent blindness. Carotidynia is a vascular disorder characterized by throbbing pain in the distribution of the external carotid artery, usually the neck and face. Palpation of the artery may reproduce the symptoms and project ipsilateral pain to the head. Other headaches that can resemble migraine may be related to many different causes of vasodilation with associated throbbing pain, i.e., altitude sickness, overexertion, dehydration, dialysis, certain allergens, caffeine, alcohol, and chemicals.

Mental Disorders

Mental disorders are conceptualized as a clinically significant behavioral or psychological syndrome or pattern that occurs in a person. It is associated with a present distress (painful symptom, disability, or with a significantly increased risk of suffering of loss). (Dworkin & Burgess, 1987). Whatever the original cause of the syndrome, it is considered a manifestation of behavioral, psychological, and/or biological dysfunction. These disorders are classified in the current edition of the DSM III R (Diagnostic and Statistical Manual, Revised, third edition, 1987). This diagnostic manual presents criteria for each disorder and is recommended by the American Psychiatric and Psychological Associations. Differential diagnostic groups include psychotic symptoms, mood disturbances, organic mental disorders, anxiety disorders, and somatoform disorders. Somatoform disorders are a class of disorders that have physical symptoms as presenting complaints but have psychological factors involved in the etiology. Somatoform disorders include somatization disorders, conversion disorders, psychogenic pain disorders, hypochondriasis, and atypical somatoform disorders. Other psychiatric disorders and symptoms include factitious disorder with physical symptoms and somatic delusions. Nonpsychiatric disorders and psychological factors affecting physical illness include malingering and chemical dependency

(Hathaway, 1988). These diagnoses are difficult to make, quite rare, and should be left to the judgement of the mental health professional. Patients with chronic pain of varying etiologies have often been unfairly labeled as psychiatric patients. Neither the style of pain presentation nor the chronicity of the problem is cause for making a psychiatric diagnosis. The presence of an irritating style or even the presence of a diagnosed psychiatric disturbance does not preclude the existence of physical pathology.

DIAGNOSTIC CLASSIFICATION OF TEMPOROMANDIBULAR DISORDERS

Defining most TMD conditions which produce musculoskeletal pain and dysfunction has been difficult due to the lack of clear etiologic factors and the lack of knowledge regarding the natural progression of TMD, as well as the lack of homogeneity of the patient population. However, as previously mentioned the American Academy of Craniomandibular Disorders had developed a well defined diagnostic classification for TMD that may be added to the Classification and Diagnostic Criteria for Headache Disorders, Cranial Neuralgias and Facial Pain by the International Headache Society (McNeill, 1990b). This effort will help emphasize the role of TMD in headache and orofacial pain. The proposed diagnostic TMD classification system for TMD is integrated with the existing medical diagnostic system, and thus, facilitates communication and shared responsibility among dentists, physicians, and allied health care providers in managing patients with TMD. However, some confusion still exists, particularly in distinguishing the muscle pain disorders (tension headache, mixed muscular vascular headache, myofascial pain, and fibromyalgia).

Temporomandibular disorders are listed in the diagnostic classification under the 11th major classification, namely, headache or facial pain associated with disorders of the cranium, neck, eyes, ears, nose, sinuses, teeth, mouth, or other facial or cranial structures (see Table III).

Temporomandibular disorders are divided into disorders of the cranial bones including the mandible, temporomandibular joint disorders, and masticatory muscle disorders. Since most disorders of the cranial bones and mandible are congenital or developmental disorders they are rarely accompanied by orofacial pain. They include agenesis, hypoplasia, condylolysis, hyperplasia, and neoplasia (McNeill, 1990b). Since they are primarily disorders that cause problems with aesthetics and/or function, the diagnostic criteria will not be presented here. Important exceptions are osteomyelitis, multiple myeloma, Pagets' Disease, and pain associated with altered function.

Table III. Recommended Diagnostic Classification For:

11.	Headache or Facial Pain Associated with Disorders of Cranium, Eyes, Ears, Nose, Sinuses, Teeth, Mouth or Other Facial or Cranial Structures
11.1	Cranial Bones Including Mandible
11.2	Neck
11.3	Eyes
11.4	Ears
11.5	Nose and Sinuses
11.6	Teeth and Related Oral Structures
11.7	Temporomandibular Joint Disorders
11.8	Masticatory Muscle Disorders

McNeill, C. (1990). Craniomandibular disorders: Guidelines for the evaluation, diagnosis and management. *Journal of Craniomandibular Disorders: Facial Oral Pain,* Special Issue.

Joint Disorders

Temporomandibular joint disorders can be divided into articular disorders related to deviation in form of the articular tissues, articular disc displacement, joint hypermobility, dislocation, inflammatory conditions, arthritides, and ankylosis (McNeill, 1990) (see table IV). These subclassifications are similar to disorders in other synovial joints in the body even though the articular surfaces of the temporomandibular joint are covered with noninnervated, avascular fibrous connective tissue as opposed to hyaline cartilage.

Deviation in Form. Deviation in form is described as irregularities or aberrations in form of intracapsular soft and hard articular tissues. It can occur because of congenital or developmental conditions, but in this category physiologic remodeling as a result of adverse loading is considered the primary etiologic factor (Moffett et al., 1964; Hansson, 1987). Adverse loading can be due to the loss of posterior tooth support, overt trauma, or microtrauma from parafunction such as tooth grinding or clenching. When the remodeling process causes a loss of integrity in the articular surfaces, a mechanical interference may result causing joint sounds on function. The condition is nonpainful and is associated with repetitive, nonvariable joint sounds that occur at the same condylar position on opening and closing of the mandible (Carlsson and Oberg, 1974).

Disc Displacement. Articular disc displacement is the most common TM joint arthropathy and is characterized by several stages of clinical dysfunction involving the condyle disc relationship (Farrar, 1972; Dolwick, 1983). Although posterior (Blankestijn & Boering, 1985) and

Table IV. Recommended Diagnostic Classification For:

11.7 Temporomandibular Joint Disorders
    11.7.1 Deviation in Form
    11.7.2 Disc Displacement
        11.7.2.1 Disc Displacement with Reduction
        11.7.2.2 Disc Displacement without Reduction
    11.7.3 Hypermobility
    11.7.4 Dislocation
    11.7.5 Inflammatory Conditions
        11.7.5.1 Synovitis
        11.7.5.2 Capsulitis
    11.7.6 Arthritides
        11.7.6.1 Osteoarthrosis
        11.7.6.2 Osteoarthritis
        11.7.6.3 Polyarthritides
    11.7.7 Ankylosis
        11.7.7.1 Fibrous
        11.7.7.2 Bony

McNeill, C. (1990). Craniomandibular disorders: Guidelines for the evaluation, diagnosis and management. *Journal of Craniomandibular Disorders: Facial Oral Pain,* Special Issue.

mediolateral (Khoury & Dolan, 1986) displacements of the articular disc have been described, the usual direction for displacement is an anterior or anteromedial direction (Isberg Holm & Westesson, 1982; Farrar & McCarty, 1982). Disc displacement is subdivided into disc displacement with reduction or disc displacement without reduction.

In the disorder of disc displacement with reduction, the "temporarily" displaced or misaligned disc abruptly reduces or improves it's structural relationship with the condyle during mandibular translation producing a joint noise (sound) described as clicking (popping). It is described as an abrupt alteration or interference of the disc-condyle structural relationship during mandibular translation, and is usually characterized by what is termed "reciprocal clicking". Reciprocal clicking refers to the reciprocal noise that is heard sometime during the opening movement and again just before the teeth occlude during the closing movement. The closing noise is usually of less magnitude and is thought to be produced by the displacement once again of the disc in the anterior or anteromedial position. Pain, when present, is precipitated by joint movement and usually occurs at the time of the disc reduction. The momentary jamming, misalignment, or displacement of the disc has been theorized to be due to articular surface irregularity, disc articular surface adherence, synovial fluid degradation, disc condyle incoordination due to abnormal muscle function, increased muscle activity across the joint, disc deformation, or gross injury resulting in stretching or tearing of the disc, ligaments, and/ or capsule of the joint. As the condition becomes more chronic or as the disc becomes further displaced, it begins to interfere later in the translating (opening) movement. Previously used terms for this condition are internal derangement, anterior disc displacement, reciprocal disc, and disc condyle incoordination.

Disc displacement without reduction is described as an altered or misaligned disc-condyle structural relationship that is maintained during mandibular translation. Thus, the disc is nonreducing or "permanently" displaced and does not improve its relationship with the condyle on translation; in fact, the relationship may become worse. It sometimes is referred to as a "closed lock". It is characterized by limited jaw motion because of a jamming or fixation of the disc secondary to disc adhesion, deformation, and/or dystrophy. Disc displacement without reduction can be acute or chronic. If the condition is acute there usually is pain precipitated by function. There is a marked limited mandibular opening due to the disc remaining anterior to the condyle. It is manifested clinically as a straight line deviation to the affected side on opening, a marked limited laterotrusion to the contralateral side, and a lack of joint noise. If the condition is chronic, it usually is not painful or, if present, the pain is markedly reduced from the acute stage. If chronic, there usually is a history of joint noise and/or limitation of mandibular opening (Eversole & Machado, 1985).

Hypermobility. Hypermobility of the TM joint, also referred to as subluxation, hypertranslation, hyperextension, and ligament laxity, defines excessive mobility of the disc and/or condyle well beyond the eminence. When present, patients may exhibit associated symptoms such as disc condyle incoordination or open condyle dislocation. Hypermobility is characterized by excessive condylar translation and excessive joint play (end feel) which is thought to be related to discal and capsular ligament laxity. Joint noise, when present, is usually not reproducible and many times occurs near the end of mandibular opening. The noise can be present with rapid mandibular movement but may disappear with routine function or superior support or loading of the mandible. Condylar hypermobility is often bilateral, asymptomatic, and insignificant.

Dislocation. Temporomandibular joint dislocation, also known as open lock or subluxation, describes a condition in which the condyle is positioned anterior to the articular eminence and/or disc and is unable to return to a closed position. It is manifested clinically as an inability to close the jaw. Dislocation may be the result of (1) a physical jamming of the disc condyle complex beyond the articular eminence that is maintained by muscular activity; (2) a true hyperextension of the disc condyle complex beyond its normal maximum translation position; or (3) failure of the disc to rotate about the condyle during jaw closure due to disc distortion and attachment elongation. The duration of dislocation can be prolonged and patients are only able to normalize jaw function with manipulation by a clinician. The condition is termed a subluxation if the patient can reduce the condyle on their own in seconds to minutes. Clinically there usually is an excessive range of motion which is not painful, but, pain can occur at the time of dislocation with residual pain following the episode.

Inflammatory Conditions. Primary inflammatory conditions of the TM joint are relatively uncommon and are associated primarily with rheumatologic disease. Inflammatory conditions, synovitis or capsulitis, frequently occur secondary to trauma or irritation and often accompany other TM joint disorders. Synovitis is described as an inflammation of the synovial lining of the TM joint, which can be due to infection, an immunologic condition secondary to cartilage degeneration, or trauma. Capsulitis is described as inflammation of the capsule related to ligamentous sprain, contusion, or tear as a result of trauma. However, the differences between synovitis and capsulitis are almost impossible to determine clinically. This also applies to the previously used terms of discitis and retrodiscitis, which are even more difficult to precisely differentiate. Synovitis is characterized by localized pain which is exacerbated by function, superior, and/or posterior joint loading. Many times there will be a fluctuating swelling due to effusion creating decreased ability to occlude on the ipsilateral posterior teeth. Capsulitis is commonly diagnosed by localized point tenderness on palpation of temporomandibular joint and by pain which is exacerbated by function especially with stretching of capsule at the end of the range of motion or manipulative distraction. Both conditions cause limited range of motion secondary to pain.

Arthritides. Arthritides of the TM joint include localized noninflammatory osteoarthrosis, inflammatory osteoarthritis, and generalized polyarthritides (Carlsson et al., 1979). Osteoarthrosis is defined as a degenerative, noninflammatory condition of the joint characterized by structural changes of the joint surfaces secondary to excessive strain in the remodeling mechanism (De Bont et al., 1985). The onset is insidious and usually not associated with systemic disease. As degeneration occurs there is a deterioration and abrasion of the articular cartilage and remodeling of underlying bone (Kopp, 1977). The process accelerates as proteoglycan depletion, collagen fiber network disintegration, and fatty degeneration weakens the functional capacity of the articular cartilage. Previous terms commonly used were osteoarthritis, arthritis, degenerative joint disease, and arthrosis deformans. Osteoarthrosis is characterized clinically by an absence of pain, possible crepitus, and usually a limited range of motion and deviation to the affected side on opening secondary to degeneration. Radiographically there is evidence of structural bony changes.

Osteoarthritis is a degenerative condition accompanied by secondary inflammation (synovitis) of the TM joint. Osteoarthritis is frequently localized to the temporomandibular joint in question but may be a part of a generalized condition (Blackwood, 1963; Toller, 1973). It is characterized by pain due to the synovitis, point tenderness on palpation, crepitus, limited range of motion with deviation on opening to the affected side, and radiographic evidence of structural bony changes. The articular changes are associated with (1) external or overt jaw trauma, (2) repetitive adverse loading, (3) infection or, (4) an idiopathic degenerative process. Although coarse crepitus can be diagnostic, confirming the diagnosis is based on joint imaging. Previously used terms were arthritis, osteoarthrosis and degenerative joint disease.

Joint inflammation and structural change caused by a generalized systemic polyarthritic condition are referred to as polyarthritides. Temporomandibular joint polyarthritides include rheumatoid arthritis, juvenile rheumatoid arthritis (Still's disease), spondyloarthropathies (ankylosing spondylitis, psoriatic arthritis, infectious arthritis, Reiter's syndrome) crystal induced disease (gout, hyperuricemia). Other rheumatologically related diseases that may affect the TM joint include auto immune disorders and other mixed connective tissue diseases (Scleroderma, Sjogren's syndrome, Lupus erythematosus). Polyarthritides are characterized by pain during acute and subacute stages, possible crepitus, limited range of motion secondary to pain and/or degeneration, and bilateral radiographic evidence of structural bony changes. This group of arthritides comprises multiple diagnostic categories which are best diagnosed with the aid of serology and managed by rheumatologists. Dental management relates to secondary complaints. Bilateral resorption of condylar structures can result in an anterior open bite (lack of overlap of the anterior teeth) in many cases.

Ankylosis. Ankylosis is defined as a restricted mandibular movement with deviation to the affected side on opening. It implies a firm, unyielding restriction due to either intra-articular fibrous or bony ankylosis and is not associated with pain. Fibrous adhesions within the TM joint are thought to occur mainly in the superior compartment of the TM joint. They produce a decreased movement of the disc condyle complex. Adhesions can occur secondary to joint inflammation resulting from macrotrauma or systemic conditions such as a polyarthrotic disease. Bony ankylosis results from the union of the bones of the TM joint by proliferation of bone cells resulting in complete immobility of that joint. No radiographic findings other than absence of ipsilateral condylar translation on opening are found with fibrous ankylosis. Bony ankylosis is characterized by radiographic evidence of bone proliferation with marked deviation to the affected side and marked limited laterotrusion to the contralateral side.

Masticatory Muscle Disorders

Masticatory muscle disorders include seven distinct disorders which are analogous to muscle disorders that can occur in other areas of the head, neck, body, and extremities. They include myofascial pain, myositis, spasm, reflex splinting, muscle contracture, hypertrophy, and neoplasm (McNeill, 1990b) (see Table V).

Table V. Recommended Diagnostic Classification For:

11.8 Craniofacial Muscle Disorders

    11.8.1 Myofascial Pain

    11.8.2 Myositis

    11.8.3 Spasm

    11.8.4 Reflex Splinting

    11.8.5 Contracture

    11.8.6 Hypertrophy

    11.8.7 Neoplasm

McNeill, C. (1990). Craniomandibular disorders: Guidelines for the evaluation, diagnosis and management. *Journal of Craniomandibular Disorders: Facial Oral Pain,* Special Issue.

Fibromyalgia, also termed myofascitis, myofibrositis, or fibrositis, is not considered a specific masticatory muscle disorder since it is manifested as a generalized, continuous, aching pain and associated with tenderness in many sites over the body, sleep disturbances and depression. It may also be associated with generalized fatigue, chronic headache, anxiety, subjective swelling, irritable bowel syndrome, and modulation of the symptoms by activity or the weather. Descriptors include pain in three of four quadrants for at least three months, tenderness in 11 of 18 specific spots, and association with normal EMG activity (Fricton & Awad, 1990).

Myofascial Pain. Myofascial pain (myalgia, trigger point pain, myofascial pain dysfunction syndrome, muscle contraction headache, and tension headache) is characterized by a regional, dull aching pain, presence of localized tender spots (trigger points) in muscle, tendons, or fascia which reproduce pain when palpated, and may produce a characteristic pattern of regional referred pain and/or autonomic symptoms on palpation (Shifman, 1984; Clark, 1985; Solberg, 1986; Fricton & Awad, 1990). The myalgia can be associated with postural hypertonicity, parafunction (bruxism), or intermittent overuse. Palpation of the "active" trigger points causes reproducible alteration of pain complaints typically to a much more extensive area that may or may not include the muscle containing the trigger points (Travell & Simons, 1983; Fricton et al., 1985). Inactivation of the trigger point area with local anesthesia, stretch, or ice relieves the larger area of pain. The pathogenesis is not well understood. Although there is some evidence that a localized ischemia may cause the characteristic trigger point sensitivity, recently interest has focused on the central nervous system including the sympathetic nervous system as the mediator of myofascial pain.

Myositis. Myositis is an acute, painful, generalized inflammation and swelling of usually the entire muscle. Clinically, the patient may exhibit a limited range of motion. Myositis is usually due to local causes such as infection or trauma. Ossification of a muscle can occur secondary to inflammation resulting in myositis ossificans. The inflammation may occur in the tendinous attachments of the muscle as well, and then the term that is used is tendinitis or tendomyositis.

Spasm. Muscle spasm (myospasm, acute trismus, or cramp) is an acute disorder and is an involuntary, sudden, tonic contraction of a muscle. A muscle in spasm is acutely shortened, grossly limited in range of motion, and painful. It is caused by overstretching of a previously weakened muscle or acute overuse of a muscle. Spasm is a continuous muscle contraction (fasciculation) and can therefore be differentiated from protective reflex splinting by clinical inspection or electromyographic (EMG) verification of sustained involuntary muscle contraction even at rest.

Reflex Splinting. Reflex splinting or protective splinting is defined as restricted or guarded jaw movement due to reflex rigidity of muscle(s) as a means of avoiding pain caused by movement of the parts (Tveteras & Kristensen, 1986). Reflex splinting is characterized by a limited range of motion, rigidity of jaw on manipulation, and pain. This problem can be further differentiated into reflex protective splinting in order to avoid a painful dysfunction such as painful TM joint clicking or traumatic trismus due to operative trauma or regional injury. Another type of reflex splinting is mediated centrally and is termed hysterical trismus, a severe restriction of mandibular motion due to acute psychological distress (Revington et al., 1985). Patients with protective splinting or trismus seldom exhibit muscle contraction when the jaw is at rest with the exception of hysterical trismus.

Contracture. Muscle contracture (chronic trismus, muscle fibrosis, or muscle scarring) is a chronic resistance of a muscle to passive stretch as a result of fibrosis of the supporting tendons, ligaments, or muscle fibers themselves. Muscle contracture is usually caused by trauma but can result from infection or any disorder resulting in hypomobility. Generally, it is not painful, but if painful, the pain decreases as fibrous scarring and hypermobility increase. Clinically there is an unyielding firmness on passive stretch.

Hypertrophy. Muscle hypertrophy is a generalized, abnormal enlargement of muscle tissue. There usually is not a limitation in the range of motion. Hypertrophy frequently involves the entire muscle and may be a benign idiopathic condition or a functional adaptation to hyperactivity. It may occur bilaterally or unilaterally. As with contracture, when hypertrophy develops over a long time, it is not usually painful.

Neoplasia. Masticatory muscle neoplasia is defined as a new, abnormal, or uncontrolled growth of muscle tissue. It can be malignant or benign and may or may not be associated with pain. An example of a muscle neoplasm is a myxoma.

EVALUATION

The goals for evaluation of TMD patients are to determine the primary and any secondary physical and/or mental diagnoses, the contributing factors, and the level of complexity of the patient's problem. However, establishing the correct diagnosis in patients with TMD and orofacial pain is difficult because of the complex psychosocial and somatic interrelationship of chronic pain. Many disorders have similar signs and symptoms and there is a high frequency of multiple diagnoses. Although individual clinicians are successful in diagnosing the more simple TMD problems, a team approach is often required for managing complex chronic TMD problems, in particular for evaluating psychological disorders that may be present. In order to ensure that all the information that may be of value in planning treatment and predicting outcome is evaluated, a multiaxial diagnostic system is suggested. A present multiaxial evaluation system model, the DSM III R model, includes: Clinical syndromes (Axis I); Developmental and Personality Disorders (Axis II); Physical disorders and conditions (Axis III); Severity of psychosocial stressors (Axis IV); and Global assessment of functioning (Axis V). This type of biopsychosocial approach to diagnosis has the benefit of combining the mental and physical disorders along with other contributing factors. The first three axes are specific diagnostic assessments and the last two provide supplementary information that may be helpful in predicting outcome. The model could be altered in order to place equal weight to the physical diagnosis and to increase the efficacy for diagnosis of orofacial pain disorders and TMD. The suggested simplified multiaxial pain classification would be as follows:

Axis I Primary clinical diagnosis using the International Headache Society's diagnostic classification for headache, cranial neuralgias, and facial pain, or the International Classification of Diseases codes (ICD.9.cm) and/or the DSM III R codes.

Axis II — Secondary clinical diagnosis(es) again using the above classification codes.

Axis III — Other physical or mental disorders and conditions that may be relevant to the understanding or management of the patient, i.e., diabetes.

Axis IV — Severity of Psychosocial stressors as coded in the DSM-III R scale of O through 6.

Axis V — Global assessment of functioning or outcome estimate (prognosis) given as a percentage.

Collection of baseline records and other diagnostic data is fundamental to the proper management of TMD since the evaluation goals are predicated on an accurate and complete evaluation. The extent to which any or all of the elements of evaluation are pursued depends upon the magnitude of the presenting complaints and the potential for the problem progressing physically or psychosocially. Screening for TMD is recommended as an essential part of all routine dental and/or craniofacial pain examinations. The screening is comprised of a questionnaire, brief history, and examination (McNeill, 1990a) (see Tables VI & VII).

The aim of screening is to determine the presence or absence of TMD signs and symptoms. If significant findings are identified and recorded, a comprehensive history and examination should be conducted (Griffith, 1983; Clark et al., 1989). The comprehensive history parallels the traditional medical history and review of systems. The comprehensive physical examination consists of a general inspection of the head and neck; a comprehensive orthopedic evaluation of the TM joint and cursory evaluation of the cervical spine; a masticatory and cervical muscle evaluation; neurovascular, neurosensory, and motor evaluation of the cranial nerves; and an intra oral evaluation including an occlusal (bite) analysis.

Imaging of the TM joint and orofacial structures may be necessary to rule out structural disorders. Panoramic and dental periapical radiographs are recommended to screen for gross tooth, periodontal, or mandibular and maxillary pathology. Special radiographic techniques, such as sialography, sinus series, radionuclide studies, and angiography may be needed in order to rule out other pathology. The extensive technology available for TM joint imaging provides clinicians with multiple options.

Radiography of the TM joint structures are prescribed primarily when the clinical examination suggests some form of joint pathology (Lindvall et al., 1976). They may include tomography or transcranial TM joint films including lateral pharyngeal, transorbital, and modified Townes

Table VI. Recommended Screening Questionnaire for TMD

1. Do you have difficulty or pain, or both, when opening your mouth, as for instance, when yawning?

2. Does your jaw get "stuck", "locked", or "go out"?

3. Do you have difficulty or pain, or both, when chewing, talking, or using your jaws?

4. Are you aware of noises in the jaw joints?

5. Do you have pain in or about the ears, temples, or cheeks?

6. Does your bite feel uncomfortable or unusual?

7. Do you have frequent headaches?

8. Have you had a recent injury to your head, neck, or jaw?

9. Have you previously been treated for a jaw joint problem? If so, when?

Note: If any one of the first three questions is answered affirmatively, the clinician should complete a comprehensive history and examination; for questions 4 through 8, two should be answered affirmatively, and for question 9, a positive answer to two other questions (4 8) is required to warrant further evaluation.

McNeill C., Mohl N., Rugh J., & Tanaka T. (1990). Temporomandibular disorders: Diagnosis, management, education, and research. *Journal of the American Dental Association, 120* :253.

views of the jaws. Corrected cephalometric tomography is the most accurate method for radiographically examining patients with suspected TM joint degenerative joint disease (Rohlin et al., 1986; Pullinger et al., 1986; Petersson & Rohlin, 1988). Computed axial tomography (C.T.) is valuable as an adjunct imaging technique in the assessment of bony abnormalities, i.e., developmental anomalies, trauma, and neoplastic conditions of the TM joint (Raustia et al, 1985; Paz et al., 1988). Magnet resonance imaging (MRI) has diverse capabilities for examination of most cases of suspected TM joint soft tissue disorders, i.e., disc displacement (Carr et al., 1987; Westesson et al., 1987; Sanchez Woodworth et al., 1988; Helms et al., 1989a, 1989b). In general, a patient should have an imaging study when the results may change treatment strategy (American Dental Association, 1984).

Basic assessment of all TMD patients should include a behavioral and psychosocial evaluation. The history should include questions to evaluate behavioral, social, emotional, and cognitive factors which may initiate,

Table VII. Recommended Screening Examination Procedures for TMD

1. Measure range of motion of the mandible on opening and right and left laterotrusion.

2. Palpate for pre auricular TMJ tenderness.

3. Palpate for TMJ crepitus.

4. Palpate for TMJ clicking.

5. Palpate for tenderness in the masseter and temporalis muscles.

6. Note excessive occlusal wear, excessive tooth mobility, fremitus, or migration in the absence of periodontal disease, and soft tissue alterations, for example, buccal mucosal ridging, lateral tongue scalloping.

7. Inspect symmetry and alignment of the face, jaws, and dental arches.

Note: Any positive finding for procedures 1 through 3 warrants consideration for a comprehensive history and examination, whereas any two positive findings for procedures 4 through 6 suggest the same consideration; procedure 7 requires two other positive findings (4-6) to suggest the same consideration.

McNeill C., Mohl N., Rugh J., & Tanaka T. (1990). Temporomandibular disorders: Diagnosis, management, education, and research. *Journal of the American Dental Association, 120*:253.

sustain, or result from the patient's condition. Comprehensive psychological inventories, such as the Minnesota Multi phasic Personality Inventory (MMPI), are not necessary for routine screening (Olson, 1982). However, the clinician should screen specifically for oral habits, signs of depression, anxiety, stressful life events, lifestyle, secondary gain, and overuse of health care. A variety of additional diagnostic studies are available for use in selected cases to assist in confirming a physical diagnosis. Diagnostic tests can include laboratory tests (blood chemistries), diagnostic injections, and diagnostic dental casts. These tests should not be considered as routine procedures, but rather be used to supplement knowledge gained during the history, examination, and imaging.

MANAGEMENT

Management goals for patients with TMD are similar to those for patients with other orthopedic or rheumatologic disorders, namely: reduce pain, reduce adverse loading, restore function, and restore normal daily activities. These goals are best achieved by a well defined program designed to treat the physical and psychological disorder(s) and reduce the contributing factors. The management options and sequencing of treatment are consistent with treatment of other musculoskeletal disorders.

Like many musculoskeletal conditions, the signs and symptoms of TMD may be transient and self limiting, resolving without serious long term effects (Mejersjo & Carlsson, 1983; Greene & Laskin, 1988). However, little is known about which signs and symptoms will progress to more serious conditions and the natural course of TMD. For these reasons, a special effort should be made to avoid aggressive, nonreversible therapy, such as complex occlusal therapy or surgery. Conservative treatment, such as patient education and palliative home care (McNeill, 1983b), behavioral modification (Rugh, 1987), physical therapy (Danzig & Van Dyke, 1983; Friedman & Weisberg, 1985), medications (Gregg & Rugh, 1988), and orthopedic appliances (interocclusal splints) (Clark, 1984) are endorsed for the initial care of nearly all TMD. The emphasis should be on conservative therapy that facilitates the musculoskeletal system's natural healing capacity and treatment that involves the patient in the physical and behavioral management of their own problem.

The majority of patients with TMD achieve good relief of symptoms with noninvasive, conservative therapy (Apfelberg et al., 1979; Greene & Laskin, 1983; Carlsson, 1985; Okeson and Hayes, 1986). Despite the success of conservative care, some patients with TMD do not improve with this strategy. The reasons for this vary considerably, but generally fall into two groups, those with pain and dysfunction due to major structural changes in the joint and those with complex chronic pain syndromes complicated by multiple contributing factors. In the first situation, TM joint surgery is often indicated (American Association of Oral and Maxillofacial Surgeons, 1984, 1988). In the second situation, a chronic pain management program with a team of clinicians is needed. With a team, various aspects of the problem can be addressed by different specialists enhancing the overall potential for success. Teams can be interdisciplinary (one setting) or multidisciplinary (multiple settings). In either approach, success is dependent on communication and integration among clinicians. Management goals are best achieved by using the optimal combination and sequence of treatment options in the context of the overall management program (Fricton & Hathaway, 1988).

Although temporomandibular disorders are a medical condition (musculoskeletal and/or rheumatologic), many physicians are not trained to treat TMD and/or complex chronic pain patients (Pilowsky, 1988), and therefore, usually prefer not to treat TMD patients. Many referrals to dentists and clinics specializing in TMD and orofacial pain come from physicians and other health professionals. This patient population, although relatively small in contrast to other dental needs, often has serious disabilities related to complicated chronic pain syndromes. Because of their training in the anatomy, function, and pathophysiology of the oral and facial structures, dentists have appropriately assumed responsibility in diagnosing and treating TMD. However, complex chronic orofacial pain, including complex chronic TMD pain, is best managed by a well trained, multi or interdisciplinary team of health professionals.

REFERENCES

American Association of Oral and Maxillofacial Surgeons. (1984). *Position paper on TMJ Surgery.* Ad hoc committees, Chicago, 1984.

American Association of Oral and Maxillofacial Surgeons. (1988). *Position paper on TMJ Arthroscopy.* Ad hoc committees, Chicago.

American Dental Association (ADA): Recommendations in radiographic practices, 1984. Council on Dental Materials, Instruments, and Equipment. *Journal of the American Dental Association, 109*:764.

Agerberg, G., & Carlsson, G. (1972). Functional disorders of the masticatory system. Distribution of symptoms according to age and sex as judged from investigation by questionnaire. *ACTA Odontologica Scandinavica, 30*:597.

Apfelberg, D., Lovey, E., Janetos. G., Maser, M., & Lash, H. (1979). Temporomandibular joint disease. Results of a ten year study. *Post Graduate Medicine, 65*:167 172.

Bell, W. (1989). *Orofacial pains. Classification, diagnosis, management* (4th ed.) Chicago: Year Book Medical Publishers.

Bell, W. (1990). *Temporomandibular disorders: Classification, diagnosis, management* (3rd ed.) Chicago: Year Book Medical Publishers.

Blackwood, H. (1963). Arthritis of the mandibular joint. *British Dental Journal, 115*:317 376.

Blankestijn & Boering (1985). Posterior dislocation of the temporomandibular disc. *International Journal of Oral Surgery, 14*:437 443.

Bonica, J. (1984). Pain research and therapy: Recent advances and future needs. (pp. 1 22) In L. Kruger & J. Liebeskind (Eds.), *Advances in pain research and therapy* (Vol. 6). New York: Raven Press.

Campbell, J. (1987). Cluster headache. *Journal of Craniomandibular Disorders and Facial Oral Pain, 1*:27 33.

Carlsson, G., & Oberg, T. (1974). Remodeling of the temporomandibular joints. *Oral Science Review, 4*:53 86.

Carlsson, G., Kopp, S., & Oberg, T. (1979). Arthritis and allied diseases. In G. Zarb & G. Carlsson (Eds.) *Temporomandibular joint function and dysfunction.* (pp. 269 320). Copenhagen: Munksgaard.

Carlsson, G. (1985). Long term effects of treatment of craniomandibular disorders. *Journal of Craniomandibular Practice, 3*:337 342.

Carr, A., Gibilisco, J., & Berquist, T. (1987). Magnetic resonance imaging of the temporomandibular joint Preliminary work. *Journal of Craniomandibular Disorders and Oral Facial Pain, 1*:89 96.

Clark, G. (1984). A critical evaluation of orthopedic interocclusal appliance therapy: Design, theory, and overall effectiveness. *Journal of the American Dental Association, 108(3)*:359.

Clark, G. (1985). Muscle hyperactivity, pain and dysfunction. In I. Klineberg & B. Sesale (Eds.), *Orofacial pain and neuromuscular dysfunction: Mechanisms and clinical correlates.* (pp. 103 111). Sydney: Pergamon Press.

Clark, G., Seligman, D., Solberg, W., & Pullinger, A. (1989). Guidelines for the examination and diagnosis of temporomandibular disorders. *Journal of Craniomandibular Disorders and Facial Oral Pain, 3*:6 14.

Cephalgia, An international journal of headache (1988). *Classification and diagnostic criteria for headache disorders, cranial neuralgias and facial pain.* Vol. 8, Suppl. 7. Oslo, Norway: Norwegian University Press.

Crook, J., Rideout, E., & Browne, G. (1984). The prevalence of pain complaints in the general population. *Pain, 18*:299 314.

Danzig, W., & Van Dyke, A. (1983). Physical therapy as an adjunct to temporomandibular joint therapy. *Journal of Prosthetic Dentistry, 49*:96 99.

DeBont, L., Boering, G., Liem, R., & Havinga, P. (1985). Osteoarthritis of the temporomandibular joint: A light microscopic and scanning electron microscopic study of the articular cartilage of the mandibular condyle. *Journal of Oral Maxillofacial Surgery, 43*:481.

Diagnostic & statistical manual of mental disorders (3rd ed.) Revised. (1987). Washington, D.C.: American Psychiatric Association.

Dolwick, M. (1983). Diagnosis and etiology of internal derangements of the temporomandibular joint. In D. Laskin, W. Greenfield, E. Gale, et al. (Eds.), *The president's conference on the examination, diagnosis and management of temporomandibular joint disorders.* (pp. 112 117). Chicago: American Dental Association.

Donaldson, D., & Kroening, R. (1979). Recognition and treatment of patients with chronic orofacial pain. *Journal of the American Dental Association, 99*:961.

Dworkin, S., & Burgess, J. (1987). Orofacial pain of psychogenic origin: Current concepts and classification. *Journal of the American Dental Association, 115*:565 571.

Dworkin, S., Hanson Huggins, K., LeResche, L., et al. (1990). Epidemiology of signs and symptoms in temporomandibular disorders: 1. Clinical signs in cases and controls. *Journal of the American Dental Association, 120*:273.

Edmeads, J. (1987). Migraine. *Journal of Craniomandibular Disorders and Facial Oral Pain, 1*:21 25.

Eversole, L., & Machado, L. (1985). Temporomandibular joint internal derangements and associated neuromuscular disorders. *Journal of the American Dental Association, 110*:69 79.

Farrar, W. (1972). Differentiation of temporomandibular joint dysfunction to simplify treatment. *Journal of Prosthetic Dentistry, 28*:629 636.

Farrar, W., & McCarty, W., Jr. (1982). *A clinical outline of temporomandibular joint diagnosis and treatment.* (7th ed.) Montgomery: Normandie.

Fields, H. (1987). *Pain.* (pp. 145 158). New York: McGraw Hill Book Co.

Fricton, J., Kroening, R., Haley, D., & Siegert, R. (1985). Myofascial pain syndrome of the head and neck: A review of clinical characteristics of 164 patients. *Oral Surgery Oral Medicine Oral Pathology, 60*:615 627.

Fricton, J., & Hathaway, K. (1988). Interdisciplinary management: Address complexity with teamwork. In J. Fricton, R. Kroening, & K. Hathaway (Eds.), *TMJ & craniofacial pain: Diagnosis and management.* (pp. 167 172). St. Louis: Ishiyaku, Euro American, Inc.

Fricton, J., Kroening, R., & Schellhas, K. (1988). Differential diagnosis, the physical disorder. In J. Fricton, R. Kroening, & K. Hathaway (Eds.), *TMJ and craniofacial pain: Diagnosis and management.* (pp. 53 65). St. Louis: Ishiyaku, Euro American, Inc.

Fricton, J., & Kroening, R. (1988). Neuralgic disorders: Peripheral nerve pain. In J. Fricton, R. Kroening, & K. Hathaway (Eds.), *TMJ and craniofacial pain: Diagnosis and management.* (pp. 131 137). St. Louis: Ishiyaku Euro America Inc.

Fricton, J., & Awad, E. (1990). Advances in pain research and therapy, Vol. 17, *Myofacial pain and fibromyalgia.* New York: Raven Press.

Friedman, M., & Weisberg, J. (1985). *Temporomandibular joint disorders diagnosis and treatment.* (pp. 124 140). Chicago: Quintessence Publishing Co.

Greene, C., & Laskin, D. (1983). Long-term evaluation of treatment for myofascial pain dysfunction syndrome: A comparative analysis. *Journal of the American Dental Association, 107(2)*:235 238.

Greene, C., & Laskin, D. (1988). Long-term status of TMJ clicking in patients with myofascial pain dysfunction. *Journal of the American Dental Association, 117*:461 465.

Gregg, J., & Rugh, J. (1988). Pharmacological therapy. In N. Mohl, G. Zarb, G. Carlsson, & J. Rugh (Eds.), *A textbook on occlusion.* (pp. 351 375). Chicago: Quintessence Publishing Co.

Griffiths, R. (1983). Report of the president's conference on examination, diagnosis and management of temporomandibular disorders. *Journal of the American Dental Association, 106*: 75 78.

Hansson, T. (1987). Temporomandibular joint anatomical findings relevant to the clinician. In G. Clark & W. Solberg (Eds.), *Perspectives in temporomandibular disorders.* Chicago: Quintessence Publishing Co.

Hathaway, K. (1988). Behavioral and psychosocial evaluation: Understanding the whole patient. In J. Fricton, R. Kroening, & K. Hathaway (Eds.), *TMJ and craniofacial pain: Diagnosis and management.* (pp. 153-166). St. Louis: Ishiyaku Euro America Inc.

Harris, L., & Associates (1985). *The Nuprin Pain Report,* Study No. 851017, New York.

Helkimo, M. (1974). Studies on function and dysfunction of the masticatory system. I: An epidemiological investigation of symptoms of dysfunction in Lapps in the North of Finland. *Proceedings of the Finnish Dental Society, 70*:37 49.

Helkimo, M. (1974). Studies of function and dysfunction of the masticatory system. II: Index for anamnestic and clinical dysfunction and occlusal state. *Swedish Dental Journal, 67*:101-121.

Helms, C., Kaban, L., McNeill, C., & Dodson, T. (1989a). Temporomandibular joint: Morphology and signal intensity characteristics of the disc at MR imaging. *Radiology, 172*:817-820.

Helms, C., Doyle, G., Orwig, D., et al. (1989b). Staging of internal derangements of the TMJ with magnetic resonance imaging: Preliminary observations. *Journal of Craniomandibular Disorders and Facial Oral Pain, 3*:93 99.

Howard, J. (1990). Temporomandibular joint disorders, facial pain and dental problems of performing artists. In R. Sataloff, A. Brandfonbrener, & R. Lederman, (Eds.), *Textbook of performing arts medicine.* New York: Raven Press.

Ingervall, B., Mohlin, B., & Thilander, B. (1980). Prevalence of symptoms of functional disturbances of the masticatory system in Swedish men. *Journal of Oral Rehabilitation, 7*:185 197.

Isberg Holm, A., & Westesson, P. (1982). Movement of the disc and condyle in temporomandibular joints with clicking: An arthrographic and cineradiographic study on autopsy specimens. *ACTA Odontologica Scandinavica, 40*:151 164.

McNeill, C. (1983b). Nonsurgical management. In C. Helms, R. Katzberg, & M. Dolwick (Eds.), *Internal derangements of the temporomandibular joint.* (pp. 193 227). University of California, San Francisco: Radiology Research and Education Foundation.

McNeill, C. (1985). The optimum temporomandibular joint condyle position in clinical practice. *International Journal of Periodontics and Restorative Dentistry - North and South America, 6*:53.

McNeill, C., Mohl, N., Rugh, J., & Tanaka, T. (1990a). Temporomandibular disorders: Diagnosis, management, education, and research. *Journal of the American Dental Association, 120*:253.

McNeill, C. (1990b). Craniomandibular disorders: Guidelines for the evaluation, diagnosis and management. *Journal of Craniomandibular Disorders and Facial Oral Pain,* Special Issue.

Magnusson, T., & Carlsson, G. (1978). Recurrent headaches in relation to temporomandibular joint pain dysfunction. *ACTA Ondontologica Scandinavica, 36*:333 338.

Magnusson, T., & Carlsson, G. (1980). Changes in recurrent headache and mandibular dysfunction after various types of dental treatment. *ACTA Odontologica Scandinavica, 38*:311 320.

Mealiea, W., & McGlynn, D. (1987). Temporomandibular disorders and bruxism. In J. Hatch, J. Fisher, & J. Rugh (Eds.), *Biofeedback studies in clinical efficacy.* (pp. 123 151). New York: Plenum Press.

Mejersjo, C., & Carlsson, G. (1983). Long-term results of treatment for temporomandibular pain-dysfunction. *Journal of Prosthetic Dentistry, 49(6)*:809 815.

Moffett, B., Johnson, L., McCabe, J., & Askew, H. (1964). Articular remodeling in the adult human temporomandibular joint. *American Journal of Anatomy,* 115:119 142.

Nickerson, J., & Boering, G. (1989). Natural course of osteoarthrosis as it relates to internal derangement of the temporomandibular joint. *Oral Maxillofacial Surgery Clinics of North America, 1*:27 45.

Nilner, M., & Lassing, S. (1983). Relationship between oral parafunctions and functional disturbances and diseases of the stomatognathic system among children aged 7-14 years. *ACTA Odontologica Scandinavica, 41*:167 172.

Nilner, M. (1983). Relationship between oral parafunctions and functional disturbances in the stomatognathic system in 15 to 18 year olds. *ACTA Odontologica Scandinavica, 41*:197-201.

Okeson, J., & Hayes, D. (1986). Long term results of treatment for temporomandibular disorders: An evaluation by patients. *Journal of the American Dental Association, 112*:473 478.

Olsson, R. (1982). *Behavioral examinations in MPD.* (pp. 104-105). In D. Laskin et al. (Eds.), *The president's conference on the examination diagnosis, and management of temporomandibular disorders.*

Paz, M., Katzberg, R., Tallents, R., et al. (1988). Computed tomographic evaluation of the density of the TMJ disk. *Oral Surgery Oral Medicine Oral Pathology, 66*:519.

Petersson, A., & Rohlin, M. (1988). Rheumatoid arthritis of the temporomandibular joint. Evaluation of three different radiographic techniques by assessment of observer performance. *Dentomaxillofacial Radiology, 17*:115 120.

Pilowsky, I. (1988). An outline curriculum on pain for medical schools. *Pain, 33*:1 2.

Pullinger, A., Solberg, W., Hollender, L., & Guichet, D. (1986). Tomographic analysis of mandibular condyle position in diagnostic subgroups of temporomandibular disorders. *Journal of Prosthetic Dentistry, 55*:723 729.

Rashkin, N., & Prusiner, S. (1977). *Carotidynia, Neurology.* (Minneapolis), 27(1):43 46.

Raskin, N., & Appenzeller, O. (1980). Cluster headache. (pp. 185-198). In *Headache: Major problems in internal medicine,* Vol. 19. Philadelphia: Saunders.

Rasmussen, O. (1981). Description of population and progress of symptoms in a longitudinal study of temporomandibular arthropathy. *Scandinavian Journal of Dental Research, 89*:196 203.

Rasmussen, O. (1981). Clinical findings during the course of temporomandibular arthropathy. *Scandinavian Journal of Dental Research, 89*:283 288.

Raustia, A., Phytinen, J., & Virtanen, K. (1985). Examination of the temporomandibular joint by direct sagittal computed tomography. *Clinical Radiology, 36(3)*:291 296.

Revington, P., Peacock, T., & Kingscote, A. (1985). Temporomandibular joint dysfunction: A case of hysterical trismus. *British Dental Journal, 158(2)*:55 56.

Rohlin, M., Ackerman, S., & Kopp, S. (1986). Tomography as an aid to detect macroscopic changes in the TMJ: An autopsy study of the aged. *ACTA Odontologica Scandinavica, 44*:131.

Rugh, J. (1983). Psychological factors in the etiology of masticatory pain and dysfunction. In D. Laskin, W. Greenfield, E. Gale, J. Rugh, P. Neff, & C. Alling (Eds.), *The president's conference on the examination, diagnosis and management of temporomandibular disorders.* Chicago: American Dental Association.

Rugh, J., & Solberg, W. (1985). Oral health status in the United States: Temporomandibular disorders. *Journal of Dental Education, 49*:398 404.

Rugh, J. (1987). Psychological components of pain. *Dental Clinics of North America, 31(4)*:579 594.

Rugh, J., & Harlan, J. (1988). Nocturnal bruxism and temporomandibular disorders. *Advances in Neurology, 49*:329 341.

Sanchez Woodworth, R., Tallents, R., Katzberg, R., & Guay, J. (1988). Bilateral internal derangements of the TMJ: Evaluation by MRI imaging. *Oral Surgery Oral Medicine Oral Pathology, 65*:281.

Schiffman, E., Fricton, J., Haley, D., & Shapiro, B. (1990). The prevalence and treatment needs of subjects with temporomandibular disorders. *Journal of the American Dental Association, 120*:295.

Schiffman, E., & Fricton, J. (1988). Epidemiology of TMJ and craniofacial pain. In J. Fricton, R. Kroening, K. Hathaway (Eds.), *TMJ and craniofacial pain: Diagnosis and management.* (pp. 1 10). St. Louis: IEA Publishers.

Shifman, A. (1984). Myofascial pain associated with unilateral masseteric hypertrophy in a condylectomy patients. *Journal of Craniomandibular Disorders, 2(4)*:373 376.

Solberg, W. (1983). Epidemiology, incidence, and prevalence of temporomandibular disorders: A review. *The president's conference on the examination, diagnosis, and management of temporomandibular disorders.* Chicago: American Dental Association.

Solberg, W. (1986). Temporomandibular disorders: Masticatory myalgia and its management. *British Dental Journal, 160*:351 356.

Sternbach, R. (1986). Survey of pain in the United States: The nuprin pain report. *Clinical Journal of Pain, 2*:49 53.

Stevens, J. (1987). Cranial neuralgia. *Journal of Craniomandibular Disorders and Facial Oral Pain, 1*:51 53.

Toller, P. (1973). Osteoarthritis of the mandibular condyle. *British Dental Journal, 134* 223.

Travell, J., & Simons, D. (1983). *Myofascial pain and dysfunction: The trigger point manual.* Baltimore: Williams and Wilkins.

Tveteras, K., & Dristensen, S. (1986). The aetiology and pathogenesis of trismus. *Clinical Otolaryngology, 11(5)*:383 387.

Wanmann, A., & Agerberg, G. (1986). Headache and dysfunction of the masticatory system in adolescents. *Cephalgia, 6*:247 255.

Westesson, P., Katzberg, R., Tallents, R., et al. (1987). CT & MR of the TMJ: Comparison with autopsy specimens. *American Journal of Radiology, 148*:1165 1171.

Chapter 13

HOSPICE, CANCER PAIN MANAGEMENT, AND SYMPTOM CONTROL

B. Eliot Cole, M. D.
Mary C. Douglass, R. N., B. S. N.

B. Eliot Cole, M. D., and Mary Douglass, R. N., provide a clear presentation of palliative care as it relates to hospice pain management. This chapter integrates information for psychological support, physical care, and spirituality within a multidisciplinary care model. Insight is gained regarding patient and family involvement and helping patients achieve death with dignity.

The authors offer practical suggestions helpful for many issues involved in hospice care including relocation issues, inpatient v. home hospice, family education, and the role of team members. Clear case examples illustrate themes presented and will help the reader generalize information for their clinical setting.

Chapter 13 ▮▮▮▮

HOSPICE, CANCER PAIN MANAGEMENT, AND SYMPTOM CONTROL

B. Eliot Cole, M. D.
Mary C. Douglass, R. N., B. S. N.

Pain is the great teacher and the great foreman, but whoso has attained the Serene Life is above pain even while under it.
Anonymous

INTRODUCTION

When finding a cure for the patient is no longer possible, the emphasis shifts to palliation (Kaye, 1989). Palliative management, the focus of hospice care, affords relief and reduces the severity of bothersome symptoms, but does not produce toxicity or hasten the death of the patient (Johanson, 1988). Palliative care becomes necessary when the patient's disease is beyond real cure, when the tumor process is the cause of symptoms, when realistic treatment goals have been established, and when clear communication exists between the treatment team, the patient, and the family regarding the treatment plan (Brescia, 1987). The goal for palliative care is to improve the quality of the patient's life, while avoiding side effects worse than the symptoms being treated. Good palliative care helps a patient avoid an untimely death while correcting unnecessary pain and suffering. To realize the goal, it is essential for the involved clinicians to believe and to assess the severity of each pain complaint.

Hospice care involves a multidisciplinary approach, and a creative process of individualized management, resulting in an empowered patient who is able to experience comfort and dignity. It integrates the best of psychological support, physical care, and spirituality for the patient directly, and provides long-term bereavement assistance for the surviving loved ones. Total pain management cannot be undertaken by an individual alone, but only by individuals working together as a team (Lack, 1984).

Hospice care has been provided in the hospital, in free-standing facilities, as well as in the patient's home. It is the experience of the authors to provide hospice care primarily in the home setting with managed hospital-based respite care. Patients electing home-based hospice care preserve their dignity through control of their own care, and avoid the sense of abandonment and solitude often associated with a hospital death.

ASSESSMENT

Certain diseases can be expected to follow a predictable course, but an individualized hospice plan of care must be completed on every new admission, and then updated continuously. This comprehensive plan of care is the task of the multidisciplinary hospice team, and is ultimately intradisciplinary in scope. It begins at the moment that the patient is referred to the hospice program, and evolves as the needs of the patient change. While the initial plan of care is the collaboration of the intake nurse, primary physician, hospice medical director, and social worker, over time the other members of the intradisciplinary team, including chaplaincy and volunteers, participate in the frequent revisions.

The referring source often has certain expectations about services for the patient, and the hospice team must rectify these wishes with the overall hospice philosophy. The orderly transition of the patient from a hospital setting to the home necessitates the close relationship between the primary physician and the hospice staff. Problems identified in the earliest stages of hospice involvement tend to reflect uncontrolled symptoms, specific equipment needs, and accessibility to the primary physician for residual therapies. Once the patient has settled into his home, a number of the hospice team members visit him to determine the longer-term needs.

Relocation issues are important considerations for home hospice care because the patient and his 24-hour-per-day caregiver have perhaps had to relocate to accommodate the care demands. Whether the caregiver has moved into the home of the patient, or the patient has moved into the home of the caregiver, there is some disruption for everyone as new routines are established. Once in a home environment, one important concern relates to safety issues. Adaptive equipment is often needed for the comfort and care of the debilitated patient. Emotional support with extensive caregiver education provides the new caregiver with the requisite confidence to take on the challenge of providing care for the terminally-ill patient. It is difficult to prepare the caregiver for the personal sacrifices that must be made to care for the very ill patient. The simplest errand takes on monumental qualities as care must be continuously provided to the hospice patient.

Trust issues appear early in the care of the homebound hospice patient. Loyalties to the primary physician must be expanded to include the hospice team. Some primary physicians are not willing to follow the patient at home and rely upon the skills of the various team members to provide the day-to-day care. The reality that most hospice patients are older and are frequently cared for by younger family members produces reversals in generational hierarchies. Daughter becomes the caregiver for mother, and mother has to adapt to this traditional role switch. Long-standing, often unresolved conflicts will reappear and can produce power struggles, especially when the caregiver assumes a strong, controlling position. Even the visit of the chaplain can evoke trust questions when the religious faith of the patient and the chaplain are significantly different.

Spirituality needs require thorough exploration from the outset of hospice care. Almost all who connect their pain with impending death review the events of their lives, and seek to determine the significance of their lives. Some return to religious values of earlier days, and others make intense demands on their faith (Lack, 1984). Rectifying previous religious traditions with present affiliations can prove problematic. When spouses are of different faith traditions, or one spouse is a relative nonbeliever, it can be difficult to provide spiritual services for the patient and the involved family members. It is not for the hospice team to resolve religious matters, but to assess and attempt to provide spiritual support for the patient and family. Symptom control has to precede spiritual support; a person cannot think about the meaning of his life while he has pain (Kaye, 1989).

Psychosocial needs are of utmost importance for the hospice patient and the family. The initial evaluation includes an assessment of the previous occupational history of the patient, present financial situation, family history and relationship patterns with the family of origin and the existing family, previous coping strategies, desire for spiritual services, wishes and plans for death, personality styles of all the parties involved, individuals at risk for bereavement, and traditional referral needs for social services. The financial profile identifies the problems associated with loss of income for the patient and the caregiver, anticipates the need for care costs, and assures the presence of an up-to-date will. Significant persons, places, and events are noted in this initial evaluation. How the patient and the family previously handled losses and deaths will best predict their response to this situation.

The nursing assessment focuses on the safety of the patient in the environment, the patient's chief complaint, use of medications, care needs over time, and developing the initial plan of care. In the assessment process, the nurse gathers information from the patient that allows her to understand his experience and its effect on his life (McCaffery & Beebe, 1989). From the outset, comfort is the highest priority, with the nurse eliciting immediate wishes from the patient. Scheduling the first home visit, and following the ideals of common courtesy set hospice nursing apart from hospital nursing. It is important to avoid making assumptions about the patient's wishes by asking the patient (Kaye, 1989). Inquiring, "How are you right now?" lets the patient know that human needs will be addressed. This must occur before trust can be established to allow screening for the long-term care requirements, such as diet, appetite, bowel function, managing unpleasant side-effects, sexual and intimacy issues, and successful pain management. Hospice nurses ensure that no patient dies alone, and work in conjunction with trained volunteers to hold a hand if there is no relative or friend to keep this vigil (Saunders, 1989).

The hospice physician primarily attends to the management of unpleasant symptoms, and serves as a supervisor for the intradisciplinary team, and acts as a liaison with the primary physician. Education of the team, support for the team members as they deal with terminal patients, and representing the hospice program before a variety of county, state, and federal agencies are key duties for this physician. A willingness to be available, often 24 hours a day, and to work collaboratively with the intradisciplinary treatment team, set the hospice physician apart from the other physicians in the community. The house call, with care provided in the home of the patient, is the preferred method of management for the hospice patient, not the office or the hospital. The hospice physician must be flexible, able to handle routine medical problems, and practice medicine without the complicated technology associated with institution-based care.

CANCER PAIN MANAGEMENT

Seventy per cent of advanced cancer patients report pain as a major symptom (Bonica, 1987). For half of them their pain is moderate to severe in intensity, while for a third of them the pain is severe to excruciating (World Health Organization [WHO], 1986). It is tragic that one in 10 cancer pain patients is difficult to control, yet 50 to 80 per cent of cancer patients fail to have their pain satisfactorily relieved because their physicians do not aggressively treat the pain problem (Bonica, 1985). With 6,000,000 newly diagnosed cancer cases in the world each year, every physician caring for cancer patients must be able to elicit a detailed pain history, and be able to bring relief for these sufferers (WHO, 1986).

The basic pain evaluation begins with the belief of the pain complaint expressed by the patient (Foley, 1988). Pain is whatever the experiencing person says it is, existing whenever the experiencing person says it does

(McCaffery & Beebe, 1989). Since all pain is very real and distressing to the patient, trying to assign relative proportions to organic or functional causes is of little value. It is more useful to determine if the pain limits the activity of the patient, or disturbs the sleep, appetite, ability to engage in productive or pleasurable endeavors. Knowing what the patient can or cannot do, what medications have or have not worked well, and what side effects the patient will or will not tolerate are key initial questions to be answered. It is vital that a language about the pain be developed between the patient, the caregiver, and the hospice team, to allow skillful management. While mild, moderate, and severe describe acute pain, excruciating, incapacitating, and overwhelming better define the pain of cancer.

There should be an assessment of the psychological state of the patient, with regard to previous illness, family response to illness, and current level of anxiety and depression. Inquiring about suicidal ideation is important, especially when large quantities of toxic medications are readily available. Ultimately, a psychological needs evaluation of the caregivers must be done since in cancer pain, as in other forms of chronic pain management, operant issues frequently make pain control more difficult. Operant describes the environmental response to emitted pain behaviors, and the likelihood that the behaviors will recur. When the environment is responsive to the pain behavior, the behavior is more likely to continue over time and the intensity of the consequent suffering escalates. If the environment responds in a more matter-of-fact fashion, pain behavior decreases and attention may shift to other issues.

To most thoroughly treat the pain, it is best to obtain the richest detail about the pain complaint that the patient and family can provide. A careful, comprehensive physical examination should be performed, and this must be global in scope, since many cancer pain patients have been recently cared for by specialists who did not provide total care for the patient. If necessary, the hospice physician should order and personally review needed diagnositic studies to better elaborate the overall problems of the cancer patient (Portenoy, 1988). Consider all of the possible methods of controlling the pain, not just pharmacological, and blend them to individualize the plan of care for the patient. Lastly, assess the level of pain control and patient satisfaction after each intervention. There is no point in frequently changing methods until compliance has occurred with what has been previously ordered. Establishing clear and reasonable goals with the patient and the family is necessary, to assure a successful outcome. Everyone must understand that analgesics are not anesthetics so absolute pain elimination is never the real goal, but improved comfort can be obtained.

With a clear understanding of the pain problem, treatment can be staged from least to most complicated. As long as the patient is able to swallow, pain should be managed with oral medications, with parenteral agents reserved for much later in the disease when swallowing is frequently compromised. The change from oral medication to injections only occurs for most hospice patients during the last 48 hours (Saunders, 1989). In the hospice setting, it is possible to create a hospital-like environment in the home, but one must be on guard to make the care within the ability of the nonprofessional caregiver who is well-meaning, but generally an unskilled family member, and to not risk caregiver burnout. A balance must be struck between the capabilities of medical science, the wishes of the patient, and the realistic abilities of the caregiver. The loss of the caregiver for the home hospice patient is a frequent cause of patients deciding to enter an extended care facility. Oral medications are administered without specialized training, easy for the nonprofessional caregiver to manage, and spare them the feeling that they are doing something painful to the patient. When it is decided that parenteral is the only route available, the use of permanent venous catheters, epidural catheters, or subcutaneous infusion systems saves many caregivers from having to give injections, and the patients from having to receive these injections from relative trainees.

Based upon the premise that oral medication is the preferred route of administration for a patient who is able to eat and take fluids orally, it is recommended that the practitioner follow the World Health Organization guidelines and progress from a nonsteroidal anti-inflammatory medication to a weak, or lower potency, opioid analgesic and then, if necessary, to a strong, or high-potency opioid analgesic (WHO, 1986). These three steps best describe the management of mild, moderate, and severe pain. At each step, adjunctive, or extra medications may be added, but similar analgesic products of the same step are unnecessary for the majority of patients. Ultimately, instead of trying to fit the patient to the medications, the medications are adjusted to the patient. The right dose of a medication becomes the dose that produces comfort and minimal toxicity. Standard textbooks of pharmacology describe analgesic dosages with respect to acute pain, but few references mention the complexities of chronic pain management. Underdosing the cancer patient is more commonly the rule (Hill, 1988), and fear about possible respiratory depression is best negated by remembering that the most potent antagonist to opioid analgesic induced depression is pain itself (Johanson, 1988). Respiratory depression is not going to be a problem until the pain is controlled.

Starting with the nonsteroidal anti-inflammatory drugs makes sense for most pain problems, since these medications work to relieve pain in the periphery where the nociceptive experience originates (Kanner, 1987). These agents interfere with the manufacture of local pain sensitizing components: prostaglandins, prostacyclins, and thromboxane,and thereby inhibit pain transmission from the periphery to the central nervous system and eventual consciousness. While aspirin significantly interferes with platelet aggregation irreversibly, most of the nonsteroidal anti-inflammatory medications decrease the platelet aggregation only while therapeutic levels are maintained (American Pain Society [APS], 1989). One notable exception would be choline magnesium trisalicylate, a nonacetylated aspirin derivative, which does not appear to have effects on the aggregation of platelets (APS, 1989, Kanner, 1987). It can be used orally, as tablets or a liquid suspension, with the same general side effects profile as aspirin, and with the ability to follow salicylate levels, but without the tendency to cause bruising or bleeding. The nonsteroidal anti-inflammatory medications produce gastric upset which can usually be controlled by taking these agents with meals, and the potential for hepatic and renal problems. It is a common occurrence in the hospice setting to encounter patients with pain that is controlled quite poorly despite high dose opioid analgesics at the time of their admission. These patients are significantly benefitted from the late addition of nonsteroidal anti-inflammatory agents without further increases in the opioid analgesics, when pain is due to bone metastases (Foley, 1985, Walsh, 1985).

Case Example

Mr. H. was a seventy-five-year-old gentleman with advanced prostate cancer with extensive bone metastases. He was initially able to control his pain with hydromorphone two (2) milligrams orally every four (4) hours. He later experienced high levels of localized pain in his lower back and pelvis. Rather than increase his opioid analgesic, he was additionally given the nonsteroidal anti-inflammatory choline magnesium trisalicylate, seven hundred fifty (750) milligrams four (4) times daily with significant improvement. As his disease progressed, he eventually required more hydromorphone to remain comfortable. His dose was adjusted to four (4) milligrams orally every four (4) hours, and he died comfortably.

If the pain is not controlled with nonsteroidal anti-inflammatory medications, the next step would be the addition of opioid analgesics. It is important to understand that all of these medications are effective analgesics if used at equianalgesic dosages (the amount of one medication which produces the same relief as another medication), and that the limiting factor for schedule three (CIII) agents used in the United States is the coanalgesic (acetaminophen or aspirin). In general, the relative potency of oral to parenteral opioid analgesics is three to one, due to the first pass effect of hepatic metabolism, which means that one must take three times more oral medication to obtain the comfort produced by intramuscular or intravenous medication. The most frequent error in working with opioid analgesics is to assume that dosages are constant despite the route of administration. It is unfortunately common to find post-operative orders routinely calling for meperidine, fifty (50) to seventy-five (75) milligrams orally or intramuscularly every four (4) to six (6) hours as needed for pain. This particular example shows pharmacologic ignorance in two areas: the equianalgesic difference between oral and parenteral routes of administration, and the duration of analgesic action (only three (3) to four (4) hours for meperidine). Most important is the use of these medications on a time contingent, by the clock basis, rather than a pain contingent, as needed method, so that comfort is maintained, not continually sought. By keeping control over the pain, most patients are able to experience a better quality of life and use less medication. From a learning theory perspective, the use of as needed medication may teach the patient to use more medication with the development of psychological craving, while the time contingent dosing pattern dissociates pill taking from pain relief, and so may prevent the most feared, but least likely, complication of opioid analgesic use — addiction. (see Table I)

In reality, very little abuse of opioid medication actually occurs among hospice patients or medical patients with legitimate use of these agents. Physical dependence does occur over time, but the need for increasing dose in cancer patients more often relates to the progression of their disease, not the rapid development of tolerance. Physical dependence is not addiction, since addiction implies that the medication is compulsively sought and utilized, while dependence simply means that a person needs the medication to prevent distressing symptoms secondary to the absence of the agent—the so called "withdrawal" or "abstinence" reaction (Hill, 1988). The cancer patient has a constant supply of medication which is used time contingently if administered correctly, and there is little drug seeking behavior seen. In fact, one of the greatest barriers to compliance with the time contingent administration of these medications when the patient is relatively comfortable is the mistaken belief by the patient that they will develop an addictive disorder (Foley & Inturrisi, 1987). The data related to the risk of addiction has been traditionally obtained by surveying known addicts, not by prospectively following legitimately prescribed opioid analgesic receiving patients. In the last 10 years it has been observed that the true incidence of opioid analgesic abuse is insignificant among patients with medically justified opioid use; only one in 700 for headache sufferers to less than one in 10,000 in burn patients (Portenoy, 1990).

Once the decision to use opioid analgesics is made, the issue becomes which one to use. For mild to moderate pain it is customary to start with the lower potency opioid analgesics like codeine or hydrocodone. In the United States these medications are commonly given as tablets containing aspirin or acetaminophen, which are often more effective than the amount of the opioid analgesic involved. When the pain is more severe, or when the lower potency opioid analgesics do not produce adequate relief, high potency opioid analgesics are recommended. The "gold standard" for these medications is morphine, and it has the distinct advantage of being available in the widest variety of routes of administration (immediate release and sustained release tablets, elixirs of varied strengths, concentrate, suppositories, preservative-containing solutions for intramuscular and intravenous use, and preservative free solutions for epidural and intraspinal techniques). All of the other opioid analgesics are equally effective in controlling pain, but none are superior to morphine, and they are typically used as alternatives when patients are allergic to morphine or experience morphine-related toxicity. The only opioid analgesic which is best avoided in cancer patients is meperidine, due to the accumulation of the active metabolite, normeperidine, which is associated with the development of irritability, myoclonic jerking, and generalized tonic-clonic seizures (Foley & Inturrisi, 1989). Since most of the cancer patients are using relatively high doses of opioid agonist medication, the combined use of a mixed agonist-antagonist is strongly discouraged because of the precipitation of opioid withdrawal and severe pain for these patients (Foley & Inturrisi, 1987).

Morphine is the analgesic "gold standard" because it is an effective, relatively inexpensive, opioid analgesic with a reasonable four (4) hour duration of action (Twycross & Lack, 1984), short half-life, and is generally available throughout the world. Unlike opioid analgesics with a long half-life (methadone and levorphanol), morphine-caused complications and toxicity are resolved within a matter of hours. The ability to convert from one route of administration to another is quite simple with equianalgesic tables. Sustained release morphine allows the patient to have uninterrupted comfort and intact sleep for the patient and the caregiver. Sublingual morphine concentrate, although variable in efficacy, allows those patients for whom it is effective to obtain pain relief without the unpleasantness of parenteral or rectal administration. The metabolite of morphine, morphine-6-glucuronide is an active analgesic with a longer duration of action and half-life than morphine (Osborne, Joel, Slevin, 1986). The accumulation of morphine-6-glucuronide probably accounts for the observation that repetitively administered oral morphine is one-third as effective as intramuscular, while single dose administered morphine is only one-sixth as effective. Opioid equianalgesic tables in pharmacology textbooks are based on acute pain models, not pain patients receiving opioids, and report the oral to parenteral efficacy as six to one.

When patients experience toxicity with morphine therapy, it is prudent to change to a synthetic opioid analgesic, rather than search for an acceptable natural opioid. Hydromorphone is frequently selected as the duration of analgesic action and plasma half-life are the same as morphine.

Table I. Opioid Analgesic Equivalency

Nonproprietary Name	Trade Name	Equianalgesic Dosage (mg)			Duration of Action (hours)	Plasma Half-life (hours)
		IM	Oral	PR		
Morphine	MS Contin Roxanol Roxanol SR RMS Supp.	10	60 acute 30 repeat	10-20	4-6 (range = 2½-7)	2-3.5
Codeine	Anexsia Empirin Tylenol Phenaphen	120	200	—	4-6	3
Heroin		5	5-60	—	3-5	0.5
Hydromorphone	Dilaudid	1.5	7.5	3	4-5	2-3
Oxymorphone	Numorphan	1-1.5	—	10	4-6	2-3
Hydrocodone	Damason Damacet Hycodan Vicodin Anexsia-D	—	5-10	—	4-8	—
Dihydrocodeine	Synalgos-Dc Compal	60-68	? 30-60	—	4-5	—

Phenanthrenes

Category	Generic	Brand					
	Oxycodone	Percodan Percocet Tylox	10-15	5-30	—	3-5	—
	Levorphanol (Morphinan)	Levo-Dromoran	2-3	4-5	—	4-6	12-16
Phenylpiper-idines	Merperidine	Demerol	75	300	—	4-6	3-4
	Alphaprodine	Nisentil	40-60	—	—	0.5-2	2
	Fentanyl	Sublimaze	0.10-0.20	—	—	1-2	5.8
Methadone-like	Methadone	Dolophine	7.5-10	20	—	3-5	15-30
	Propoxyphene weak K	Darvon Darvocet Dolene Wygesic	—	300-400	—	4-6	8-24
Agonists-Antagonists	Pentazocine	Talwin	60	180	—	4-6	2-3
	Nalbuphine	Nubain	10	—	—	4-6	5
	Buprenorphine	Buprenex	.4	—	—	4-6	—
	Butorphanol	Stadol	2	—	—	4-6	2.5-3.5

B. Eliot Cole, M.D.

Traditionally less nauseating and constipating than morphine, hydromorphone is also available in oral tablets, suppositories, and injectable solutions, including ten (10) milligrams per milliliter which is quite useful for end-stage cancer pain management where high dose parenteral infusions are common. Other synthetic opioid alternatives include the long half-life medications, methadone and levorphanol, which require careful titration to prevent toxic accumulation (Twycross & Lack, 1984).

Case Example

Mr. C. was a seventy-year-old gentleman with advanced lung cancer complicated by sacroiliac and fifth lumbar vertebral metastases. He experienced severe pain in his left thigh with muscular wasting. He had previously tried oral morphine with an unclear "reaction". Although he was able to tolerate oral fluids and solids without any difficulty he was quite anxious about taking any oral analgesics. Since he was cared for by a daughter who was a registered nurse, it was possible to consider the use of parenteral analgesics. He had already been started on intravenous hydromorphone in the hospital before coming home to the hospice program. The hospice nursing staff maintained a patent intravenous access with a heparin peripheral port, and his daughter gave him every three (3) hour doses of five (5) or six (6) milligrams of hydromorphone with good relief of his pain for the first week on the program. He was able to sleep well, and developed a good appetite. By the second week his pain was beginning to bother him much more. A home pain management evaluation was done and it was decided to add the anti-inflammatory choline magnesium trisalicylate, at seven hundred fifty (750) milligrams orally four (4) times daily with food, and to maintain the intravenous hydromorphone at six (6) milligrams every three (3) hours. Through the next week he felt much better but developed the need for increasing doses given at decreasing intervals by the fourth week. When his intravenous hydromorphone reached eleven (11) milligrams every two and a half hours he developed considerable nausea and vomiting, associated with anxiety about the ability to ever control his side effects and pain simultaneously. He was given sublingual haloperidol one (1) to two (2) milligrams every four (4) hours as needed and had relief of his nausea and vomiting. In the final and fifth week on the program, he continued to increase the use of the hydromorphone, eventually reaching twenty (20) milligrams every three (3) hours, yet remained alert, active, and involved with his family and care needs. The family was grateful that they could maintain meaningful dialog with him and complete much of the anticipatory bereavement work. On the day before he died he met with the funeral director to plan the details of his own funeral, and with a close friend to help prepare the eulogy that would be delivered. Later that day he went to sleep and died during the night. Although he had miotic pupils suggesting an opiate effect throughout his participation on the hospice program, he never developed any respiratory depression except as an agonal event.

The practice of combining opioid analgesics to provide better patient comfort is confusing for the patients, their caregivers, and even the prescribing physicians, and is not justified under most circumstances. Often there is misuse of multiple opioid medications because few appreciate that pill size has little to do with relative potency, or that sustained release tablets do not adequately control pain until proper titration has occurred over two (2) to three (3) days. It is necessary to provide additional immediate release opioid medication for pain breakthrough at certain times, especially when the base opioid analgesic is a sustained release preparation. In that way, unanticipated changes in pain can be effectively managed on an immediate basis, with day-to-day tailoring of the overall opioid analgesic medication by observing the use of these additional doses. Monitoring the 24 hour total usage is essential for keeping up with the opioid analgesic medication needs of the patient.

The major complication of opioid analgesic therapy is constipation, and must be vigorously managed from the initiation of treatment. Failure to correct opioid induced constipation can lead to intractable nausea, vomiting, and abdominal discomfort. Respiratory depression, significant central nervous system dysfunction, and the risk of chemical dependency are insignificant in comparison. Although nausea and vomiting are initially common with opioids, once acclimated to these medications, later appearing nausea and vomiting more often result for unrecognized and ineffectively treated constipation.

Case Example

Mr. F. was sent home from the hospital with advanced prostate cancer and widely-spread bone metastases, but no bowel movement for one week prior to entering the hospice program. He was fairly comfortable from a pain perspective, although experienced increasing abdominal fullness and discomfort felt to be due to opioid analgesic induced constipation. Digital examination of the rectum found significant hard, impacted stool that was manually decompressed. Once free of the impaction he was started on an oral laxative and stool softener combination, and developed bowel regularity within two days. There were no further episodes of impaction, and his bowel integrity was maintained with the same daily laxative/softener combination.

When opioid analgesics fail to provide relief of significant pain desp te clear toxicity (respiratory or central nervous system depression), it is necessary to remember that these agents are not generally effective for deafferentation pain due to nerve involvement, viscus or muscle spasm, or extreme psychological distress. It is the use of the adjunctive medications that is warranted, not further opioid analgesics.

Adjunctive medications include antidepressants, antipsychotics, anticonvulsants, and anxiolytics. These useful materials may be added at any step in the continuum of cancer pain management, and often save the patient from progression to high potency opioid analgesics. The adjunctive medications manipulate the neurochemistry of the nervous system, and augment the overall effectiveness of the nonsteroidal anti-inflammatory and opioid analgesic combinations.

The antidepressants are remarkable agents with the ability to block the presynaptic reuptake of noradrenaline and serotonin, resulting in elevated levels of these important neurotransmitters in the brain (Botney & Fields, 1982, Hendler, 1982). The benefit of enhanced serotonin centrally is the consequent periaquaductal release of endogenous opioid peptides with a dampening effect on pain perception (Frier, 1985). These agents correct the depression (which is so common with persistent pain), stabilize sleep, and improve appetite, energy level, concentration, and ability to experience pleasure. The ability of antidepressants to relieve pain is independent of the antidepressant effect (Feinmann, 1985). Although antidepressants generally used for pain management are serotonin enhancing, the noradrenaline enhancing agents are often useful when a psychomotor retarded depression is more of the problem. Antidepressants are not habit forming, have little effect on respiration when used in therapeutic doses, but are associated with a number of annoying anticholinergic side effects which may limit their usefulness unless the patient is forewarned about them.

Case Example

Mr. D., a seventy-five-year-old gentleman, had severe lability of affect, impaired sleep, and advanced pulmonary cancer leaving him short of breath and in need of continuous oxygen therapy. He had used diazepam for many years as a bedtime hypnotic, but the hospice staff was concerned about the cumulative respiratory depression of diazepam and sustained release morphine. Rather than administer diazepam with the sustained release morphine at sixty (60) milligrams twice daily, he was started on doxepin hydrochloride, ten (10) milligrams at bedtime, which was eventually adjusted upward to twenty (20) milligrams the next week with improvement in sleep, stabilization of his mood, loss of affective lability, and a better management of his chest wall pain.

Antipsychotic medication, more commonly referred to as neuroleptics or major tranquilizers, blocks the post synaptic dopamine receptors and prevents the transmission of neuronal information. The consequence of these agents is the functional disconnection of the limbic system, the modern day equivalence of a frontal lobotomy, with the patient relatively unconcerned about the pain problem. This effect often permits the rapid tapering of high dose opioid analgesic medication, especially intravenous, when the patient is trying to leave the hospital to return to the home setting. With the antipsychotic medications, it is possible to significantly decrease the opioid dosage, and maintain the patient in a relaxed state. Antipsychotic agents are also powerful antiemetics, and control nausea and vomiting (Hanks, 1984, Johanson, 1988). The high potency medications, droperidol and haloperidol, are particularly noteworthy because they work with minimal effect on the cardiovascular system. Droperidol is only available as a parenteral agent, but haloperidol is available as oral tablets and an oral concentrate (two (2) milligrams per milliliter) which can be used sublingually (Johanson, 1988). The low potency medications, chlorpromazine and thioridazine, are relatively toxic for the cardiovascular system, and are best avoided in the seriously ill patient. Extrapyramidal reactions do occur with the high potency medications, but can be easily managed with the anticholinergic agents, benztropine and diphenhydramine.

Case Example

Ms. M. was a forty-five-year-old woman with end stage human immunodeficiency virus infection. She did not experience significant pain, but suffered from intractable nausea and vomiting which was not relieved with standard antiemetics used orally or rectally. She was given sublingual haloperidol, one (1) milligram every four (4) hours with good control of her symptoms.

Anticonvulsants stabilize nerve cell membranes and inhibit spontaneous discharge resulting in seizures centrally, or neuropathic pain peripherally (WHO, 1986). The most commonly used agents are clonazepam, carbamazepine, and phenytoin, and have been employed in the management of lancinating or stabbing dysesthetic pain (Lack, 1984). Clonazepam is a potent benzodiazepine with a relatively greater anticonvulsant effect than its congeners (Hanks, 1984). Clonazepam is the least difficult to use in the home hospice setting due to the ability to use it without the need for blood level monitoring. It does tend to accumulate, causes a moderate degree of sedation, and for this reason is often avoided in the severely ill patients. The long half-life of clonazepam allows effective once daily dosing for most patients. Carbamazepine with the relative risk of bone marrow suppression, gastric upset, and the need for blood level monitoring, is unattractive as an anticonvulsant for in the home hospice patient. It is the preferred medication for trigeminal neuralgia, and for other supraclavicular pain problems. Phenytoin has the reputation of being the anticonvulsant for infraclavicular pain, but has the distinct disadvantage of requiring days of therapy before improvement is noted unless initially given as an intravenous loading dose, and must be followed with blood levels. In general, the anticonvulsants are frequently the only effective oral medications for deafferentation pain, nerve injuries, and pain characterized by burning, tingling, or paroxysms (Swerdlow, 1986).

Benzodiazepines, although not thought of as analgesics, have a limited role in the management of cancer pain. Anxiety, depression, fear, sleeplessness, and restlessness may all lower a patient's pain tolerance (Hanks, 1984). Most patients in a hospice sleep well but as these patients near the end of their lives they sometimes have recurrent nightmares (Saunders, 1989). When pain so interferes with the normal sleep pattern that little or no stage four, delta wave sleep occurs, the addition of a short-acting agent is beneficial. It appears that without the deepest stage of sleep, muscles do not completely relax, and muscular pain may spontaneously develop causing the patient widespread discomfort. By improving stage four sleep, this diffuse muscular ache that many cancer patients experience also as a consequence of their debilitation and malnutrition, can be lessened. When the patients are morbidly anxious about their condition, the addition of a benzodiazepine medication may significantly improve their anxiety. The long half-life benzodiazepine medications are preferable with maintained blood levels by time contingent dosing over the short half-life medications which are more likely to produce wide swings in blood levels and consequent rebound anxiety.

Certain anesthetic techniques are often used prior to the patient coming to the home hospice, including the celiac plexus block for abdominal pain, the stellate ganglion block for upper quarter pain, the lumbar sympathetic block for lower extremity pain, the intraspinal neurolytic block for bilateral lower body pain, and the epidural use of opioid analgesics (Cousins & Mather, 1984, Foley, 1985). As patients deteriorate, it is not uncommon to progress from one procedure to another, to maintain their comfort.

Case Example

Ms. N. was a fifty-year-old woman with ovarian and abdominal carcinomatosis, colectomy, and colostomy. She suffered from extreme abdominal, upper and lower back, and pelvic pain. Despite ten (10) to twenty (20) milligrams of intravenous morphine per hour she was never able to achieve effective control of her pain. She was not convinced that further chemotherapy was going to help her condition and elected the hospice program for her management. She was initially recommended for an epidural catheter, and after it was placed had reasonable control of her abdominal and pelvic pain components using hydromorphone, five (5) to ten (10) milligrams every five (5) hours. This was supplemented with oral methadone, ten (10) milligrams every five (5) hours to control the upper back pain not well managed by the epidural catheter. Later, as her disease spread, she experienced more abdominal pain and a celiac plexus block was done, giving her very good relief and a reduction of her methadone to just five (5) milligrams every six (6) hours, with the epidural hydromorphone at ten (10) milligrams every six (6) hours. Although she was finally comfortable with this complex management, her course was punctuated over the last two months of her life by good days and bad, impaired appetite and sleep, and then a pervasive depression. With the addition of twenty-five (25) milligrams of amitriptyline at bedtime she quickly improved these symptoms. She became more emaciated over the time she spent on the hospice program, yet tolerated both of the invasive procedures without significant adverse outcome. As she began to actively die, she spent her final hours in the arms of her husband, and communicated to him her wishes for the music at her funeral.

The celiac plexus block provides good abdominal analgesia for several months, and is perhaps the ideal management approach for pancreatic (Parris, 1985), hepatic, intestinal cancer and abdominal carcinomatosis from ovarian malignancy. Sixty to 90 per cent of patients report a significant reduction in pain after this block (Foley, 1985, Verrill, 1989), and if survival extends beyond several months, the block can be repeated, although frequently with a less successful outcome.

The stellate ganglion block is useful for sympathetically mediated pain involving the scalp, face, neck, arm, and upper chest (Campbell, 1989). It is frequently used in the management of upper quarter pain related to brachial plexus involvement by lung cancer, or highly invasive breast cancer. Often a single block is useful, but commonly a series of these blocks is performed to modify the discomfort. When effective, the results of this block can be quite impressive and startling.

Case Example

Ms. W. was a tragic thirty-seven-year-old woman who had suffered with widely metastatic breast cancer for three years when she was first seen for pain control. She had moved from a small town in the Midwest to become a prostitute in one of Nevada's legal brothels, and when she developed her breast cancer, she saw it as punishment sent to her by God. She talked a great deal about getting well, yet could accept no real involvement in her own care, and waited to be rescued. Over many months she had been tried on several different analgesic medications, both nonsteroidal anti-inflammatory and even steroidal agents, along with different oral and parenteral opioid analgesics. She never developed overt dysesthetic pain, but antidepressants and anticonvulsants failed to relieve her horrible right chest and arm pain. A series of hypnotic sessions proved to be the most useful, and allowed her to rest for a short time, but only brought relief from her suffering while she was profoundly relaxed in the session. Otherwise, her pain was too severe to allow her to rest comfortably. It was decided to try a stellate ganglion block to see if her pain might be sympathetic in origin, when the right arm began to swell quite rapidly. The block was done late in the afternoon, and upon return to her room, she was smiling and reporting very little overall discomfort. She drifted off to sleep, for the first time in days, and died peacefully a few hours later without awakening. The first reaction of the anesthesiologist upon learning of the sudden demise of Ms. W. was to assume that there had been an adverse outcome from the technically well done stellate ganglion block. It was clear that she was finally able to experience comfort for the first time in years, and was able to let go and die in her sleep.

Intraspinal neurolysis is a highly destructive technique used for intractable pain when lower body motor function, along with bowel and bladder control is lost, usually due to a spinal cord tumor or invasion of the spine by metastatic lesions. It involves the deliberate chemical coagulation of the remaining cord structures by placing alcohol or phenol in the subdural space (Ferrer-Brechner, 1989). The end result is absolute anesthesia below the level of the completed cord destruction.

Case Example

Mr. A. was an unfortunate sixty-five-year-old gentleman with a widely metastatic prostate cancer that had invaded his lumbar spine anteriorly and left him paralyzed below the level of the lesion, without bowel or bladder control, but in constant excruciating pain in his lower body. Despite adequate trials of nonsteroidal anti-inflammatory medication, low and high potency opioid analgesics, and transcutaneous electrical nerve stimulation, nothing seemed to relieve his suffering. After consultation with an anesthesiologist, it was decided to complete his cord lesion with intraspinal alcohol. This was done with the patient's informed consent, and quickly produced complete resolution of his lower body pain. He still required some anti-inflammatory and opioid analgesic medication for his upper body pain, but was much improved and relatively comfortable after the spinal neurolysis.

Epidural administration of opioid analgesics is quite effective when the pain is fairly localized, especially if it is entirely below the level of the nipples. By placing the opioid analgesics into the epidural space there is relatively little cognitive impairment experienced by the patient, and while the pain is significantly relieved, normal sensation is preserved. Once the catheter is in place the opioid, usually morphine or hydromorphone, is administered by continuous infusion or by bolus injections. The availability of small, light weight, battery-powered portable infusion pumps allows the hospice nursing staff to provide a 24 to 48 hour supply of medication to the patient without the risk of catheter infection due to poor injection technique by the nonprofessional caregiver.

In some hospice patients, all of the pain management techniques are used, due to a variety of complications, personal requests, and personnel available. The last ditch stand of hospice is usually the use of intravenous opioid infusions, but this requires a patent intravenous access, frequently unavailable in the end stage patient. An alternative for the home hospice patient is the use of subcutaneous high potency opioid analgesics delivered by a portable infusion pump through a small needle inserted into the abdominal wall.

Case Example

Ms. T. was a sixty-year-old woman with advanced hepatic cancer with pelvic metastases. She had delayed chemotherapy to allow for a long hoped for trip to Europe, and when she first presented to the hospice program she was experiencing severe bilateral hip pain with radiation into her thighs. There were bothersome muscle spasms complicating her pain problem. She was a suspicious and guarded woman who did not have much faith in her physicians, who did not want to take any medication, and who desperately wanted to avoid being hospitalized. She was initially treated for her pain with intravenous morphine at twelve (12) milligrams per hour, but was successfully converted to oral morphine in a sustained release form at three hundred (300) milligrams every eight (8) hours. Once she went home she began to need more morphine and was quickly using one hundred fifty (150) to one hundred eighty (180) milligrams of immediate release morphine every day in addition to the sustained release morphine. It was observed by the hospice staff that she used more morphine when her family members were around, but relatively little when the nurses, aides, and physician visited. Due to the wide fluctuations in her comfort level, and her increasing belief that the oral medications would never entirely control her discomfort, she was returned to the hospital for the placement of an epidural catheter, and the use of epidural opioid analgesics. She was given epidural hydromorphone, one (1) milligram per hour via a compact infusion pump, as this medication was available in a high potency preparation and would avoid the large volumes needed when using preservative-free morphine. The epidural hydromorphone proved to be quite effective for her, and she was able to discontinue the oral morphine. Once back in her home, she did well until she accidentally pulled out her catheter about a week later. She was again hospitalized and another epidural catheter was placed and subcutaneously tunneled. Back home she did well for another week, requiring more hydromorphone and eventually reaching three (3) milligrams per hour and then mysteriously this second catheter was lost. Because she was quite debilitated by this point it was decided to use subcutaneous hydromorphone, one (1) milligrams per hour with as needed bolus doses of 0.5 milligrams every thirty (30) minutes, but not to return her to the hospital for further catheter placement. Using a small, subcutaneously placed needle she was able to receive hydromorphone by infusion pump. She remained fairly comfortable with this technique, eventually using two (2) milligrams of hydromorphone per hour, until her death one week later. It was learned from her daughter after her death that she could never resolve things, and died the best that she could.

Cancer pain is also managed by a number of nonpharmacological methods, including cognitive therapy, hypnosis, transcutaneous electrical nerve stimulation, radiation therapy, physical and occupational therapy services, and the involvement of the clergy. For prominent muscle spasm, predictably painful procedures, depression and anxiety, the cognitive techniques are useful (Cleeland, 1987). Hypnosis can augment pain control, but rarely completely relieves the pain. Providing orthotics or prosthetics, assistive devices, range of motion exercises, and bedside stretching can keep the remaining activities of daily living available for the patient. Radiation therapy and transcutaneous electrical nerve stimulation are often the most effective management for bone metastases and pathologic fractures (Howard-Ruben, McGuire, Groenwald, 1987, Bosch, 1984). Transcutaneous electrical nerve stimulation requires the participation of the patient, while radiation therapy can be performed on those who are quite debilitated. Involvement of the clergy can produce significant comfort for patients who are actively dying, and should not be forgotten with those on the home hospice program.

To successfully manage the terminal cancer pain patient, the issues must be globally addressed. The etiology of the pain is accurately defined to direct the therapy. The analgesics progress from nonsteroidal anti-inflammatory agents to opioids, but with the clear understanding that the medications are titrated. Realistic goals must be set, and clear communication maintained with all of the parties involved. Education of the patient and the family regarding the use of resources and decision making for choices of therapy are part of the process (Ferrer-Brechner, 1984). The emotional and spiritual needs of the patient are as important, and as aggressively managed as the somatic needs.

PROBLEM SYMPTOMS

Besides pain, hospice patients, especially those with cancer, are bothered by constipation, nausea and vomiting, poor appetite and weight loss, seizures, difficulties with oral care, hydration, skin integrity, and itching. These symptoms are bothersome and steal from the patient quality comfort so they must be as aggressively managed as pain itself.

Constipation is the expected consequence of opioid analgesic management, and must be anticipated and preventatively controlled from the moment pain is treated. Most patients should be given a diet high in fiber or a bulk laxative, and if ineffective in two or three days, additional laxatives are needed (Portenoy, 1987). Bowel care products are available in a variety of groups, including stool softeners which prevent excessive drying, irritants which increase mucosal secretion and peristalsis, causing movement of fecal material, and combination products. The goal is to maintain bowel regularity, and keep stool texture like that of toothpaste. In that way, even the weakest patient is able to still expel stool with little straining or effort.

Nausea and resulting vomiting may initially be due to the opioid analgesics, but over time, constipation, metabolic abnormalities, or bowel obstruction may be likely causes. If a correctable process is the culprit, it is best to manage the symptom by focusing on the pathology. When this is not possible, then the routine use of antiemetics is justified. High potency antipsychotic medications, droperidol and haloperidol, either oral, sublingual, or parenteral, are effective for nausea and vomiting (Johanson, 1988). The lower potency antipsychotic medications, the typical antiemetics, generally are more sedating than the high potency agents, and are more likely to produce unpleasant side effects such as dry mouth, constipation, urinary hesitancy, and hypotension. Until vomiting is well controlled, most patients experience high levels of discomfort, presumably due to electrolyte imbalance and dehydration.

Appetite loss and declining weight leave most hospice patients weak, listless, and susceptible to skin breakdown. As a result of chemotherapy, radiation therapy, surgery, and the overall debilitation of chronic illness, many patients cannot experience any pleasure associated with eating. With swallowing difficulties and the risk of choking or aspiration, some patients even become anxious about eating. The involvement of a dietician to assist with food preferences, or a communication therapist to improve swallowing can be quite useful. Small, frequent portions are better tolerated than large, traditional meals. If chemotherapy has left the patient with little sense of taste, altering the diet to include highly seasoned or spicy foods, or serving the meals as colorfully as possible may help to stimulate the appetite (Kaye, 1989).

Case Example

Ms. A. was a severely emaciated woman with advanced ovarian and abdominal carcinomatosis. She had undergone extensive surgical resection of her tumor, radiation therapy, and several courses of chemotherapy.

She had lost most of her appreciation for taste, and consequently found all food to have the taste and texture of oatmeal. It was hard for her to maintain her weight without motivation to eat. She began to experiment with different foods and found that spicy Mexican and Chinese meals were satisfying and helped her remain motivated to eat, when the more traditional oral nutrition supplements were being refused. She enjoyed the cold and creamy quality of vanilla ice cream over any other dessert type food.

Seizures are a significant concern for patients with metastatic brain lesions, and cause a great deal of distress for their family members who must witness seemingly unrelenting convulsions. Although fairly easy to control with oral anticonvulsant and steroidal medication, seizures occurring near the end of life are problematic because the patients often are no longer able to swallow effectively. A useful alternative to the use of crushed tablets or liquid suspensions via a feeding tube, is the injectable benzodiazepine, lorazepam. Lorazepam provides seizure control for three to four hours (Leppik, et al., 1983), does not significantly accumulate since it has no active metabolites, and is rapidly absorbed from intramuscular injection sites unlike the other benzodiazepines. As seizures are often an agonal event, giving a few intramuscular injections is rarely a problem for the caregivers once they understand that the patients are not going to experience significant pain.

Case Example

Ms. H. was a sixty-five-year-old woman with ovarian cancer which had metastasized to her right brain producing a left hemiplegia and motor seizures. Her pain did not appear to be cancer-related, but involved her right hip and was thought to be due to a previous total hip replacement. She was a remarkably angry woman who, while being mildly dysphasic in her speech, was actually electively mute at times. Initially, phenytoin three hundred (300) milligrams at bedtime controlled her seizures, and oral naproxen two hundred fifty (250) milligrams three (3) times daily managed her hip discomfort. Later, one (1) milligram of clonazepam was added at bedtime to control sleep and reported spasm, along with thirty (30) milligrams of sustained release morphine twice daily. This produced marked daytime agitation which was felt to be due to the benzodiazepine, and it was replaced by oral haloperidol, two (2) milligrams every two (2) hours as needed. She lost control of swallowing and stopped taking any oral medications, fluids, or foods in the last week of her life. This resulted in more frequent and severe motor seizures resulting in secondary generalization. As her daughter was able to administer intramuscular injections, she was managed for the last two days of her life with intramuscular lorazepam, one (1) to two (2) milligrams every four (4) hours with good control of her seizures. Although she steadily deteriorated she did not appear to experience significant pain, and was able to remain seizure-free with the lorazepam. Parenteral phenytoin was not used because she had poor vascular access, and an intravenous line could never be established.

Skin care is vitally important for hospice patients, especially those who are bed bound. Changes in body position, with frequent turning, proper padding with heel and ankle protectors, and the use of a thick foam mattress cover should be done to prevent decubitus ulceration. Once ulcers are established they are difficult to treat due to the poor wound healing of the malnourished and debilitated patients. Bowel and bladder incontinence will produce skin breakdown if the patient is not kept relatively clean and dry. While powders are helpful in keeping the patient dry, the use of a barrier ointment can be quite effective once skin is irritated.

Case Example

Ms. K. was an eighty-year-old woman with pancreatic cancer and secondary liver failure who developed skin breakdown of her buttocks due to frequent diarrhea. Cleansing of her buttocks and perineum was associated with burning pain due to extensive irritation. She became progressively more fearful of any type of bowel activity, and would allow herself to remain in a fecal and urine soaked bed rather than request appropriate care. To relieve her condition, and her resulting anxiety about hygiene, she was given a topical material made from equal parts of zinc oxide ointment, Vitamin A and D ointment, and dibucaine one (1) percent ointment, to be applied to the involved area every four (4) to six (6) hours. Within the first few applications immediate comfort was obtained, and significant healing occurred over the next week.

Itching can be quite serious for patients with extremely dry skin, and is often a complication of hepatic failure. Applying topical moisturizers may be helpful for skin dryness, but for protracted, distressing itch, the use of antihistamines, diphenhydramine and hydroxyzine, or low dose antidepressants may provide relief (Johanson, 1988, Kaye, 1989). One particularly useful agent for itching is the antidepressant, doxepin hydrochloride, which is a potent antihistamine (about 800 times more antihistaminic than diphenhydramine) producing moderate sedation (Richelson, 1979).

Oral care is routinely performed by healthy individuals and sadly forgotten in some terminal patients. With dehydration due to decreased oral intake, coupled with mouth breathing as death approaches, it is common for the oral membranes to become dry and caked with debris. Cleansing the mouth with small quantities of water, wiping the mouth with a lemon-flavored glycerine swab, and applying a lip balm is soothing for these dying patients (Kaye, 1989). Whether or not intravenous fluids should be started and maintained until death is more debatable, with most hospice patients prospectively requesting that such measures not be undertaken as they die.

There are interesting family problems that emerge over the course of several weeks on the hospice program. A common scenario involves the patient as the central focus of the tragedy, cared for by a designated martyr, who is constantly criticized by the family. Despite all of the caregiver's best efforts and intentions, nothing seems to please the family about the management of the patient, and none will help with the care requirements.

Case Example

Mr. B. was a sixty-five-year-old gentleman with advanced lung cancer, and terrible bilateral leg pain thought to be due to bone metastases. He was cared for by his daughter who had some nursing experience. Several members of the family lived in the same household, and although two of his sons were large, strong men, only his petite daughter provided his care. Whenever she attended to his needs, or tried to assist him with transfers, the sons would offer criticism about her technique, drink beer, and watch television, but would never offer to help her. She was never able to do anything to their satisfaction, and yet mastered the proper aseptic technique for the administration of her father's epidural morphine. She lovingly cared for her father, kept him on the schedule that was provided for his oral and parenteral medications, and saw to it that he never developed a bed sore or other complication. She was always exhausted but never complained about her work load.

In hospice literature the patient and the caregiver merge to become the hospice unit, because treatment involves not only the identified patient, but also those who care for him (Adams, 1984). The caregiver as part of the hospice unit requires our skilled attention. The care of the family is an integral part of the treatment plan, and a contented family increases the likelihood of a contented, pain-free patient (Lack, 1984). The relief of the caregiver's pain and suffering is brought about by the same interventions that we provide our patients: concerned listening, education, sharing, touching, and caring by the hospice team. The caregiver in the patient's life becomes the bereaved upon the patient's death.

Bereavement, a separation or loss through death, derives from the Old English bereafian, which means "to rob," "to plunder," or "to dispossess" (Burnell & Burnell, 1989). Every caregiver has loss experiences that color how they handle subsequent losses, and these losses need acknowledgement in preparation for healthy grieving with the loved one's death. Soon after the death, or often through the dying process, the caregiver must look for new ways of establishing an identity. The caregiver may experience an initial sense of relief, and simultaneously with the death of the patient, feelings of emptiness, and times when old ways have not yet been replaced with new ways. This caregiver confusion arises from the focus on the needs of the patient, throughout the course of the illness.

Many caregivers report how much of their day is centered around the dying patient, attending to positioning, feeding, bathing, and medicating. The care needs of the patient direct the life of the caregiver. Although appropriate and encouraged during the patient's hospice care, upon the death of the patient, the routine is radically altered for the caregiver. This loss of activity and fulfillment of nurturing needs should be acknowledged as part of the emptiness experienced after death. Hospice programs provide bereavement support, and maintain continued involvement with the caregiver, through the professional staff headed by the medical social worker in coordination with chaplaincy, nursing, and supported by the program volunteers. These volunteers, often drawn from the pool of past caregivers, are trained people who demonstrate the hospice philosophy of care and communicate, "I have been there, you will get through this."

CONCLUSION

Hospice home care is not for every patient, family, or health care provider (Jacobsen, 1984). It requires a special commitment on the part of the caregiver, and the support of a skilled hospice team. We use personal illustrations in this chapter from actual cases effectively managed by the home hospice program. The stories are deliberate human experiences as they serve as our best teachers. Our hospice work with pain and symptom management is enriched by the patients who believe in our program, and provide us with the opportunity to participate in their deaths. There is no single or best way to control any particular symptom, but the coordinated efforts of the intradisciplinary team eventually brings effective relief for physical, emotional, and spiritual discomfort. Although the team members would like to feel clever and take credit for a successful outcome, the patients remind us that hospice management is not finite, but is evolving and that the individualized care is absolute. Only our patients and their families are able to judge our effectiveness as a hospice team.

REFERENCES

Adams, A. B. (1984). Dilemmas of hospice: A critical look at its problems. *Ca — A Cancer Journal for Clinicians, 34,* 9-16.

American Pain Society (1989). *Principles of analgesic use in the treatment of acute pain and chronic cancer pain: A concise guide to medical practice* (2nd ed.). Skokie, IL: American Pain Society.

Bonica, J. J. (1985). Treatment of cancer pain: Current status and future needs. In H. L. Fields et al., (Eds.), *Advances in pain research and therapy,* Vol. 9 (pp. 589-616). New York: Raven Press.

Bonica, J. J. (1987). Preface — A short course on the management of cancer pain. *Journal of Pain and Symptom Management, 2,* S3-4.

Bosch, A. (1984). Radiotherapy. *Clinics in Oncology, 3,* 47-53.

Botney, M., & Fields, H. L. (1982). Amitriptyline potentiates morphine analgesia by a direct action on the central nervous system. *Annals of Neurology, 13,* 160-164.

Brescia, F. J. (1987). An overview of pain and symptom management in advanced cancer. *Journal of Pain and Symptom Management, 2,* S7-11.

Burnell, G. M., & Burnell, A. L. (1989). *Clinical management of bereavement.* New York: Human Sciences Press.

Campbell, J. N. (1989). Pain from peripheral nerve injury. In K. M. Foley & R. M. Payne (Eds.), *Current therapy of pain* (pp. 158-169). Toronto: B. C. Decker.

Cleeland, C. S. (1987). Nonpharmacological management of cancer pain. *Journal of Pain and Symptom Management, 2,* S23-28.

Cousins, M. J., & Mather, L. E. (1984). Intrathecal and epidural administration of opioids. *Anesthesiology, 61,* 276-310.

Feinmann, C. (1985). Pain relief by antidepressants: Possible modes of action. *Pain, 23,* 1-8.

Ferrer-Brechner, T. (1984). Treating cancer pain as a disease. In C. Benedetti, et al., (Eds.), *Advances in pain research and therapy:* Vol. 7 (pp. 575-591). New York: Raven Press.

Ferrer-Brechner, T. (1989). Anesthetic techniques for the management of cancer pain. *Cancer, 63,* 2343-2347.

Foley, K. M. (1985). The treatment of cancer pain. *The New England Journal of Medicine, 313,* 84-95.

Foley, K. M., & Inturrisi, C. E. (1987). Analgesic drug therapy in cancer pain: Principles and practice. *Medical Clinics of North America, 71,* 207-232.

Foley, K. M. (1988). Pain syndromes and pharmacologic management of pancreatic cancer pain. *Journal of Pain and Symptom Management, 3,* 176-187.

Foley, K. M., & Inturrisi, C. E. (1989). Pain of malignant origin. In K. M. Foley & R. M. Payne (Eds.), *Current therapy of pain.* Toronto: B. C. Decker.

Frier, J. W. (1985). Therapeutic implications of modifying endogenous serotonergic analgesic systems. *Anesthesia Progress,* Jan./Feb., 19-22.

Hanks, G. W. (1984). Psychotropic drugs. *Clinics in Oncology, 3,* 135-151.

Hendler, N. (1982). The anatomy and psychopharmacology of chronic pain. *Journal of Clinical Psychiatry, 43,* 15-21.

Hill, C. S. (1988). Narcotics and cancer pain control. *Ca — A Cancer Journal for Clinicians, 38*, 322-326.

Howard-Ruben, J., McGuire, L., & Groenwald, S. L. (1987). Pain. In S. L. Groenwald (Ed.), *Cancer nursing principles and practice*. Boston, MA: Jones & Bartlett.

Jacobsen, G. A. (1984). Hospice: What it is not. *Ca — A Cancer Journal for Clinicians, 34*, 28-29.

Johanson, G. A. (1988). *Physicians handbook of symptom relief in terminal care* (2nd ed.). Sebastopol, CA: Home Hospice of Sonoma County.

Kanner, R. M. (1987). Pharmacological management of pain and symptom control in cancer. *Journal of Pain and Symptom Management, 2*, S19-21.

Kaye, P. (1989). *Notes on symptom control in hospice and palliative care*. Essex, CT: Hospice Education Institute.

Lack, S. (1984). Total pain. *Clinics in Oncology, 3*, 33-44.

Leppik, I. E., et al., (1983). Double-blind study of lorazepam and diazepam in status epilepticus. *Journal of the American Medical Association, 249*, 1452-1454.

McCaffery, M., & Beebe, A. (1989). *Pain, Clinical manual for nursing practice*. St. Louis, MO: C. V. Mosby Company.

Osborne, R. J., Joel, S. P., & Slevin, M. L. (1986). Morphine intoxication in renal failure: The role of morphine-6-glucuronide. *British Medical Journal, 292*, 1548-1549.

Parris, W. C. V. (1985). Nerve block therapy. *Clinics in Anesthesiology, 3*, 93-109.

Portenoy, R. K. (1987). Constipation in the cancer patient. *Medical Clinics of North America, 71*, 303-311.

Portenoy, R. K. (1988). Practical aspects of pain control in the patient with cancer. *Ca — A Cancer Journal for Clinicians, 38*, 327-352.

Portenoy, R. K. (1990). Chronic opioid therapy in nonmalignant pain. Journal of *Pain and Symptom Management, 5*, S46-62.

Richelson, E. (1979). Tricyclic antidepressants and histamine H1 receptors. *Mayo Clinic Proceedings, 54*, 669-674.

Saunders, C. (1989). Pain and impending death. In P. D. Wall & R. Melzack (Eds.), *Textbook of Pain* (2nd ed.). (pp. 624-631). Edinburgh: Churchill Livingstone.

Swerdlow, M. (1986). Anticonvulsants in the therapy of neuralgic pain. *The Pain Clinic, 1*, 9-19.

Twycross, R., & Lack, S. (1984). *Oral morphine in advanced cancer*. Beaconsfield, Bucks, England: Beaconsfield Publishers.

Verrill, P. (1989). Sympathetic ganglion lesions. In P.D. Wall & R. Melzack (Eds.), *Textbook of pain* (2nd ed.). (pp. 773-783). Edinburgh: Churchill Livingstone.

Walsh, T. D. (1985). Common misunderstandings about the use of morphine for chronic pain in advanced cancer. *Ca — A Cancer Journal for Clinicians, 35.*

World Health Organization (1986). *Cancer pain relief.* Geneva: World Health Organization.

Chapter 14

REFLEX SYMPATHETIC DYSTROPHY

Verne L. Brechner, M. D.

Dr. Brechner traces the history of our understanding of Reflex Sympathetic Dystrophy and provides the clinician a review of symptom presentation as well as an organized treatment approach to this problem. Symptoms include hypersensitivity to light touch, persistent burning, redness, sweating, and swelling. If untreated, many patients become depressed and even suicidal.

Relief of pain may occur with sympathetic blockaide. Mechanical stimulation and TENS may increase sympathetically maintained pain. A sub group of patients may be candidates for surgical sympathectomy. Oral medication, i.e., Prednisone and tricyclic antidepressants may be of benefit. Psychological support, such as counseling and biofeedback, is often useful for treating patients with Reflex Sympathetic Dystrophy.

Chapter 14 ████████████

REFLEX SYMPATHETIC DYSTROPHY

Verne L. Brechner, M. D.

It is a few years more than four score and twenty since Weir Mitchell published his classical description of the phenomena of burning pain associated with nerve injury (Mitchell, 1864, 1872). His patient's were civil war soldiers who had received penetrating wounds to nerve roots and peripheral nerves. They developed a previously unrecognized sequence of symptoms. While they had the expected neurological deficits of a traumatized nerve root or peripheral nerve, there was, in addition, the phenomena of hypersensitivity to light touch, and persistent agonizing burning pain involving most of the extremity. Elaborate precautions were taken by these patients to protect the extremity from the most trivial of mechanical contact or stimulation which would initiate a painful episode. These precautions included wrapping the extremity in cotton, wool, or silk, and avoiding the approach of any person who might touch the extremity. They eventually developed hostility to any individual coming within close proximity. Emotional depression developed to such degree that suicide was the final outcome in many cases. Physical observations throughout the course of this syndrome involved, initially, blushing or redness of the extremity. This soon was followed by episodes of cyanosis and blanching, excessive sweating, and the occurrence of swelling throughout the extremity. There was excessive hair length because of the guarding phenomena and also excessive length of fingernails. Water, in some form either warm or cold, usually relieved the pain temporarily. Some of these veterans were said to have filled their boots with water to ease the pain in a lower extremity. Soaking the hand in water was a common pain relieving procedure.

From Weir Mitchell's initial description has evolved the recognition of a family of conditions included under a broad umbrella of "Sympathetic Maintained Pain". There are a variety of synonyms which are employed, such as: major causalgia, minor causalgia, shoulder-hand syndrome, Sudex atrophy, reflex sympathetic dystrophy, post traumatic pain syndrome, post traumatic vaso motor disorder, post traumatic spreading neuralgia, and post traumatic painful osteoporosis (Kozin, McCarty, Sims, & Genant, 1976).

It must also be recognized that included in this spectrum of patients are those in whom the final diagnosis is that of hysteria. The separation of these patients, with mainly hysterical components, from those with more classical sympathetic dystrophy is a major diagnostic problem.

These definitions are clearly separated in the *Classification of Chronic Pain Descriptions of Chronic Pain Syndromes and Definitions of Pain Terms* as prepared by the International Association for the Study of Pain subcommittee on taxonomy (1986). In this classification there are two diagnoses: (1) causalgia (Mitchell, 1872, Mitchell, Morehouse, & Keen, 1864, Kozin, McCarty, Sims, & Genant, 1976, International Association for the Study of Pain, 1986) and (2) reflex sympathetic dystrophy (Mitchell, 1872, Mitchell, et al., 1864, Kozin, et al., 1976, International Association for the Study of Pain, 1986, Blumberg, Griesser, & Homyak, 1990). The major difference separating these categories is that causalgia involves a disruption of the somatic nerve or nerve root as well as the other phenomena which we associate with sympathetically maintained pain. Reflex sympathetic dystrophy does not involve the disruption of a nerve trunk or a peripheral nerve. Causalgia (Mitchell, 1872, Mitchell, et al., 1864, Kozin, et al., 1976, International Association for the Study of Pain, 1986) is associated with physical findings of nerve disruption, such as numbness or anesthesia throughout a dermatomal or peripheral nerve distribution and appropriate muscle weakness. On the other hand, in reflex sympathetic dystrophy these neurological findings are not present and the syndrome may evolve after a relatively minor soft tissue trauma in the extremity, although the trauma may include a fracture. With causalgia (Mitchell, 1872, Mitchell, et al., 1864, Kozin, et al., 1976, International Association for the Study of Pain, 1986), the onset of the burning pain is usually immediately after the nerve injury. In reflex sympathetic dystrophy (Mitchell, 1872, Mitchell, et al., 1864, Kozin, et al., 1976, International Association for the Study of Pain, 1986, Blumberg, et al., 1990), the pain follows the trauma, but not necessarily immediately, and there is no demonstrable nerve injury. Trophic changes and phenomena associated with altered sympathetic activity, such as blushing of the skin followed by cyanotic cold sweating extremities, are noted in both. Demineralization of bone, particularly in the juxtarticular area, occurs in both conditions. Relief of pain by sympathetic block is diagnostic of sympathetically maintained pain. In both causalgia and reflex sympathetic dystrophy the condition may progress to dysfunction and disuse of the involved extremity and profound emotional depression and chronic pain behavior may occur. Treatment of these emotional responses is of equal importance to any somatic remedy.

Now it is time to enumerate the objective physical findings that can be associated with sympathetically maintained pain (Blumberg, Greisser, & Homyak, 1990, Kozin, Genant, Bekerman, & McCarthy, 1976, Davidoff, 1988). First of all, the findings are general throughout the extremity and not dermatomal or peripheral nerve distribution related. Prominent among the findings is reduced mobility of the extremity. There are also obvious changes in skin temperature. Swelling or increase in limb volume is a universal finding, and indeed, measurement of the volume of the extremity may be used as a sensitivity predictor of the success or failure of applied treatment. As successful treatment progresses, the swelling inevitably reduces. Abnormal sweating and muscle weakness is also a consistent companion of the syndrome. Abnormal temperature complaints, such as burning sensations or cold feelings, occur in about 95% of the patients. Objective measurement of surface temperature of the fingers reveals significant difference in the involved side compared to the noninvolved. The MMPI is not diagnostic but simply reflects the profile of chronic benign pain (DeGood, Shutty, Adams, & Anderson, 1990, Ray, Kelly, Cannella, & McConn, 1990).

Upper extremity sympathetic dystrophies may follow cervical spine injury (Wainapel, 1984, Cremer, Maynard, & Davidoff, 1989). Twenty percent of patients with shoulder-hand syndrome may have a spondylosis of the cervical spine, and 20 percent of quadriplegics will develop Sudex atrophy. Twelve percent of patients with hemilateral stroke paralysis develop shoulder-hand syndrome. The reflex sympathetic dystrophy which follows spinal cord injury must be separated from dysesthetic pain of central origin or radicular pain. Reflex sympathetic dystrophy, of course, is diffuse and involves the distal portion of the limb and is associated with edema and vaso motor instability. It is also noted that TPBS (Three Phase Tinactin Bone Scan) is positive appearing in patients with sympathetic dystrophy during the first six months following spinal cord injury. Mechanical stimulation and stimulation with transcutaneous electrical nerve stimulators (TENS) provoke intense pain in sympathetically maintained pain. Thermal stimulation, however, to the sympathetic dystrophic extremity provokes no more pain than when the same intensity of stimulus is applied to the contralateral normal extremity. Swelling, trophic skin changes, such as atrophy, hyperhydrosis, hypertrichosis, and fingernail changes along with vaso motor instability are all prominent features of the causalgia or sympathetic dystrophic extremity. In patients with shoulder-hand syndrome shoulder, ROM of shoulder is reduced as well as the grip strength. Extremity circumference measurements which correlate with volume changes are of significant importance is far as diagnosis is concerned. There is also point tenderness in the articular areas and synovial biopsy reveals edematous and proliferative lining cells with fibrous and perivascular infiltration of inflammatory cells. The radiological findings are those of patchy osteoporosis, juxtarticular demineralization, and erosion of subchondral bone. Sintography with technetium is positive in these patients.

Early diagnostic features of the disease can be described as a triad of swelling, abnormal sweating, and diminished muscle strength (Blumberg, et al., 1990). This is accompanied by spontaneous diffuse pain, hyperasthesia, abnormal temperature sensation, and observable differences in the temperature of the fingertips of the symptomatic hand compared to the temperature of the normal hand.

The exact mechanism by which a sympathetic system becomes involved in perpetuating a burning type pain and the development of trophic signs and sympathetically maintained pain is not precisely known. Recent evidence points to the participation of spinal wide dynamic range (WDR) neurons in perpetuating the painful sensation (Roberts, & Toglesong, 1988). It is suggested that nociceptor response associated with trauma can produce prolonged sensitization of these (WDR) neurons. It is also suggested that low threshold myelinated mechanoreceptors participate in afferent activity which activates sympathetic efferent. Chronic sympathetically maintained pains are mediated by activity in low threshold myelinated mechanoreceptors. This afferent activity results from sympathetic efferent actions upon the receptors, or upon afferent fibers ending in a neuroma; and these afferent fibers evoke sufficient activity in sensitized spinal WDR neurons to produce a painful sensation (Roberts, 1976). This suggests that anesthetizing sympathetic ganglia removes the sympathetic excitation of A fiber mechanoreceptors and a reduction in the mechanoreceptor activity following sympathetic block results in defacilitation of the WDR neurons. This defacilitation reduces hyperpathia and allodynia.

Analysis of noradrenaline in venous blood from a dystrophic limb, compared to that from a nondystrophic limb, in the same individual reveals a concentration of noradrenaline lower in the dystrophic limb than in the nondystrophic—particularly if allodynia is present (Drummond, & Finch, 1990). It is concluded that sympathetic outflow is lower in the dystrophic limb than in the nondystrophic. The phenomenon of sweating and of vascular change in the dystrophic limb may be a result of hypersensitivity to circulating neurotransmitters.

The main thrust of therapy is intervention of efferent sympathetic activity at some level between the central neuraxis and the peripheral sympathetic activity. The most popular and accepted site of attack is at the sympathetic ganglia (Luh, & Nathan, 1978, Wang, Johnson, & Ilstrup, 1985). Anesthesia blockade at these sites (stellate ganglia, or lumbar paravertebral) provides diagnostic criteria in that if stigmata of sympathetic blockade is accompanied by pain relief, diagnosis is confirmed. If the pain is not relieved, although stigmant of sympathetic neuroblockade are observed, then the diagnosis is invalid. There are several groups of response from sympathetic ganglian blockade. The first of these is that the duration of pain relief outlasts by many hours the duration of anticipated anesthesia from the local anesthetic injected. It also is noted in this group the return of pain is at a considerable less intensity than the pain suffered prior to the sympathetic block. With each successive injection, this phenomenon continues so that eventually duration of pain relief is extensive and intensity of pain return is insignificant. The author feels that when this sequence of events is recognized, the early institution of biofeedback and supportive psychotherapy as well as appropriate physiotherapy accelerate the progression of the beneficial results.

A second group of patients are those that respond dramatically to the sympathetic ganglian blockade in that there is a marked reduction in their pain associated with signs of sympathetic block. However, the duration of pain relief is consistent with the duration of activity of the local anesthetic injected. With each successive sympathetic block the duration of pain relief remains the same and the intensity of pain when it returns also is unaltered. These patients are candidates for surgical sympathectomy.

There are other logical sites of intervention of sympathetic activity aside from the sympathetic ganglia. In the upper extremity, median nerve block at the cubital fossa may provide results identical to those of a stellate ganglian block (Wassef, 1990). Most of the sympathetic innervation to the hand is of the median nerve. If the regional anesthesia therapist is more comfortable providing median nerve block than a stellate ganglian block, the therapeutic results may be anticipated to be identical and a median nerve block is an acceptable alternative.

For the lower extremity, epidural injection of a small quantity of local anesthesia at the L2 3 level will provide sympathetic denervation of the entire lower extremity bilaterally (Brechner, 1990). This will be accompanied by somatic anesthesia, but if the quantity of local anesthetic injected is restricted to 5cc one may observe somatic anesthesia limited to the L2 dermatome. Again, if the therapist is more comfortable with this particular type of block than paravertebral lumbar sympathetic block, it is thoroughly acceptable.

It is the author's opinion that if paravertebral lumbar sympathetic block is to be employed, it should be done under image intensification or fluoroscopic control, with certain identification that the site of injection is along the anteralateral border of lumbar 3 vertebral body.

An alternative method of therapy is to use a terminal sympathetic block with the injection of the Bier technique of either reserpine or bretylium (Ford, Forrest, & Eltherington, 1988). It is the author's preference to avoid this type of therapy for the pragmatic reason that insertion of an intraveneous needle in the dystrophic edemetous limb is difficult and painful. Also painful is the extraction of blood from the dystrophic limb with Eschmare bandage and the application of tourniquets as is necessary to produce this type of block.

A nonprocedural method of treating sympathetic dystrophy is the use of high dosage Prednisone orally for a brief time (Kozin, Soin, Ryan, Carrera, & Wortman, 1981). This consists of the use of 60 80 mg per day for two weeks and then tapering the dosage over an ensuing two-week period.

In all of the above mentioned methods of therapy it is of the utmost importance that physiotherapy be applied to improve range of motion and enhance muscle strength. Indeed, one of the major purposes of providing a period of pain relief by whatever method, is to allow the physiotherapy to be instituted during the pain-free period. It should also be stressed that appropriate psychological supports, treatment of depression and the use of biofeedback be employed along with the somatic intraventive procedures. Biofeedback is particularly appropriate in that if properly instructed the patient can, by the use of biofeedback, generate many of the conditions that result from a sympathetic block. It is quite possible for a patient to receive several sympathetic blocks and then, with appropriate biofeedback training, be able to replicate the conditions following the block by his own thought intervention. This places the patient in the position of being his own therapist. Also, the use of biofeedback allows a psychotherapist an easy approach to providing other psychotherapeutic methods in treatment of the psychological traumas that accompany sympathetic dystrophy.

REFERENCES

Blumberg, H. Griesser, H. J., Homyak, M. (1990). Early bedside diagnosis of reflex sympathetic dystrophy in upper extremities. Abs. slide #945. *Pain Suppl. 5.*

Brechner, V. L. (1990). Management of pain by conduction anesthesia techniques. *Youman's neurological surgery* (3rd ed.), Vol. 6, Chap. 150, 4007-4025. Philadelphia: W. B. Saunders Co.

Cremer, S. A., Maynard, F., Davidoff, G. (1989). The reflex sympathetic dystrophy syndrome associated with traumatic myelopathy. *Pain, 37*:187-192.

Davidoff, G. (1988). Pain measurement in reflex sympathetic dystrophy syndrome. *Pain, 32*:27-34.

DeGood, D., Shutty, M., Adams, L., & Anderson, C. (1990). Psychosocial behavior distress pattern of reflex sympathetic dystrophy patients is not different from that of low back patients. Abs. Poster #19, Abs. #823. *Pain Suppl. 5.*

Drummond, P. D., & Finch, P. M. (1990). Autonomic function in reflex sympathetic dystrophy. Abs. Poster #805. *Pain Suppl. 5.*

Ford, S. R., Forrest, W. H., & Eltherington, L. (1988). The treatment of reflex sympathetic dystrophy with intravenous regional bretylium. *Anesthesiology, 68*:139-140.

International association for the study of pain subcommittee on taxonomy classification of chronic pain. (1986). *Pain Suppl. 3*:51-5225.

Kozin, F., McCarty, J., Sims, J., Genant, H. (1976). Reflex sympathetic dystrophy syndrome I. *American Journal of Medicine, 60*:321-331.

Kozin, F., Genant, H. K., Bekerman, C., & McCarthy, D. J. (1976). The reflex sympathetic dystrophy syndrome II. *American Journal of Medicine, 60*:332-338.

Kozin, F., Soin, J. S., Ryan, L. M., Carrera, G. F., & Wortman, R. L. (1981). Reflex sympathetic dystrophy syndrome III. *American Journal of Medicine, 70*:23-30.

Luh, L., & Nathan, P. W. (1978). Painful peripheral states and sympathetic block. *Journal of Neurology and Psychiatry, 41*:664-671.

Mitchell, S. W. (1872). *Injuries of nerves and their consequences.* Philadelphia: J. B. Lippincott Co.

Mitchell, S. W., Morehouse, G. R., & Keen, W. W., Jr. (1864). *Gunshot wounds and other injuries of nerves.* Philadelphia: J. B. Lippincott Co.

Ray, P. P., Kelly, J. F., Cannella, S. J., & McConn, K. (1990). Multidisciplinary assignment and management of reflex sympathetic dystrophy. Abs. Poster #6, Abs. 810, *Pain Suppl. 5.*

Roberts, W. A. (1986). A hypothesis on the physiological basis for causalgia and related pains. *Pain, 24*:294-311.

Roberts, W. I., & Toglesong, M. E. (1988). Spinal recordings suggest that wide dynamic range neurons mediate sympathetically maintained pain. *Pain, 34*:289-304.

Wainapel, S. F. (1984). Reflex sympathetic dystrophy following traumatic myelopathy. *Pain, 18*:345-349.

Wang, J. K., Johnson, K. A., & Ilstrup, D. (1985). Sympathetic blocks for sympathetic dystrophies pain. *Pain, 23*:13-17.

Wassef, M. R. (1990). Management of reflex sympathetic dystrophy syndrome of the hand with very low dose mepivacaine. Median Nerve Block Slide #946. *Pain Suppl. 5.*

Chapter 15

MYOFASCIAL PAIN SYNDROME

Clinical Evaluation and Management of Patients

Michael Margoles, M.D., Ph.D.

Michael Margoles, M.D., Ph.D. captures the essence and brings to the reader, a clear review of Myofascial Pain Syndrome. Doctor Margoles builds upon the seminal work of Travell and Simons in aiding the clinician to understand how to conduct a physical evaluation and manage patients suffering from Myofascial Pain Syndrome. This chapter provides the reader with a number of forms which can be reproduced for use in practice.

The perpetuating factors, which prolong the experience of Myofascial Pain, are clearly described with advice given for implementing a step-wise approach toward their elimination. Doctor Margoles also provides a brilliant taxonomy relating severity of Myofascial Pain Syndrome to length of treatment and preclusions for work.

A deposition on this is included in the Appendix section entitled, "Depositions."

Chapter 15

MYOFASCIAL PAIN SYNDROME

Clinical Evaluation and Management of Patients
Michael S. Margoles, M.D., Ph.D.

ABSTRACT

Myofascial Pain Syndrome(MPS) is a frequent basis of acute and chronic pain in any muscle location of the body. Awareness of its existence is growing. Specifics of clinical diagnosis are well-defined and have been published in texts and magazines. Proper evaluation of the patient with MPS requires: (1) a thorough history, emphasizing detailed analysis of the mechanism of injury(MOI), (2) physical examination employing analytic techniques that are specific for MPS, and (3) search for perpetuating factors. Perpetuating factors are mechanical, physiological, psychological, biochemical, metabolic, hormonal, and infectious elements that, if abnormal, promote chronicity in MPS; and cause it to become resistant to many types of therapy. Management is a complex procedure that must be properly sequenced to ensure success in the recovery of the MPS patient. Clarification of International ICD-9-CM coding is presented. Grading of MPS severity is discussed to enhance professional communication and promote better understanding of MPS. Staging of therapy is broken into 10 stages to simplify management sequencing.

INTRODUCTION

The work that follows is intended to compliment the seminal works of Travell and Simons (Travell and Simons, 1983) (Travell, in press). The reader is referred to their texts for more comprehensive reading about Myofascial Pain Syndrome (MPS) (Myofascial Syndrome) ICD-9-CM = 729.1.

A great deal of the most common, persistent, and disabling pains are of musculoskeletal origin (Fields, 1987).

MPS is pain and/or altered sensation (tingling, numbness, burning, goose flesh, swelling, tightness, tension, and other paresthesias) referred

from active myofascial trigger points (TrP), and may occur in the immediate area about a TrP or as referred pain 1 to 3 feet away from the source.
The pain of MPS can vary from mild to severe and incapacitating. MPS
occurs most commonly in single muscles. However, it can spread to
involve many other adjacent and distant muscles. Myofascial trigger
points may occur in any of the 500 muscles in the body.

Historically, MPS has been intermingled with numerous other terms
used to describe soft tissue pain problems such as fibrositis, fibromyalgia,
fibromyositis, non-articular rheumatism, paucy-articular rheumatism,
psychogenic rheumatism, psychogenic pain, myogelosis, lumbago, and
other clinical pain syndromes characterized by the terms such as
"functional overlay," "symptom magnification," etc. The result of all this
varied terminology has been confusion.

Although MPS is common, and not too difficult to diagnosis, many
therapists are unaware of it existence (Fields, 1987). There are some who
claim that there is a paucity of "objective signs." They say nothing of significance can be detected on the X-ray, CT, and MRI scans, and that diagnostic laboratory testing is lacking. This has the appearance of adding
more confusion to confusion.

MPS is diagnosed by clinical assessment and augmented by appropriate laboratory testing. The criteria for diagnosing MPS have been published by Travell and Simons (1983).

In an era where "high tech" is "in," proper evaluation and management
of MPS requires astute comprehensive skills in clinical evaluation. The
"hands on" approach to MPS patients is still the only way that a proper
diagnosis can presently be made. It is critical to determining the extent
and complexity of MPS in order to decide what management approaches
will be necessary to manage the patient.

Lack of an adequate physical examination, geared specifically to evaluation for MPS, is probably the most common reason that physicians fail to
make the diagnosis. Diagnostic evaluation for MPS must be performed
by clinicians with proper skills and training. The evaluations are ardu-
ous, technical, and time-consuming.

While evaluating a patient with a soft tissue pain problem keep the following formula in mind:

MYOFASICAL TRIGGER POINTS + TAUT BANDS + PERPETUAT-
ING FACTORS = MYOFASCIAL PAIN SYNDROME

CLINICAL POINTS OF IMPORTANCE

Clinical Examination

Adequate physical examination of the grade 2, 3 and 4 (see Appendix 3
at the end of this chapter for grading of severity and definitions) patients

may require up to one to two hours. This is in addition to the history taking. With each increased grade of severity the amount of time to complete an adequate history and physical examination (consisting of routine and myofascial elements) increases.

Preeminent Themes in the History

1. Mechanism of onset (MOO) may be injury, trauma, strain, sprain, or spontaneous onset. The patient may be vague about the exact date of onset (Fields, 1987).

2. Etiology.
   a. Muscle overload (the muscle is usually strained in a shortened position) (Baker, 1986) may be one of a number of the important components here.
   b. Excessive or repeat traumas.
   c. Sleep disorder.
   d. Unknown.

3. Complaints of pain in a distribution that is regional and does not follow spinal segmental nor single peripheral nerve distribution.
   a. Myofascial pain occurs in classic Tp reference zones (Travell and Simons, 1983; Travell and Simons, in press).
   b. The referred pain of myofascial origin is frequently confused with radicular pain of spinal disc origin.
   c. The pain of MPS is deep and/or aching in quality, and can be felt in joints, muscles, or any place in the body.
   d. Tp's can generate paresthesias, autonomic symptoms (burning and goose flesh), proprioceptive dysfunction and weakness.
   e. The distribution of pain and/or altered sensations is usually not coextensive with the Tp's producing it.
   f. Symptoms from MPS may begin at the time of injury, or may occur minutes, hours, days, weeks, or months after an initiating incident.
   g. Once initiated, an MPS can become progressively worse over a period or days, weeks, months, or years.

4. Complaints of dysfunction.
   a. Weakness of the effected limb.
      1. Unexpected giving away of the leg.
      2. Dropping things with the hand on the pain side.

5. The severity of symptoms from myofascial Tp's ranges from painless restriction of motion due to latent Tp's so common in the aged, to agonizing incapacitating pain caused by very active Tp's (Travell and Simons, 1983).

6. Pain may be aggravated by:
   a. Changes in weather.
   b. Emotional stress.
   c. Physical stress.
   d. Premenstrual syndrome.

7. Difficulty finding a comfortable sleeping position is common in the more severe cases.

8. Dizziness may occur in cases where there is involvement of the head and neck.

9. Absence of other diseases to account for the symptoms.

10. Study of pain charts (Also called a "symptom chart." The pain chart is an important diagnostic tool that helps determine the extent of the MPS and its severity.) preferably filled out by the patient at each visit, provides clues to the location of trigger points causing the specific pain patterns (Margoles, 1983).

11. Pain may switch sides.
    a. Generally over a period of months.
    b. Occasionally within a few weeks.
    c. Rarely on a daily or every other day cycle.

12. Pain from one trigger point may mask that from another.

Physical Examination — Trigger Points

All patients with persistent pain or aching should be examined for myofascial trigger points and MPS (Fields, 1987). It must be emphasized that the evaluation of patients with Myofascial Pain Syndrome is not a casual endeavor. The clinician attempting to diagnose the more complex cases must be specifically trained in the evaluation techniques of Myofascial Pain Syndrome (Travell and Simons, 1983; Travell, in press) and/or should be supervised by a therapist expert in the proper techniques of evaluation and management. A "shot in the dark" approach is no substitute for training, skill, and acumen.

I. The essential aspects of the examination for myofascial trigger points consist of the following major and minor criteria that have been adapted from Simons (personal communication). To make the diagnosis the findings should include five major criteria and at least one of the three minor criteria.

Major Criteria
1. Regional pain complaint.
2. Pain complaint or altered sensation in the expected distribution of referred pain from a myofascial trigger point.

3. Taut band palpable in muscles that are accessible. The accessibility to palpation of a taut band in a muscle is variable depending on the thickness of adipose tissue, turgor, and tension of the subcutaneous tissue, thickness, and tension of overlying muscles, and tension on the muscle fibers being examined.
4. Exquisite spot tenderness at one point along the length of the taut band, in the muscle belly. This is usually the location of the trigger point.
5. Some degree of restricted stretch range of motion, when measurable, for the primary function of that muscle. For example, a trigger point in the levator scapulae muscle will cause decrease lateral rotation of the neck.

Minor Criteria
1. Reproduction of clinical pain complaint, or altered sensation, by pressure on the tender spot. The tender spot must cause referral of pain (or change in sensation) at a distance of at least 2 cm beyond the spot of local tenderness. Pain referral or altered sensation is elicited in response to pressure applied to the tender spot for 10 seconds before considered negative. "Altered sensation" may be described by the patient as a tingling, numbness, or "unusual feeling."
2. Elicitation of a local twitch response by transverse snapping palpation at the tender spot in the taut band.
3. Pain alleviated by elongating (stretching) the muscle, or by injecting the tender spot (trigger point).
4. Restricted range of motion of the body part or joint effected by the myofascial trigger points bearing on it. Restricted range of motion of a joint gives clues to the location of trigger points. For example, decreased active abduction of the shoulder may be due to an infraspinatus trigger point, or any of the five other muscles that can cause a similar problem about the shoulder.
5. Patients frequently give a startled response (jump sign) when sufficient pressure is applied to the trigger point (Travell and Simons, 1983). See definition of a jump sign at the end of the chapter.
6. The trigger point occurs at a classic location. (See Appendix 6.)

Physical Examination — Other Myofascial

I routinely examine other body areas, unrelated to the patient's presenting problem(s), as part of my usual evaluation of MPS patients. I do this to determine the extent of the myofascial problem. I want to know if the patient has a simple (a single muscle MPS) or complex problem (multiple muscle MPS). A quick and easy way to do this is to palpate an area that is easily accessible in all patients whether thick or thin. The paraspinal muscles in the back extending from the base of the occiput to the end of the sacrum are ideal for this purpose.

To accomplish this:

1. The patient is prone on the exam table.
2. The neck is positioned in flexion by having the patient's neck and chin hung over a pillow at one end of the exam table.
3. The patient's arms dangle over the sides of the exam table to move the scapulae away from the paraspinal muscles.
4. All the paraspinal muscles from the base of the skull to the fifth sacral segment are palpated along both sides of the spine. Beginning 2 to 3 inches away from the midline flat palpation (Travell and Simons, 1983) is used to check for taut bands, local twitch responses, trigger points, jump signs, and unusual tenderness.
5. In the more severe cases I encounter an increased frequency of abnormal findings. Prognostically this means slower response to appropriate management and a longer amount of time to recover.
6. Even if the back is the main area of involvement it is rare that the entire back from C1 to S5 is involved. Therefore, the uninvolved areas can be examined to determine if overall involvement is greater than the presenting problem.
7. Results of this testing can be accurately logged onto the sheet marked "paraspinal muscle assessment" (See Table I).

Physical Examination — Problems Caused by Myofascial

Trigger points can cause dysfunction and other problems in the muscles they inhabit. This may manifest as weakness. The patient may have an abnormal JAMAR grip strength test. There may be decreased strength on manual muscle testing (MMT) in one or a number of muscles affected by any myofascial trigger points anywhere in the body.

Some muscles will demonstrate breakaway weakness (BAW) (Baker, 1986) when manual muscle testing (MMT) is carried out. This occurs as the muscle is being resisted through its normal range of motion. About half way through the muscle arc of motion there is a sudden "breakaway." The muscle quickly loses strength, and the patient may experience pain in the muscle being tested. The suddenness of the breaking away addresses the presence of a trigger point. On the other hand, if the muscle being tested is diffusely tender and painful, the MMT procedure will show a generalized weakness throughout its entire range of motion. Functionally, the BAW can cause problems of dropping silverware, pots, dishes, and other potentially dangerous objects. It can cause the hip, leg, or knee to give away without warning.

Another manifestation of dysfunction related to trigger points is decreased range of motion of a limb, joint, neck, or back. At times, involvement of the shoulder(s) can be so severe as to cause a "frozen shoulder" that clinically looks identical to that of a bony fusion. The pain may be agonizing, especially when the patient attempts to move the shoulder.

Table I. Prone position back muscle examination. This is a routine part of the comprehensive MPS examination.

Coding: Tenderness: 0 = none; 1 = mild; 2 = moderate; 3 = intolerable.
Taut bands: 0 = none; 1 = thin; 2 = thick
Jump sign (involuntary withdrawal, wriggling, or twitch 'jump')
 Use a check mark if present.
Local twitch response
 Use a check mark if present.

Segment	Tenderness (paraspinal muscles)		Taut band (paraspinal muscles)		Trigger point (paraspinal muscles)		Jump sign[1] (paraspinal		Local Twitch response muscles)	
	Left	Right	Left	Right	Left	Right	Left	Right	Left	Right
C1										
C2										
C3										
C4										
C5										
C6										
C7										
T1										
T2										
T3										
T4										
T5										
T6										
T7										
T8										
T9										
T10										
T11										
T12										
L1										
L2										
L3										
L4										
L5										
S1										
S2										
S3										
S4										
S5										

[1] In some of the grade 2 patients, and most of the grade 3 and 4 when adequate pressure is applied as the taut band is snapped, the jump sign is such that the patient all but jumps off the examination table.

Other dysfunction (s) may present as tendonitis and bursitis. The effected tendon, bursae, or joint may even appear slightly swollen.

Trigger points that are active cause pain and pain patterns that are frequently confused with "arthritis." Careful study of the pain chart, physical examination, and X-rays usually reveal the myofascial nature of the problem. Even though the X-rays may show some degenerative changes Myofascial Pain Syndrome may still be the cause of the pain and not the joint changes. One of my patients had fairly advanced rheumatoid arthritis of her hands. She did secretarial work. Typing activities caused pain in her hands. With proper myofascial management her myofascial hand pain was resolved. Her hands became painless, but the rheumatoid deformities remained. Everyone that has a limp does not have arthritis of the hip or leg. A frequent cause of limping are trigger points in the gluteus minimus, medius, or maximus muscles. Limping can be caused by a trigger point in almost any muscle of the leg.

Paresthesias associated with active trigger points can be very distressing. At times the numbness produced in the fingers and finger tips may cause the patient to get burned because of impaired perception to heat in the effected hand(s).

Proprioceptive dysfunctions are annoying. Trigger points in muscles cause faulty spatial orientation messages to be sent to the brain. Because balance is adversely effected distances are misjudged. This is commonly manifested by bumping into furniture or doorways. In some of the worst cases patients have reported walking into walls.

The net result of the dysfunctions caused by myofascial trigger points or Myofascial Pain Syndrome (MPS) may be overall decreased physical functioning for activities of daily living such as job duties, bathing, hygiene, sleeping, sexual activity, etc. The greater the number of trigger points that scatter throughout the body, the more sizable is the degree of physical impairment.

Physical Examination — MPS - PTM

As part of my routine examination of the grade 2, 3, and 4 patients I perform a pressure threshold meter test (Available from Pain Diagnostics and Thermography, Inc. 233 East Shore Road, Suite 108, Great Neck, New York, 11023, (516) 829-9469). This hand-held, pressure sensitive gauge can be used quickly and easily. Testing is carried out in all or some of the muscles on the graph in Appendix 9. The meter can be used for three purposes:

1. To assess the presence of generalized tenderness in a patient that presents with what appears to be a localized problem.
2. To pick up trigger points in the classic MPS locations.
3. To document that the trigger point has been eradicated after being

treated. After the trigger point is adequately treated the abnormal tenderness changes back to normal.

Normative data is not available for all the muscles on the graph.

Perpetuating Factors and Laboratory Evaluation

This is a vital part of the evaluation and management of patients with MPS, yet many clinicians pay little or no attention to it. Perpetuating factors (PF) are a number of essential elements of MPS that prolong the pain and dysfunction. They make MPS resistant to "usual and customary" methods of management (Margoles, 1983; Margoles, in press; Margoles, 1987; Rask, 1980; Simons, personal communication; Travell and Simons, 1983; Travell, 1976; Travell, personal communication). They impede the patient's progress of recovery, and confound the patient and the therapist.

If only short-term or incomplete relief is obtained after the application of an appropriate physical management (trigger point injection (TPI), stretch and spray (S&S), (Lewitt stretch, etc.), the patient has to be reevaluated for perpetuating factor problems.

In the more complex cases (grade 3 or 4) this must be done routinely as part of the initial comprehensive evaluation and management (see Fig. 1).

The well-known perpetuating factors include:

I. Mechanical problems:
1. Repeated injuries or accidents.
2. Structural problems (Travell and Simons, 1983).
   a. Short leg.
   b. Short hemi-pelvis.
   c. Long 2nd metatarsal(s) and short first metatarsal(s).
   d. Short upper extremity(s).
3. Ruptured cervical or lumbar disc (Margoles, 1987).
4. Brassiere straps that are too tight and/or support heavy breasts.
5. Persistent muscular over-exertion (abuse of muscles).
6. Abnormalities of dental structures including teeth, bones, joints, and/or muscles (Mackley, in press).

II. Physiological problems:
1. The stress of a surgical procedure.
2. Chronic fatigue.
3. Lack of restorative and/or restful sleep.
4. Malabsorption syndrome.

III. Psychological problems:
1. Too much nervous tension and emotional stress.
2. Drug overdoses.
3. Chronic anxiety and/or worrying.

4. The Myofascial Pain Syndrome, with its associated pain and dysfunction, is a source of stress, anxiety, and depression.
5. Behaviors that promote abuse of muscles.

Laboratory Assessments for Perpetuating Factors

Utilization of specific laboratory testing (Travell and Simons, 1983)
and appropriate interpretation of results are some of the most important
means of detecting perpetuating factors. Currently, many clinicians are
skeptical about the role of correcting the metabolic abnormalities cited in
chapter 4 of Travell and Simons (1983). Correct adjustment of the biochemical, metabolic, and hormonal perpetuating factors is crucial to a
satisfactory outcome in the management of patients with MPS.

IV. Biochemical:
　　1. Vitamin problems:
　　　　a. Too little (insufficient, less than optimal, or deficient) serum
　　　　　　levels of:
　　　　　　　　B1 Thiamine
　　　　　　　　B2 Riboflavin
　　　　　　　　B3 Niacin
　　　　　　　　B5 Pantothenate
　　　　　　　　B6 Pyridoxine
　　　　　　　　Bc Folic Acid
　　　　　　　　B12 Cobalamin
　　　　　　　　Vitamin C Ascorbic Acid
　　　　　　　　Vitamin D Cholecalciferol

Less than optimal is defined as a blood test level below the upper 75%
of the normal range. For example, a blood test for a perpetuating factor
had a normal range of 10 to 50 units. If the range is broken up into quar-
tiles the plotting would look like Fig. 7. If the patient's result is below 40
the blood test level is less than optimal. A practical example would relate
to a tire on your car. If its air content gets down to less than 75% of usual,
the car does not handle well, and may even be dangerous to drive. The tire
functions best at between 75 and 100% of the manufacturer's recommended inflation. The same holds true for adjusting the blood test results
in the management of patients with MPS.

　　　　b. Too much
　　　　　　1. Vitamin A:
　　　　　　　　a. Vitamin A toxicity from intake of Vitamin A supple-
　　　　　　　　　　ments or excess carotene conversion, in the body, to vita-
　　　　　　　　　　min A (Margoles, in press).
　　　　　　　　b. Eating foods too high is vitamin A or carotene.
　　　　　　2. Mineral problems:

      a. Too little (less than optimal serum levels of):
          Potassium
          Calcium
          Magnesium
          Iron and ferritin

V. Metabolic:
    a. Relative or absolute hyperuricemia (Travell and Simons, 1983).
    b. Low grade or frank anemia.

VI. Hormonal: (Barnes, 1976)
    a. Hypometabolism (low thyroid function) (Travell and Simons, 1983)
    b. Insufficient estrogen supply.

VII. Infections:
    a. Acute and chronic virus, bacterial, and other organism infections of the lungs, kidneys, bones, sinuses, teeth, and gums.

Blood testing for biochemical, metabolic
and hormonal

PERPETUATING FACTORS

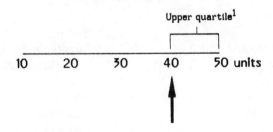

Figure 1

If the patient blood tests below the arrow pointing to the 40 units, he/she has a less than optimal blood level of that perpetuating factor.

[1] This represents the optimal part of the normal range.

LABORATORY TESTING

I routinely order the testing listed below on all MPS patients with suspected biochemical perpetuating factors. The patients with grade 2, 3, or 4 are routinely tested before their first visit. Some of the tests take 7 to 10 days to get results back. In the grade 1 cases the patient is first seen and examined to determine whether the blood testing seems necessary as part of their evaluation.

"PANEL" Test (or equivalent)	Additional Initial Testing to Order
Includes:	ferritin
HEMATOLOGY	magnesium
CBC	calcium, ionized
DIFF	Endocrinology
ESR	T4 by RIA
Chemistry	T3 by RIA
bicarbonate	12 Vitamin panel from
calcium	Vitamin
chloride	Diagnostics
creatinine	Vitamin B12
glucose	Folic Acid
iron	Vitamin B6
phosphorus	Thiamin
potassium	Niacin
sodium	Biotin
urea nitrogen	Riboflavin
uric acid	Pantothenic Acid
Liver function	Vitamin A
Protein, total	Vitamin C
Bilirubin, total	Vitamin E
LDH	Beta-Carotene
Alk Phosphatase	
SGOT(AST)	
SGPT(ALT)	
GGTP	
Lipids	
Cholesterol	
Triglycerides	
Urinalysis	

The ionized calcium test measures the unbound calcium in the blood. It is not the same as the routine serum calcium test. MANY LABS GET THE TWO TESTS MIXED UP.

NOTE: Special arrangements have to be made to ship the blood for vitamin levels to Vitamin Diagnostics. If you are interested in the specialized vitamin tests call Susan Feingold at Vitamin Diagnostics. Vitamin Diagnostics, Route 35 and Industrial Drive, Cliffwood Beach, New Jersey, 07735. (201) 583-7773

SPECIAL STUDIES

X-ray, CT, MRI, etc.

At present there are no predictable findings in X-ray, CT, MRI, Bone scan, or EMG studies that consistently support the diagnosis of MPS. Instead, it is the absence of significant bony, disc, and nerve pathology that helps point the clinician in the direction of MPS as the cause of the patients presenting complaints. On the other hand, a positive result in any of the above mentioned tests does not rule out MPS.

Figures 2 through 7 give the 9 crucial states of therapy in the management of Myofascial Pain Syndrome(MPS), plus the optional stage 10 for advanced therapeutic management. They are a summary of the text that appears in the section about management of MPS patients.

MANAGEMENT

Management – Introduction

The management of MPS may be an endeavor that is complex and challenging for both the therapist and the patient. There may be frustration for both sides of the management team. Certain of the perpetuating factors take time to correct. For example, muscles that have been thrown out of balance, along the spine, neck, and other areas need time to come back into balance once the proper lift is prescribed for the shoe on the short leg side. Less than optimal serum potassium levels require time, effort, and retesting of the blood levels until the serum potassium reaches the optimal part of the normal range. The multiplicity of factors involved are shown in Figures 2 and 3, stages 1-3.

The patient may have a number of etiologies for his or her pain complaints. For example, there may be pain radiating down the leg. There may be trigger points about the low back, hip, or buttock that, when stimulated, reproduce the leg pain. The patient may also have an absent achilles reflex and a MRI scan positive for a herniated disc on that side. The MPS can mimic the disc rupture. Therefore, in the absence of an acute paralysis from the ruptured disc, it is important to treat the MPS first.

Rehabilitation of the (MPS) patient is a progressive endeavor. Starting the therapy program for a grade 2, 3, or 4 patient, with stage 10 (See Fig. 7) physical therapy will fail. Prescribing a NSAID to a grade 3 or 4 patient

MPS STAGING OF MANAGEMENT

FOUNDATIONAL STAGES

STAGE 1

CORRECT ALL PERPETUATING FACTORS

Structural (all anatomical problems including dental), Mechanical, Endocrine Biochemical, Physiological, any infectious problems regardless of location in the body

May require 6-12 weeks to accomplish. Check and adjust serum potassium levels every 10-14 days for the first 6 weeks. Some of the grade 1 and 2 MPS patients will recover merely by correction of their perpetuating factors.

STAGE 2

NORMALIZE SLEEP

Behavioral techniques are used first. Next, mild muscle relaxers and antihistamines are used to to induce sleep (Benadryl, Elavil[1], Klonopin, Soma, or similar medication.
May require 6-12 weeks to stabilize.

[1] Brand name is preferred here

Figure 2

MPS STAGING OF MANAGEMENT

FOUNDATIONAL STAGES
FOUNDATIONAL STAGES

STAGE 3

CORRECT PSYCHOLOGIC PERPETUATING FACTORS

Reduce tension, stress and anxiety. Correct behaviors that promote abuse of muscles. Correct dysfunctional thinking. Cognitive restructuring.

May require up to three months of therapy.

STAGE 4

PAIN SYMPTOM CONTROL

Begin with NSAID's[1] and Tylenol. Progress to Darvon, Talwin, and finally to the narcotic containing or narcotic medications. Dosing is time contingent. Aim for 30-50% relief or to the point where the medication "takes the edge off" of the pain.

[1] Nonsteroidal antiinflammatory drugs

Figure 3

MPS STAGING OF MANAGEMENT

INTERMEDIATE STAGES
INTERMEDIATE STAGES

STAGE 5

MEDICATIONS TO FACILITATE PHYSICAL RECOVERY

These are used to combat muscle soreness as physical activity level increases. NSAID's are useful here. Injectable NSAID[1] can be used in patients who have gastric intolerance. Patient is given home stretching program and encouraged to increase overall physical activity level.

[1] Sodium thiosalicylate I.M. or Colchicine I.V.

STAGE 6

FACILITATE RECOVERY

This is important for the grade 3 and 4 patients. A Registered Occupational Therapist is consulted to expedite activities of daily living. The patient is given a disability parking sticker to encourage return to normal activity levels.

Figure 4

MPS STAGING OF MANAGEMENT

INTERMEDIATE STAGES
INTERMEDIATE STAGES

STAGE 7
MOBILIZATION

Begin formal physical therapy. Stretch and spray. Trigger point injections. Lewitt stretch. Chiropractic. Low impact aerobics. "Tube" exercises. Williams and McKinzie exercises. Massage. Low resistance stretching. Partial range of motion stretching. NOTE: patient may only be able to tolerate therapy twice per week.

Begin to get rid of *BARRIER* trigger points.

Nerve blocks and epidural injections can be attempted at this stage. If there is no significant improvement after three attempts, these injections should be deferred to stages 8 or 10.

Figure 5

MPS STAGING OF MANAGEMENT

FINAL STAGES

STAGE 8

IMPROVE FLEXIBILITY, STRENGTH AND ENDURANCE

Back school. Work hardening program. Aggressive physical therapy. Trigger point injections. Stretch and spray. Lewitt stretch. Chiropractic. Swimming. Jogging. Full range of motion stretching. Work out BARRIER trigger points. Medium load stretching against resistance.

STAGE 9

VOCATIONAL REHABILITATION

Vocational testing and vocational rehabilitation. Slowly work the patient back into the job market. In addition, a comprehensive ergonomic analysis is carried out to ensure compatability with the patient's new or old employment.

Figure 6

MPS STAGING OF MANAGEMENT

ADVANCED STAGES

STAGE 10

ADVANCED PHYSICAL THERAPY (APT)

NOTE: this stage of the program is only for those MPS patients wishing to pursue a career or avocation that calls for maximum physical performance. All of the listed components can be utilized.

1. Work hardening program - more aggressive than in stage 8.
2. Aggressive aerobic workouts.
3. Progressive weight training.
   a. Weights can be used.
   b. Cybex or similar can be used.
4. Parallel bars.
5. Proprioceptive reeducation, neuromuscular timing and and coordination - "fine tuning"
6. Running and improving cardiac endurance.
7. Use of pressure threshold meter to measure progress and set further goals.
8. Work out all remaining BARRIER trigger points.

Figure 7

and injecting a single trigger point, followed by stretch and spray to the injected muscle may net very limited results. Recovery is a "step wise" undertaking (See stages 1-10, figures 2-7).

At times, an interdisciplinary team of pain management specialists are necessary for treating the recalcitrant cases. This team needs to be coordinated by a physician knowledgeable in MPS.

Timing and staging of therapeutic interventions is crucial to the patient's advancement toward recovery. This is shown in Figures 2-6. For example, taking a grade 3 MPS patient and starting the therapeutic program with him or her in an aggressive, sports-oriented, physical therapy program (stage 10) will net disaster and frustration. It is unrealistic to treat MPS patients as purely mechanical problems. It is sad to see MPS patients condemned as malingerers when they fail a purely mechanical physical therapy rehabilitation program. This situation prevails with therapists who do not understand the limits and restrictions that MPS imposes on the myofascial muscles. Given proper management and management staging, the MPS patient can be brought to the stage where they can begin to work out the kinks and stiffness (stage 7). However, if that same patient is taken through all the proper stages and staging of therapy listed below, and then put into the same Advanced Physical Therapy (APT) program, the patient is more likely to succeed and become rehabilitated. Stretch and spray (S&S) or trigger point injections (TPI), if poorly timed, may appear to backfire, resulting in frustrating pain flare-ups and disappointment. When they are properly sequenced in the management staging the results can be impressive.

When setbacks occur, if the clinician CAN COMPREHEND that more perpetuating factors need to be sought out and corrected before further physical therapies are attempted, the situation is salvageable.

FOUNDATIONAL STAGES

Management — Staging of Therapy

STAGE 1 (Fig. 2): Correct all Pf's (Travell and Simons, 1983).

    a. This must be done, in most cases (some of the grade 1 and 2 patients, and all of the grade 3 and 4 patients) before the physical therapies of stages 7, 8, 9, and 10 are attempted.

    b. Special attention must be given to meticulously "cleaning up" all the Pf's (Travell and Simons, 1983).

    c. When all these are corrected the MPS will either resolve spontaneously or will become more responsive to the next stages of management.

    d. Special note about some of the biochemical problems:

1. An easy program of oral replacement therapy is given in Appendix 5. It can be implemented, without the use of recommended blood testing, in all of the grade 1, and some of the grade 2 patients. Patients can order the products from Bronson, or you can stock the products in your office. It can be used in the grade 3 and 4 patients, but I recommend that the complete panel of blood testing be ordered first. Reason: once the patient is on oral B-complex vitamins for as little as three days, it distorts the blood test results. If you think you may need a panel of vitamin tests, to orient your management regimen, have the testing done before you begin to supplement whatever the patient is taking.

2. Taking vitamins by mouth does not guarantee an optimal blood level. There is no way to guess the vitamin nutriture from the clinical picture and complaints. Currently, the only accurate way to assess this is to get the 12 vitamin panel from Vitamin Diagnostics (see section on blood testing below). Vitamin Diagnostics also offers cellular vitamin assays. Consult Goodhart, R., 1980 for listings of the symptoms of deficiency and inadequacy of the various vitamins.

3. Some patients need a course of high potency (Margoles, 1989) B-complex injections. The composition of the injections is:

Syringe #1

Fortaplex or B-Plex 100 .... 1/2cc
Riboflavin 50mg/ml 1/2cc
2% Xylocaine (lidocaine) or
Novocaine (procaine) w/o epi. 1/2cc

Syringe #2

DPAN (Dexpanthenol 250mg/ml) 1cc
Hydroxocobalamin 1,000mcg/ml 1/4cc
Folic acid (5 or 10mg/ml) 1/4cc

Separate syringes are used because Folic Acid precipitates the B1 and B6 in the Fortaplex or B-Plex 100. Depending on the vitamin blood test results, patients are given the above injections once or twice per week. Patients with the lower blood test levels are given the injections twice per week. In the severely depleted patients the contents of each syringe can be doubled during the second and following weeks, to increase the effectiveness of the B-complex injections. See Appendix 1 for suppliers of the recommended products.

4. Some of the low normal hemoglobin, hematocrit, RBC, and Ferritin levels are resistant to many of the commonly available

iron tablets. The therapist may have to resort to Feosol elixir, and if that fails, a short course of low dose iron-dextran injections may be necessary to bring the hemoglobin, hematocrit, and RBC count up to a satisfactory part of the normal range.

5. Some patients are intolerant of the magnesium tablets that will be used to bring their serum magnesium levels into the optimum part of the normal range. In those cases giving 3 mg of boron p.o. may help (Travell and Simons, 1983).

6. Some of the patients may require up to 60 to 100 meq. of oral potassium per day. The need for potassium seems to vary directly with the severity of the disease. The low normal serum potassium levels are responsible for both the cramping and Charlie horses these patients complain of, and much of the myofascial muscular irritability. A simple formula for oral replacement is found in Appendix 6.

STAGE 2 (Fig. 2): Normalize sleep (Margoles, in press)

a. MPS patients need 6 to 8 uninterrupted hours of restful and restorative sleep.
b. Therapy is initiated with behavioral techniques.
c. Medications are added as the need arises.
   1. Tailored to meet the needs of the patient.
   2. Tricyclic antidepressant (TCA), Benadryl, muscle relaxer (Soma, Ativan, Klonopin). Brand name medications are preferred. Intermittent use is preferred. The more severe grades of MPS, patients have a higher tolerance for these medications. I believe this is a reflection of their altered biochemistry, and usually corrects as the patient progresses through all the stages of recovery (Margoles, 1989).

STAGE 3 (Fig. 3): Correct psychological perpetuating factors

a. Reduce tension, stress, and anxiety.
b. Correct behaviors that promote abuse of muscles.
c. Correct dysfunctional thinking.
d. Cognitive restructuring.
e. Correction of "Good sport syndrome" behavior (Travell and Simons, 1983).

STAGE 4 (Fig. 3): Pain symptom control (Margoles, in press; Margoles, 1984).

a. Some patients can benefit from behavioral approaches to pain symptom control.

1. Cognitive therapy.
2. Biofeedback.
3. Therapies mentioned in stage 3 can be beneficial for pain symptom control.
   b. Additionally, some of the more severely afflicted patients can benefit from the adjunctive use of adequate analgesic medications.
      1. Medication is used strictly to improve overall physical functioning, social interaction, and returning to gainful employment.
      2. Medications are given on a time contingent (TC) basis (Margoles, in press).
         a. Begin with the least potent analgesics such Tylenol, nonsteroidal anti-inflammatory drugs (NSAID), or Darvocette-N-100, and then progress up to the stronger analgesics as the need arises: Tylenol with codeine, Vicodin, Anexia 7.5, Percodan, Demerol, Morphine, etc. (Margoles, in press; Margoles, 1984; Meyers, 1987; Tennent, 1983; Smith, 1983 & 1989; Jaffe & William, 1985; Foley & Portnoy, 1986; Goodman, Gilman, & Goodman, 1980; Houde, 1974; Porter & Jick, 1980; Stimmel, 1985).

Use of this medication is contingent upon:
1. The clinician's "comfort level" in dealing with these meds.
2. The patient's pain severity, cooperation, initiative, complexity, chronicity, tolerance, psychologic status, and motivation towards appropriate goals.
3. With the use of the recommended vitamin program patients slowly develop a negative tolerance to narcotics, narcotic-containing analgesics, and most other controlled substances, as management progresses (Margoles, in press).

INTERMEDIATE STAGES

STAGE 5 (Fig. 4): Medications to facilitate physical recovery (Margoles, in press).

a. Nonsteroidal anti-inflammatory drugs (NSAID) to control stiffness and muscle soreness as activity level is increased. Use sparingly because the chronic complex MPS patients frequently have gastric intolerance to many of the NSAID medications.
   1. Useful in controlling post-exercise stiffness.
   2. Useful in decreasing morning stiffness.
      a. The patient takes a long-acting NSAID at HS with a snack.

3. In some cases of NSAID intolerance it is possible to use small doses of oral and intravenous Colchicine (Margoles, 1988; Margoles, in press; Rask, 1980 & 1985). Intravenous Colchicine (Available through Merit Pharmaceuticals. See Appendix 1.) can produce dramatic pain relief and improved physical function in some of the grade 2 and 3 MPS patients. It can be given I.V. once or twice per week for 3 to 6 weeks or more. Obtain a CBC every 6 to 12 weeks while the patient is taking Colchicine.

4. In patients intolerant to oral NSAID's the patient or spouse can be taught to give 1-2 cc injections of sodium Thiosalicylate (Arthro 5023 (Salsalate) B.i.d., or T.i.d.

Use of Physical Approaches and Physical Therapies

STAGE 6 (Fig. 4): Facilitate recovery

a. Registered Occupational Therapist is called in.
1. Comes in to facilitate activities of daily living with respect to household work, work outside the home, driving automobile, etc.
2. Facilitate hygiene.
   a. Bathing.
   b. Showering.
   c. Use of bathroom and toilet.
   d. Other.
3. Makes recommendations for adaptive devices.
   a. Toilet.
   b. Shower and bath.
   c. Kitchen.
   d. Gardening.
   e. Automobile.
   f. Dressing and undressing.
   g. Other.
b. Disability parking sticker.
1. Helps with banking, shopping, getting to work, etc.
2. If in doubt, the physician should give one to patient to see if it encourages increased functioning.
3. Encourages the patient to get out and get back into society.
4. Effective in return to work.
c. Correct abuse of muscles.
1. Avoid excessive bending, lifting, and twisting.
2. Avoid lifting loads that are too heavy.
3. Avoid the "Good Sport Syndrome" (Travell and Simons, 1983).

4. Don't carry luggage or bags that are too heavy.
5. Avoid clothing that is too tight.
6. When travelling long distances get up every 20 to 30 minutes to stretch and relieve tension on muscles.

STAGE 7 (Fig. 5): Mobilize (Margoles, in press)

a. To improve range of motion.
b. To decrease dysfunction.
c. To improve pain by getting muscles back to normal resting length.
d. This is accomplished by:
    1. Stretch and spray (S&S) (Travell and Simons, 1983)
    2. Trigger point injection (TPI) (Travell and Simons, 1983)
    3. Begin to work on BARRIER trigger points (See Appendix 10)
    4. Lewitt stretch.
    5. Chiropractic.
    6. Specific physical therapy.
        a. Low impact aerobics.
        b. "Tube" exercises (Margoles, in press).
        c. Williams flexion exercises.
        d. McKinzie extension exercises.
        e. Low load stretching (against resistance).
        f. Partial range of motion stretching.
        g. Low resistance stretching.
    7. Swimming.
    8. Nerve blocks, epidural injections, and sympathetic blocks. These can be attempted at this stage. If no positive results with 2 to 3 procedures, these can be attempted again at stages 8 or 10.

FINAL STAGES

STAGE 8 (Fig. 6): Improve flexibility, strength, and endurance (Margoles, in press)

a. Back school program.
b. Work hardening.
c. Aggressive physical therapy.
d. This is enhanced by:
    1. Stretch and spray (S&S) (Travell and Simons, 1983).
    2. Trigger point injection (TPI) (Travell and Simons, 1983).
    3. Lewitt stretch.
    4. Chiropractic.
e. Swimming.

f. Jogging.
g. Full range of motion stretching.
h. Medium load stretching (against resistance).
i. Get rid of more BARRIER trigger points (Appendix 10)
j. Manipulation under anesthesia.

STAGE 9 (Fig. 6): Vocational rehabilitation

a. Vocational testing.
b. Ergonomic analysis.
>   1. This relates to energy requirements to perform specified tasks.
>   a. An example would be measurement of the amount of energy and range of motion to perform a strenuous work task, which could then be compared to the patient's current work capacities.
>   2. At present this is not an exact science.
c. Vocational counseling.
d. Vocational training and rehabilitation.
e. Vocational placement.

Prognosis

a. Grade 1 and 2 MPS patients should be able to get back to either their usual work or modified usual work.
b. Grade 3 patients will have to be retrained to lighter work, and only if they can tolerate it.
>   1. If the patient can be retrained, he or she should be phased back into active employment slowly. This is advised because of unavoidable muscle atrophy when they are off work for 8 weeks or more. An approximate return to work schedule would be: 4 hours per day for 2 to 4 weeks; 6 hours per day for 2 to 4 weeks; 8 hours per day for 2 to 4 weeks; then they can begin to do overtime work.
>   1. Patients who have been off work for a year or more would be the ones needing the 4-week intervals for shifting up to longer work hours.
c. There is no predictable recovery for the grade 4 patients at the present time.

ADVANCED STAGES

STAGE 10 (Fig. 7): Advanced physical therapy (Margoles, in press)

Note: this program is only for those MPS patients who have a professional career or avocation that calls for maximum performance. This relates to athletes, dancers, and the like. It may necessitate extra "fine tuning" of all perpetuating factors that were picked up on the initial and subsequent exams.

    a. Work hardening program.

    b. Aggressive aerobics.

    c. Progressive weight training.

    d. Parallel bars.

    e. Proprioceptive reeducation.

    f. Aggressive rehabilitation of neuromuscular timing and coordination.

    g. Fine tuning of muscular coordination.

    h. Running.

    i. Improving cardiac endurance.

    j. Use of pressure threshold meter (PTM) to measure progress and set further goals.

    k. Use of Cybex or similar to set aggressive goals to spur recovery.

    l. Work out all remaining BARRIER trigger points.

Conclusion:

The speed of recovery at each stage must be adjusted to the patient's fortitude in achieving each level of accomplishment.

Management: Conclusion

Some patients will respond to the simplest of interventions such as massage or gentle pressure applied on the Tp. The more severely afflicted patients will require an extensive and complex therapy program that requires a number of years to accomplish substantial recovery. Some of the grade 3 and grade 4 patients will only obtain partial recovery with a year or more of therapy. Some of the more complex cases, such as the grade 3's, will not be able to make it past stage 7. Most of the grade 4's will not be able to make it past stage 6.

Many of the MPS patients will not tolerate physical therapy at three times per week. These patients will do better if the physical therapy is kept to twice per week.

As management progresses the metabolic, biochemical, mineral, and hormonal perpetuating factors need to be rechecked at least every 6 to 12 weeks. This will ensure that the blood levels remain in the optimal part of the normal range. In most cases the potassium needs to be rechecked every 10 to 14 days during the first 8 to 12 weeks of therapy. In many of the grade 3 and 4 patients difficulty may be encountered in attempting to bring the serum potassium level to the optimal part of the normal range (Margoles, in press).

Some of the grade 1 patients will have to be on their vitamin and mineral supplements for the rest of their life. All the of the grade 2, 3, and 4 patients should be on permanent (ongoing) correction of all perpetuating factors for the rest of their lives.

The effectiveness of sleep normalization should be assessed every 2 weeks. Patient's needs for behavioral techniques and medications change frequently during the first 6 months of management in the grade 3 and 4 patients. As they improve it takes less and less medications to effect an adequate sleep pattern. There is no one technique or medication that works for all of the MPS patients.

For most of the grade 4 cases there are perpetuating factors that are yet to be discovered to help reclaim these most challenging cases.

At every stage of recovery extensive teaching of patients must be carried out so they can learn self-management techniques. This will help them "stay out of trouble" in the future. They must be taught "early warning signs" to know when to return for help. Some of these include:

1. Return of pain.
2. Disrupted sleep patterns.
3. Can't find a comfortable sleeping position.
4. Persistent aches.
5. Unexplained weakness.

PROGNOSIS

Once a myofascial, always a myofascial. Myofascial pain patients are not treated and cured, they are managed (Travell, personal communication). In some patients, after the initial incident in which the MPS became active, the tendency to recurrences of trigger point related problems remains for life. The second, third, and fourth episodes of MPS may occur in areas different from the original problem, and differing from each other.

Many of my patients relate that a close relative such as their mother, dad, or sibling, and, in some cases, their child or children have problems that sound like a Myofascial Pain Syndrome.

To date, there has been no conclusive proof that the problem is genetically transmitted or that the tendency to generate a Myofascial Pain Syndrome predated any given accident. However, I believe that tendency to Myofascial Pain Syndrome is inherited. I also believe that some people are predisposed to it for an as yet unknown reason.

Future studies (Texidor and Margoles, in press) will assess some of the genetic problems that are felt to be relevant to MPS.

Some patients will discontinue the treatment(s) used to correct their perpetuating factors. For most of the grade 1 and 2 patients this may not have an adverse effect. However, this may be different for some of the grade 3 and 4 MPS patients. After a few months or years pass they may trigger another flare-up of MPS pain and dysfunction that is worse than the original problem. With prompt treatment these subsequent episodes can usually be managed quicker than the original problem.

Many of the Grade 1 patients will respond to just the correction of the perpetuating factor problems. The higher the grade of severity (i.e., grade 3 or grade 4) the more complex and prolonged the management program becomes.

Overall prognosis for full recovery and return to normal life-style:

Grade 1: Excellent: up to 100% of pre-MPS functioning.

Grade 2: Good: up to 75% recovery.

Grade 3: Fair: up to 50% recovery.

Grade 4: Poor: up to 25% recovery.

Some relative time-tables for response to appropriate therapy:

Grade 1: Usually 2 to 4 weeks of treatment. One to four office visits.

Grade 2: Up to 12 weeks of therapy. Visits are every 1 to 2 weeks.

Grade 3: Six months to 3 years. Weekly visits for the first 6 weeks. Every 2 weeks for the next six weeks, and every 2 to 4 weeks after that. Even after the 3 years, patients may have to be seen every 1 to 6 months for an indefinite period of time.

Grade 4: These patients will require all the therapy indicated for the grade 3 patient, and the management may need to go on indefinitely. After the first 6 to 12 weeks of therapy patients need to be seen at 2 week to 3 month intervals. This group of patients are prone to mishaps such as falling when a weak leg gives out. A minor auto accident can cause an acute flare up that may last 6 to 12 weeks, requiring weekly or every other week visits for 6 to 12 weeks.

Treatment Costs

The cost of management for the grade 1 and 2 patients is usually no more than that incurred in the treatment of an acute arthritis or an acute back or neck strain.

Cost of treating the grade 3 patients is similar to that of treating an acute arthritis problem that goes onto chronicity. Medication costs would be less expensive for the MPS patient.

When the grade 4 patients are analyzed for cost of therapy two issues must be kept in mind:

1. These patients have historically been MPS patients who were mistaken for a patient with a ruptured disc. At present, all costs associated with lumbar or cervical surgery run about $20,000. This cost is unfortunate. Had the patient been recognized as having a referred pain of a ruptured disc instead of radicular pain of a ruptured disk, the savings are obvious. The surgery compounds the MPS problem by possibly adding scar tissue and other surgery-related problems.

2. The cost of chronic ongoing therapy in the treated versus the untreated patients.

   a. Without treatment the grade 4 patient may remain unavoidably disabled. The problem may remain static for years, or until adequate therapy is instituted.
   b. The best hope for recovery and relief of disability is an active treatment program. In the long-run this is a less expensive way to treat the grade 4 MPS patients.

CONCLUSION

MPS should be suspected in all cases of unexplained pain. It is relatively easy to diagnose once the clinician has proper training.

MPS is a complex problem. It is a manageable condition. Proper procedures must be followed in the staging of therapy. In the treatment of MPS, resolution of the perpetuating factors is a critical step of prime importance to the rest of the recovery program.

MPS is broken up, in this chapter, into gradations of severity. The prognosis for complete recovery decreases as the grade of severity increases.

Suggestions are made for minor changes in the ICD-9-CM coding of MPS (Appendix 4) to enhance the overall ability to record and report MPS.

BARRIER trigger points are presented as one of the many unique features of MPS. The concept of BARRIER trigger points explains some of the more frustrating aspects of treating patients with MPS.

GLOSSARY OF TERMS

Dysfunction

Lack of proper function. Abnormal function. Weakness of a limb. Dropping things with the hand on the effected side. The leg gives out unpredictably on the effected side.

Jump sign

A general physical response to a unanticipatedly painful stimulus. Like a recoil, flinch, or startle. The patient may unexpectedly wince, cry out, withdraw, or "jump" in response to the painful stimulus. This is frequently a response that occurs to pressure applied to an active trigger point. It may also be noted when a taut band is a muscle is snapped either by pincer palpation or flat palpation (Travell and Simons, 1983). A general response that occurs so rapidly and spontaneously that the patient has no time to prepare for it.

Local twitch response

Transient contraction of the group of muscle fibers that contains a trigger point. The trigger point is usually in a taut band. Palpation must be specific. The muscle is palpated at right or oblique angles to the trigger point containing a taut band. The contraction of fibers is in response to stimulation (usually by snapping palpation or needling) of the same, or sometimes of a nearby trigger point (Travell and Simons, 1983). The contraction may occur locally at the site of the trigger point, such as occurs in the infraspinatus muscle. It may occur to 1 feet away from the trigger point, but within the fibers of the muscle, such as occurs when the Iliocostalis thoracis is strummed by flat palpation at T9 and causes a "twitch" in the Iliocostalis lumborum at L2, L3, L4 or L5.

Myofascial trigger point — active

A focus of hyperirritability in a muscle or its fascia that is symptomatic with respect to pain; it refers a pattern of pain at rest and/or on motion is specific for the muscle. An active trigger point is always tender, prevents full lengthening of the muscle, weakens the muscle, usually refers pain on direct compression, mediates a local twitch response of muscle fibers when adequately stimulated, and often produces specific referred autonomic phenomena, generally in its pain reference zone. To be distinguished from a latent myofascial trigger point. (Travell and Simons, 1983).

Myofascial trigger point — latent

A focus of hyperirritability in a muscle or its fascia that is clinically quiencent with respect to spontaneous pain; it is painful only when palpated. A latent trigger point may have all the other clinical characteristics of an active trigger point, from which it is to be distinguished (Travell and Simons, 1983).

Paresthesias

Abnormal sensations in the effected area such as tingling, numbness, sense of ants crawling on or in the area of problem. Is broadly defined as an abnormal sensation, but will in the present context be restricted to mean an altered quality of sensation other than allodynia and dysesthesia. It is usually difficult to describe paresthetic sensations, because specific words are lacking, and the patient uses metaphorical expressions like "crawling," "running water," "tingling," "tightness," etc., or simply stated "different from normal" (Lindblom, 1985). Refers to crawling, burning, or "pins and needles" feelings that arise spontaneously (Dorland's, 1985).

Pro-prioception

Sense of position. Spatial orientation. Perception mediated by proprioceptors or proprioceptive tissues. (Dorland's, 1985). Receiving stimuli within the tissues of the body, as within muscles and tendons (see proprioceptor) (Dorland's, 1985). Sensory nerve terminals which give information concerning movements and positions of the body; they occur chiefly in the muscles, tendons, and the labyrinth (Dorland's, 1985).

Taut bands

(palpable band, or nodule) The group of taut muscle fibers that is associated with a myofascial trigger point and is identifiable by tactile examination of the muscle. Contraction of the fibers in this band produces the local twitch response (Travell and Simon). This is an objective finding. The patient has no control over the presence or absence of the taut band. These are present up to the point of onset of rigor mortis.

"Trick"   Substituting or using uneffected muscles and/or
                         joints for (instead of) movements   the ones that are
                         painful or restricted by the presence of an active or
                         latent trigger point.

APPENDIX 1: SUPPLIERS OF INJECTABLES

Suppliers of B-complex Injection Products

Because of FDA intervention products listed below are not always available from the listed distributor. You may have to contact a number of distributors listed in order to obtain the indicated product.

Product	Brand Name	Distributor
Riboflavin (B2)	Various @ 50 mg/ml	Kripps (6)
		Merit (1)
Dexpanthenol (B5)	D-PAN 250 mg/ml	Merit (1)
	Dexpanthenol	Schein (3)
		Adria
Folate (Bc)	Folvite 5 mg/ml	Lederle (4)
	Folic acid 10 mg/ml	Merit (1)
Hydroxocobalamin (B12)	Various @ 1,000 mcg/ml	Merit (1)
		IDE (2)
		Schein (3)

B-Complex Products

Fortaplex (10cc)	Per cc	Kripps (6)
Thiamine (B1)	100 mg	
Riboflavin (B2)	10 mg	
Pyridoxine (B6)	10 mg	
Panthenol (B5)	10 mg	
Niacinamide (B3)	100 mg	
Cyanocobalamin (B12)	100 mcg	

B-Plex 100 (30cc)	Per cc	Merit (1)
Thiamine (B1)	100 mg	
Riboflavin (B2)	2 mg	
Pyridoxine (B6)	2 mg	
Panthenol (B5)	2 mg	
Niacinamide (B3)	100 mg	

27 ga. 1" or 1½" needles	MPL (5)
30 ga. 1" or ½" needles	MPL (5)

(1) Merit Pharmaceuticals
    2611 San Fernando Road
    Los Angeles, CA 90065
    213-227-4831

(2) Interstate Drug Exchange, Inc.
    1500 New Horizons Blvd.
    Amityville, NY 11701
    800-626-DRUG

(3) Henry Schein, Inc.
5 Harbor Park Drive
Port Washington, NY 11050
800-772-4346

(4) Obtain through local drugstore.

(5) Smith + Nephew MPL
1820 West Roscoe St.
Chicago, IL 60657
312-248-3810
604-687-2564

(6) Kripps Pharmacy Ltd.
994 Granville Street
Vancouver, B.C.
Canada V6Z 1L2

APPENDIX 2: ABBREVIATIONS USED IN THIS PAPER

MMT = Manual Muscle Testing
1. Muscle testing that is done manually by the evaluating therapist.
2. Does not refer to Cybex, etc. testing.

ROM = range of motion
1. This can be done visually with an estimate.
2. Can be done with a goniometer or flexometer.
3. Can be done with electronic goniometer.

BAW = breakaway weakness (Baker, 1986)
1. Refers to sudden giving way of the part being manually tested.
   a. Usually points up the presence of a trigger point in the muscle being tested.

LTR = local twitch response

PF = perpetuating factors

JS = jump sign

TB = taut band

TPI = trigger point injection

APPENDIX 3: CLINICAL CLASSIFICATION OF SEVERITY

MPS includes persons in whom all pain is soft tissue in nature. MPS refers specifically to trigger point problems relating to muscles, and not other types of soft tissues such as ligaments, tendons, and skin. The following is a classification of MPS based on (1) extent of geographic involvement, (2) severity of pain and altered sensation (3) presence of perpetuating factors, and (4) extent of physical impairment.

Format followed for each grade of MPS:

1. Extent of or geographic involvement.

2. Presence of perpetuating factors.

3. Severity of pain and altered sensations.

   Pain severity is graded as follows:

   P1: Physical impairment: Minimal.
   Intensity: Mild.
   Patient appears uncomfortable: No.
   Pain affects psyche: No.
   Frequency of pain: Intermittent.
   Patient is aware of pain during activity: No.
   Pain is aggravated by activity: Minimal.
   Need to change position for comfort: No.
   Pain is present while resting: No.
   Pain interferes with sleep: No.
   Other: Pain is forgotten during activity.

   P2: Physical impairment: Minimal.
   Intensity: Mild.
   Patient appears uncomfortable: Occasionally.
   Pain affects psyche: Mild.
   Frequency of pain: Intermittent.
   Patient is aware of pain during activity: Mild.
   Pain is aggravated by activity: Occasionally.
   Need to change position for comfort: No.
   Pain is present while resting: None.
   Pain interferes with sleep: No.
   Other: Mild interference with activity.

   P3: Physical impairment: May prevent some activities.
   Intensity: Moderate.
   Patient appears uncomfortable: Occasionally.
   Pain affects psyche: Mild.
   Frequency of pain: Intermittent, and frequent.

Patient is aware of pain during activity: Yes.
Pain is aggravated by activity: Yes.
Need to change position for comfort: Yes, occasionally.
Pain is present while resting: Mild.
Pain interferes with sleep: No.
Other:

P4: Physical impairment: Prevents that patient from doing many activities.
Intensity: Moderate to severe.
Patient appears uncomfortable: Frequently.
Pain affects psyche: Moderate.
Frequency of pain: Constant and varies little with activity.
Patient is aware of pain during activity: Yes.
Pain is aggravated by activity: Yes.
Need to change position for comfort: Frequently.
Pain is present while resting: Bothersome.
Pain interferes with sleep: Frequently. Can find no comfortable sleeping position.
Other: Marked handicap. Pain may cause outcries.

P5: Physical impairment: May prevent almost all activities.
Intensity: Severe.
Patient appears uncomfortable: Frequently to constantly.
Pain affects psyche: Severe.
Frequency of pain: Constant.
Patient is aware of pain during activity: Yes.
Pain is aggravated by activity: Constantly.
Need to change position for comfort: Frequently.
Pain is present while resting: Constantly.
Pain interferes with sleep: Constantly.
Other:

4. Degree of physical impairment. This consists of evaluation of physical functioning in the following categories:
    1. Routine job-related activities.
    2. Work around the home.
    3. Socialization activities.
    4. Getting up or down out of a chair.
    5. Sports activities.
    6. Hobbies.
    7. Sexual activity.
    8. Sleep function.
    9. Hygiene (shower, grooming, shampooing, toilet, etc.)
    10. Eating and feeding functions.

11. Chewing (food, etc.).
12. Dressing and undressing.
13. Driving a vehicle.
14. Overall strength and endurance.

5. Other pertinent comments.

Grade 1 Mild:

1. A single muscle (see Appendix 7 for trigger point locations). Unilateral.
2. None.
3. Frequently P1 and on occasion may go to P4.
4. General impairment is mild. May preclude heavy lifting.
5. Altered sensations are low intensity. Once treated there is usually no recurrence of symptoms.

Example: A 32-year-old female patient presents with pain in the shoulder and arm. She is found to have an infraspinatus trigger point of the shoulder. It causes a slight decrease of range of motion with accompanying pain when she brushes her hair to a point past her ear on the ipsilateral side. The problem is easily relieved with a trigger point injection (TPI) plus stretch and spray (S&S).

Grade 2 Moderate:

1. Bilateral involvement of the same muscle (e.g., deltoid on both sides, gluteus maximus on both sides, etc.).
2. A few are active: for example, a short leg or arm, and a less than optimal serum potassium level.
3. Frequently P2 and on occasion may go to P4.
4. As much as 50% for physical work. Precludes heavy lifting repeated bending and stooping. Occasional absence from work (one to two days of missed work per six-week period).
5. One of the trigger points usually produces more of the total symptom picture than the mirror image partner. Both must be treated to obtain a successful outcome. A moderate amount of problems with altered sensations.

Example: A 27-year-old male patient presents with dizziness and headache after a rear end automobile accident. He has a "whiplash" injury of the neck. The headaches and dizziness prevent him from driving to work occasionally. Examination reveals symptom producing trigger points in the Sternocleidomastoid muscles on both sides. He has a short hemipelvis on the left. The problem is corrected with a one centimeter butt lift under the left buttock, and TPI to both of his Sternocleidomastoid muscles, followed by stretch and spray (S&S). There is no recurrence of symptoms.

Grade 3 Severe:

1. Multiple single muscle Myofascial Pain Syndromes in numerous areas of the body. Some are active unilaterally, and some are active bilaterally (see Appendix 7).
2. Many perpetuating factors are detectable, both from the physical examination, and comprehensive blood testing.
3. Severity may vary with different regions of the body. Some may be P1, some P2, some P3, and some P4. P3 and P4 are most frequent.
4. Impairment of activities of daily living is severe, resulting in limited employment (either unemployment because of the pain problem, or limited to very light type work) and hardship. Depending on the overall clinical picture, some of these patients will be limited to light work whereas others may only be able to do sedentary work.
5. In the instances of bilateral activation of trigger points one of the pair usually produces more of the total symptom picture than the mirror image partner. Both must be treated to obtain a successful outcome. There is a moderate amount of altered sensations and dysfunction related to the trigger points. The numerous perpetuating factors complicate the recovery.

A grade 3 patient may present with a moderate to severe, intermittent, myofascial low back pain. It may appear that only one muscle, such as the longissimus thoracis or one of the glutei is responsible for the problem. However, in reality, in the grade 3 patients, any of a number of the following muscles may be contributing to the problem (the contribution of symptoms usually comes from paired muscles such as right and left longissimus thoracis, right and left iliocostalis lumborum, and right and left quadratus lumborum, to mention only a few):

Coccygeus	Obturator internus
Gluteus Maximus	Piriformis
Gluteus Medius	Quadratus lumborum
Gluteus Minimus	Rectus Adominis
Iliocostalis Lumborum	Rotatores Brevis
Iliopsoas	Rotatores Longus
Iliocostalis thoracis	Sphincter Ani
Levator Ani	Soleus
Lower latissimus dorsi	Serratus post. Inferior
Longissimus thoracis	Vastus Lateralis
Multifidus	

The grade 3 complex may produce a significant physically disabling clinical picture. Mild to moderate reflex sympathetic dystrophy may occur in any of the painful extremities. Intense referred extremity pain may be mistaken for the radicular pain of a ruptured disc.

Example: A 45-year-old woman is struck on the driver side of her car while going through an intersection. Impact is greatest at the driver's door. The door is caved in, breaking her left pelvis. Her seat belt is torn away, and she's thrown about in the front of the car. She sustains muscle trigger points in the right trapezius, sternocleidomastoid muscle, scalenus anterior muscle, muscles acting upon the jaw, both infraspinatus, both quadratus lumborum, right gluteus medius, right pyriformis, and right gluteus minimus muscles. She has constant headaches on the right, radicular pain down the right arm and leg. She has not been able to work for two months since the injury. She also has postconcussion syndrome (PCS) and Post-traumatic stress disorder (PTSD). She spends 6 weeks in a pelvic sling in the hospital to heal the pelvic fracture, which also disrupted her pubic symphysis. Once ambulatory all the above pains are still problematic. Examination reveals one inch of shortening of the left leg. This is corrected with a shoe lift of one inch. Her pelvis is now short on the left side, and this is corrected with a butt lift. Blood testing reveals less than optimal levels serum of blood count, potassium, ionized calcium, iron, magnesium, thiamin, pyridoxine, pantothenate, folic acid, and cobalamin. The biochemical problems are corrected with oral supplements, and a few weeks of twice-weekly balanced B-complex injections. She is put through a program of stretch and spray (S&S), trigger point injections (TPI), Lewitt stretch, and limbering and strengthening exercises. By six months postinjury she has made 50% recovery of physical function and 50% relief of pain. At that point she can return to her routine secretarial work, but finds that she can't work any overtime, and misses up to 2 days of work per week because of pain and fatigue problems. She is able to do only 50% of her usual housework.

Grade 4 Severe and Complex:

In this group is seen all of the grades 1-3. Restricted range of motion of a joint gives clues to the location of trigger points. For example, decreased active abduction of the shoulder may be due to an infraspinatus trigger point, or any of the five other muscles that can cause a similar problem about the shoulder. However, because the referred pain of Myofascial Pain Syndrome (MPS) has been mistaken for radicular pain of a ruptured disc, or a surgically treatable mechanical back problem, these patients will have had one or more surgical attempts to remedy the problem. In my practice I have seen such patients who have had as many as 20 surgical attempts to remedy the pain and dysfunction. One patient had five cervical disc removals and fusions, five lumbar disc removals and fusions, and five surgeries on each of his shoulders to attempt to remedy his myofascial pain and dysfunction problems.

1. Same as for grade 3.
2. Numerous and extensive.
3. Moderate to severe in most areas. Constant in most areas. Varies between P4 and P5.
4. Totally disabled for all work.
5. The multiple surgeries add another dimension to the overall problem, and that is sizable amounts of scar tissue. This often makes it impossible to obtain meaningful remedies to the problem. Moderate to severe reflex sympathetic dystrophy may occur in any of the painful extremities and may significantly compound the problem of management. These patients are totally disabled.

Example: For our example here, we will pick up on the 45-year-old woman from the example given in the grade 3 section above. Twelve months post trauma, becoming weary of the unrelenting pain radiating down her right leg, she searched out a reputable neurosurgeon for a second opinion. A CT and a myelogram show a "bulging disc" at L4-5 and L5-S1. She's desperate and pleads with the surgeon, "Do something, the pain is driving me crazy!" Surgery is performed. Pain is significantly relieved for three months. Then the pain returns "with a vengeance." She asks for further surgical options, and a fusion is performed. This time there is no relief of the pain at all. She is left an invalid who can not work at any gainful employment.

APPENDIX 4: ICD-9-CM CODING OF MPS

I propose that the following be adopted for coding MPS:

Under 729.1 "Myalgia and myositis, unspecified"
  729.10 = is specific for Myofascial Pain Syndrome (MPS)

The following fifth-digit subclassification is used to designate site of involvement:

  0 = Head and neck
  1 = Shoulder region
  2 = Upper arm
      a. Elbow to humerus
  3 = Forearm
      a. Radius to the wrist
  4 = Hand including fingers
  5 = Pelvic region and thigh
      a. Low back, buttock, hip, femur
  6 = Lower leg
      a. Knee joint to just above the ankle
  7 = Ankle and foot
      a. From the ankle to the toes
  8 = Other specified sites
      a. Ribs, trunk, vertebral column, upper back, mid-back
  9 = Multiple sites

The following sixth-digit subclassification is used to designate
grade of severity:

  1 = Mild
  2 = Moderate
  3 = Severe
  4 = Severe and complex

The following seventh-digit subclassification is used to designate whether the MPS is occurring on only one side or both (MPS that is bilateral represents a more complicated and difficult to treat condition):

  1 = Unilateral
  2 = Bilateral

Therefore, if a patient is coded as 729.1532 it means that the patient has a severe bilateral Myofascial Pain Syndrome of the low back.

APPENDIX 5: ORAL REPLACEMENT PROGRAM

It must be kept in mind that the use of vitamin and mineral therapy acts as a compliment to a well-planned management program.

The management suggestions made here are based upon answers obtained in a study within my practice (Margoles, in press), clinical experience with 1,500 patients, and recent medical literature on the subject (Jeppsson, 1983; Margoles, 1983; Margoles, in press; Travell & Simons, 1983; Travell, 1976; Farmer, 1985).

Individual variability may exist from patient to patient with respect to absorption of orally administered vitamins and minerals.

The body does not recognize any differences between vitamins that are "organic," "natural," or "synthetic" in origin. They all work equally well.

The various vitamins and minerals are all interdependent. To attack the deficiencies and insufficiencies one by one, in a consecutive series of time frames, would be impractical, expensive, and time-consuming.

A trial of vitamin and mineral supplements is initiated for 6 to 12 weeks. It usually takes that long to decide whether the therapy will have a positive effect on the patient's Myofascial Pain Syndrome.

I recommend vitamins and minerals from Bronson Pharmaceuticals vitamins and minerals for oral use because the products are:

1. Pharmaceutical grade.
2. Hypoallergenic.
3. Well-formulated by recognized authorities and biochemists.
4. No unusual ingredients used.
5. Inexpensive.
6. Available throughout the world by mail or telephone order from the following location:

Bronson Pharmaceuticals
4526 Rinetti Lane
La Canada, California 91011-0628

Note: If you are ordering from countries outside the U.S.A. put: "Attention Ellen" on your correspondence.

In California: 800-521-3323
Outside California: 800-521-3322
International: Dial the United States of America. Then dial: (818) 790-2646. When the phone is answered ask for extension #37. When answered, place your order. Specify your name, address, and country. You will be given additional instructions by the person at Bronson.

Product recommendations: (Bronson)

B-complex with C and E (non-time release)

Begin one tablet daily for 10 days, then go to one tablet twice per day. Next, go to 2 in the AM and one in the afternoon for 10 more days. Finally, go to 2 tablets twice per day.

Note: Nerve regeneration may occur with the recommended dosing of the B-complex vitamins.

If you do not want to work with the Bronson product, obtain a B-Complex with C, but without zinc or iron, that has the following formulation or close to it:

Per tablet:

B-1 (Thiamine Mononitrate)............................... 15mg
B-2 (Riboflavin) 10mg
B-6 (Pyridoxine Hydrochloride) 10mg
B-12 (Cobalamin Concentrate)............................. 5mcg
Niacinamide 100mg
D-Calcium Pantothenate 20mg
Folic Acid ....0.4mg) 400mcg
Biotin 200mcg
C (Ascorbic Acid)... 500mg
E (Alpha Tocopherol) ....30 I.U

Mineral Insurance Formula

Three per day. Or, if you don't want to use the Bronson, obtain a complete mineral supplement that has:

Per three tablets:

Calcium 250mg
Phosphorus 250mg
Magnesium 200mg
Iron.. 15mg
Zinc.. 15mg
Copper 2mg
Iodine 150mcg
Manganese 5mg
Molybdenum 100mcg
Chromium.. 200mcg
Selenium 20mcg

Calcium, Minerals, and Vitamin D

One twice per day. Or, if you don't want to use the Bronson, obtain a calcium supplement that has:

Per tablet:

Calcium 275mg
Vitamin D . . . . .100 I.U
Phosphorus 110mg
Magnesium 135mg
Iron 2.5mg
Iodine 0.03mg
Copper 0.1mg
Zinc 1.5mg
Manganese 0.5mg

Potassium 98 mg tablets

One twice per day or as dictated by the blood testing (Appendix 6).

Although it is generally recommended to take vitamins with meals or food, some people can take them on an empty stomach without problems.

While on this program the patient should avoid any vitamin A supplements, or supplements of Beta-carotene, unless there is blood testing proof that the patient is low in either one.

APPENDIX 6: MANAGEMENT OF POTASSIUM PROBLEMS

Potassium is replenished based on the serum potassium level. This is demonstrated in figure 8.

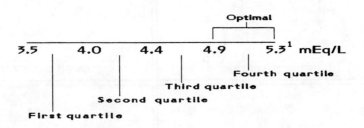

Blood testing for serum potassium level

Potassium is replaced at the dosing of 10 mEq for each quartile away from the optimal part of the range. Therefore, if the patient has a blood test level of 3.8, 30 mEq of potassium is the initial dose, given in divided dosing throughout the day. When the serum potassium is repeated, 7-10 days later, the same formula is used to bring the blood test level to the optimal part of the normal range. If the patient retests at 4.5 mEq/L 10 more mEq of potassium are given per day, for a total of 40 mEq of supplemental potassium per day.   Time release products are preferred, but KCL-Elixir, or K-Lyte type products do equally well.   Some of the more complex cases may eventually   need as much as 50-100 mEq per day.

[1]Values for serum potassium may vary from lab to lab.

Figure 8

APPENDIX 7: CLASSIC TRIGGER POINT LOCATIONS (Simons, 1984).

Figures 9–15 from Basmajian, J.V. and Kirby, L.: *Medical Rehabilitation*. Baltimore, Williams and Wilkins Company, 1984. Reproduced with permission.

HEAD AND NECK PAIN

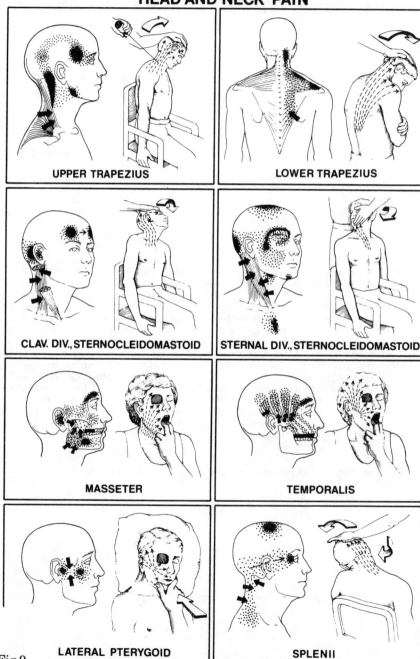

UPPER TRAPEZIUS

LOWER TRAPEZIUS

CLAV. DIV., STERNOCLEIDOMASTOID

STERNAL DIV., STERNOCLEIDOMASTOID

MASSETER

TEMPORALIS

LATERAL PTERYGOID

SPLENII

PAIN PATTERN ■ TRIGGER POINT ➡

Fig.9

HEAD AND NECK PAIN (CONTINUED)

SHOULDER AND UPPER EXTREMITY PAIN

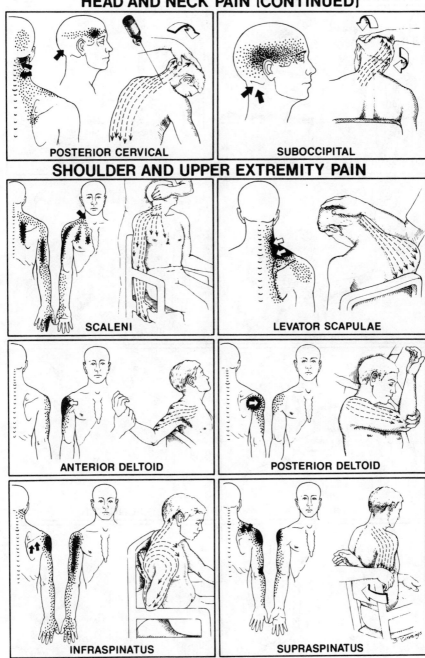

POSTERIOR CERVICAL

SUBOCCIPITAL

SCALENI

LEVATOR SCAPULAE

ANTERIOR DELTOID

POSTERIOR DELTOID

INFRASPINATUS

SUPRASPINATUS

PAIN PATTERN ░ TRIGGER POINT ➡

Fig. 10

SHOULDER AND UPPER EXTREMITY PAIN (CONTINUED)

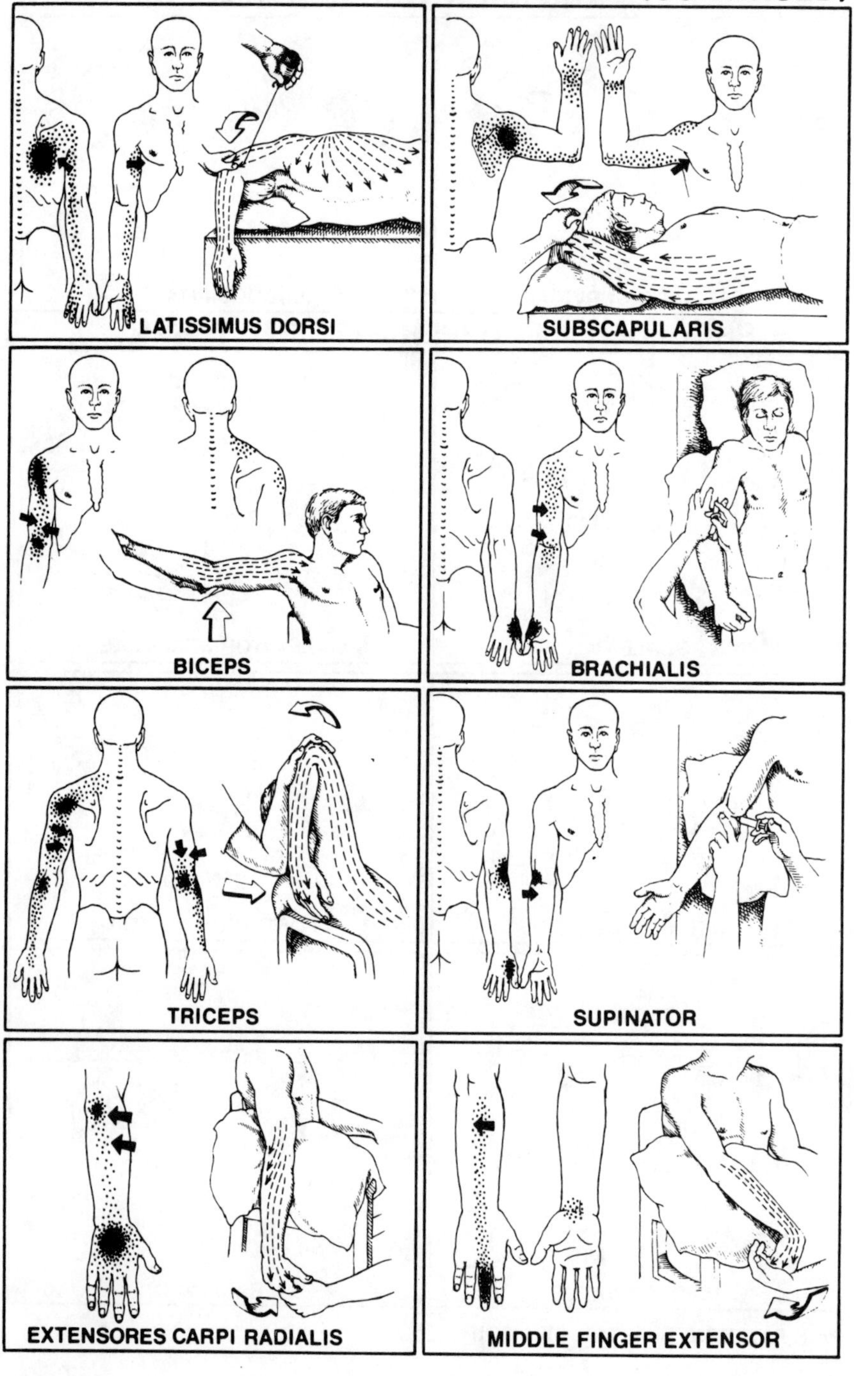

LATISSIMUS DORSI

SUBSCAPULARIS

BICEPS

BRACHIALIS

TRICEPS

SUPINATOR

EXTENSORES CARPI RADIALIS

MIDDLE FINGER EXTENSOR

Fig. 11

SHOULDER AND UPPER EXTREMITY PAIN [CONT.]

TRUNK AND BACK PAIN

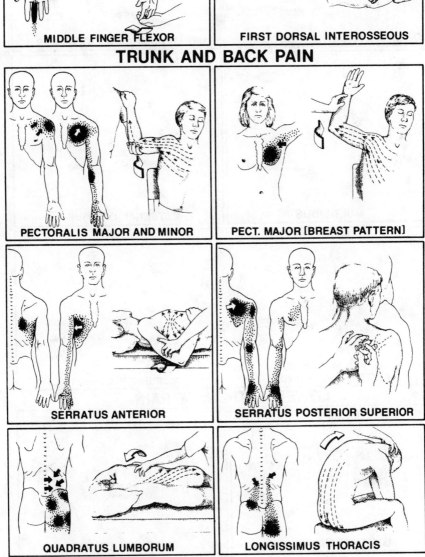

MIDDLE FINGER FLEXOR

FIRST DORSAL INTEROSSEOUS

PECTORALIS MAJOR AND MINOR

PECT. MAJOR [BREAST PATTERN]

SERRATUS ANTERIOR

SERRATUS POSTERIOR SUPERIOR

QUADRATUS LUMBORUM

LONGISSIMUS THORACIS

PAIN PATTERN ⬛   TRIGGER POINT ➡

Fig. 12

TRUNK AND BACK PAIN (CONTINUED)

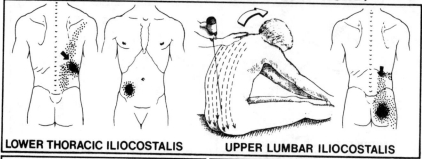

LOWER THORACIC ILIOCOSTALIS   UPPER LUMBAR ILIOCOSTALIS

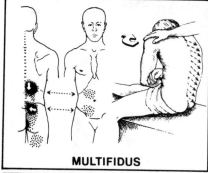

MULTIFIDUS

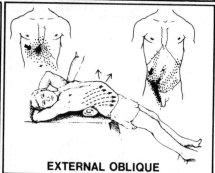

EXTERNAL OBLIQUE

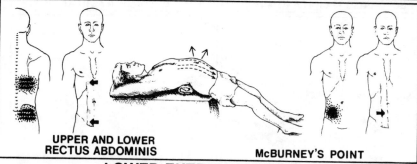

UPPER AND LOWER
RECTUS ABDOMINIS   McBURNEY'S POINT

LOWER EXTREMITY PAIN

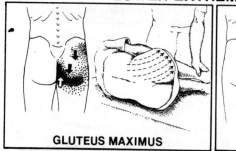

GLUTEUS MAXIMUS

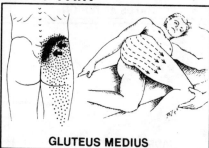

GLUTEUS MEDIUS

PAIN PATTERN ▨ TRIGGER POINT ➡

Fig. 13

LOWER EXTREMITY PAIN [CONTINUED]

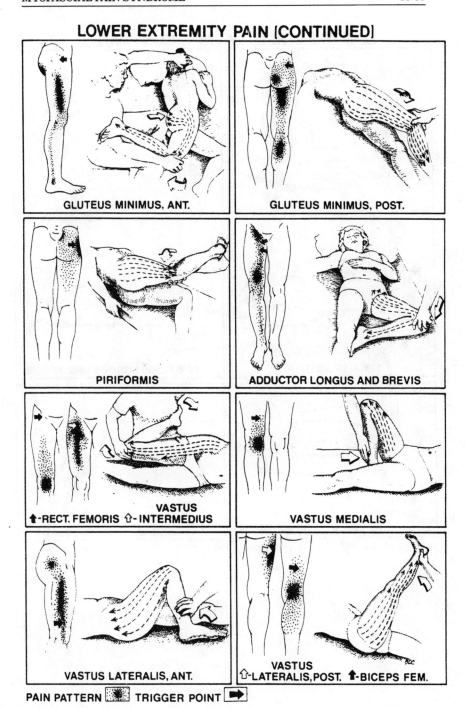

GLUTEUS MINIMUS, ANT.

GLUTEUS MINIMUS, POST.

PIRIFORMIS

ADDUCTOR LONGUS AND BREVIS

VASTUS
⬆-RECT. FEMORIS ⇧-INTERMEDIUS

VASTUS MEDIALIS

VASTUS LATERALIS, ANT.

VASTUS
⇧-LATERALIS, POST. ⬆-BICEPS FEM.

PAIN PATTERN ▨ TRIGGER POINT ➡

Fig. 14

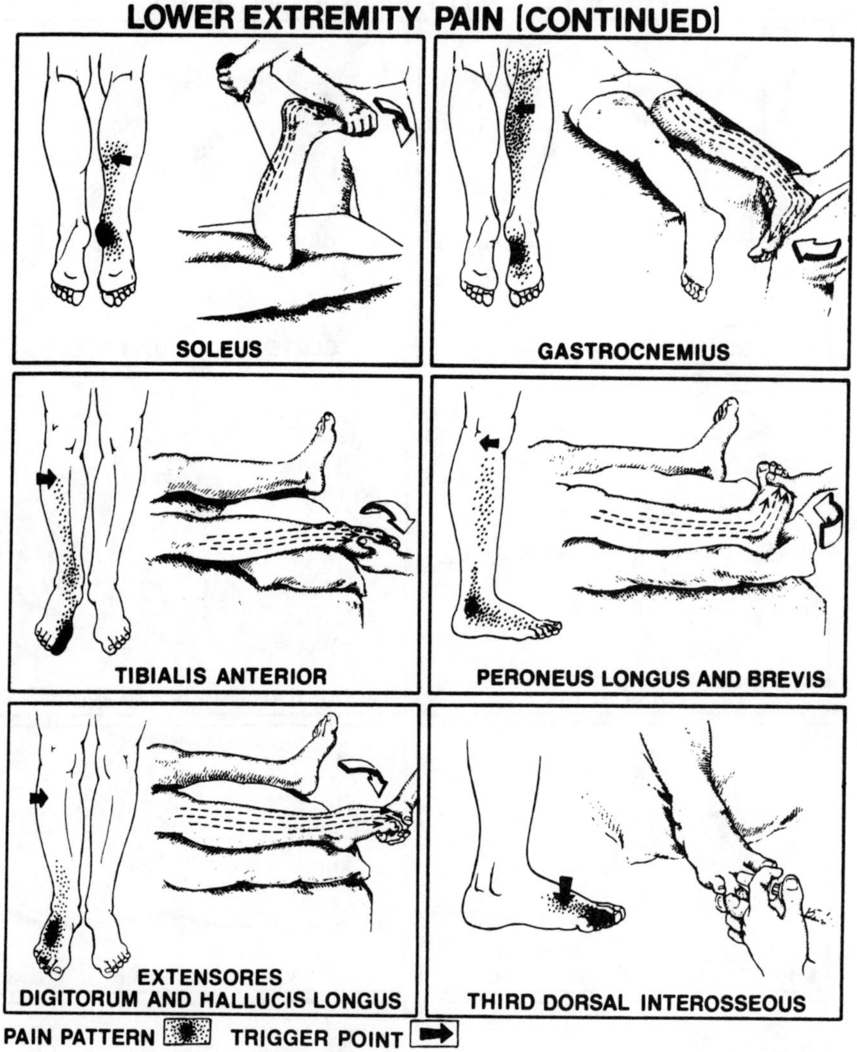

LOWER EXTREMITY PAIN (CONTINUED)

SOLEUS

GASTROCNEMIUS

TIBIALIS ANTERIOR

PERONEUS LONGUS AND BREVIS

EXTENSORES
DIGITORUM AND HALLUCIS LONGUS

THIRD DORSAL INTEROSSEOUS

PAIN PATTERN ▨   TRIGGER POINT ➡

Fig. 15

APPENDIX 8: MUSCLES AFFECTED BY TRIGGER POINTS

Abdominis obliqui
Abdominis transversus
Adductor pollicis
Anconeus
Biceps brachii
Brachialis
Coracobrachialis
Deltoid
Digastric, posterior
Extensor carpi radialis
Extensor carpi ulnaris
Extensor digitorum
Extensor indicis
Flexor carpi ulnaris
Flexor digitorum
Flexor policis longus
Frontalis
Gastrocnemeus
Gluteus maximus
Gluteus medius
Gleuteus mninimus
Hamstring
Iliacus
Iliocostalis lumborum
Iliocostalis throacis
Iliopsoas
Infraspinatus
Interosseus of the hand
Lateral pterygoid
Levator ani
Levator scapulae
Longissimus thoracis
Lower latissimus dorsi
Masseter
Medial pterygoid
Multifidus
Obliqi inferior
Obliqi superior
Obterator internus
Occipitalis
Omohyoid
Opponens pollicis
Orbicularis oculi

Palmaris longis
Paraspinal muscles
Pectoralis major
Pectoralis minor
Peroneus longus
Piriformis
Platysma
Pronator teres
Psoas
Pyramidalis
Quadratus Lumborum
Rectus abdominis
Rectus capitus post maj.
Rectus capitus post min.
Rotatores longus
Scalenus anterior
Scalenus medius
Scalenus minimus
Scalenus posterior
Scbclavius
Semispinalis capitis
Semispinalis cervicis
Serratus posterior inferior
Serratus posterior superior
Soleus
Sphincter ani
Splenius capitus
Splenius cervicis
Sternalis
Sternocleidomastoid
Subscapularis
Supinator
Supraspinatus
Temporalis
Teres major
Teres minor
Tibialis anterior
Trapezius
Triceps brachii
Upper latissimus dorsi
Vastus lateralis
Vastus medialis
Zygomaticus major

APPENDIX 9: PRESSURE THRESHOLD METER LOG SHEET

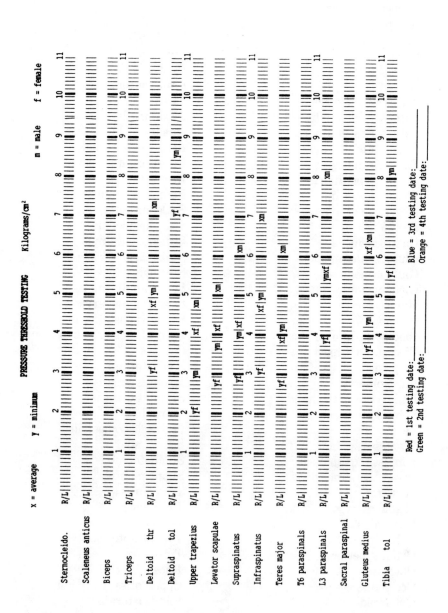

APPENDIX 10: BARRIER TRIGGER POINTS

To highlight one of many problems that are unique to MPS I have employed the term BARRIER TRIGGER POINT.

BARRIER trigger points produce trigger point barriers. A BARRIER trigger point is any trigger point, active or latent, that prevents an MPS patient from obtaining desired physical activity goals. They appear as a silent encumbrance. They are perceived by the patient as a wall, snag, or impasse. It's a message that the patient gets in the back of their mind, that if they push their physical activity level too far they may suffer and pay dearly, and possibly for a long time. At times BARRIER trigger points have the appearance of a boundary that must not be crossed. It's part of the stress and frustration that exasperates many Myofascial Pain Syndrome patients.

Along the way from step to step and stage to stage of recovery BARRIER trigger points may be encountered. As soon as one myofascial trigger point is gotten rid of, it paves the way for more action, motion, and activity. However, other trigger points may be activated as the MPS patient tries out his/her new freedom.

When asked how they are doing, established patients will frequently say they are doing fine. A new patient when asked if their pain problem is getting better, worse, or staying the same may say that their pain problem is presently unchanged. What they are frequently saying is that as long as they don't try to traverse their BARRIER trigger points they have no problems.

They give the appearance of being back to "business as usual." However, if you ask a few more questions often you'll find out they are holding back for fear of bringing on an attack of pain and disability by triggering a BARRIER trigger point.

For example: a woman likes to bowl. Before the onset of her Myofascial Pain Syndrome she could bowl 5 lines before getting tired or feeling a bit achy. Now she says she can bowl one line, but if she goes more than that she will experience a pain flare up for 3 weeks. That is something she can't risk because of her job and family responsibilities. This woman may have a problem with trigger point BARRIERS.

Then there's the company executive who no longer flies in a plane for more than an hour because of the fear of triggering off a disabling low back pain problem.

Not all BARRIER trigger points will become painful when activated. Some may only appear to the patient as mild stiffness or a short-lived ache as he or she steps up their activity level and breaks through a barrier.

A case example will be used to illustrate the concept of BARRIER trigger points. The case that is being related below assumes that all perpetuating factors have been brought under control in order to keep the focus on the BARRIER problem.

Example: Before management 32-year-old Mary Smith had a painful and totally frozen right shoulder, for 6 months, because of subscapularis trigger points. This problem resulted from a fall at work. It represented the first, or major, BARRIER to her recovery from her MPS. She also had pain in the right side of her neck and interscapular area from T3 to T7. She was graded at a 3.

Pain prohibited her from work, housework, bowling, and skiing. Management resolved the problem. She was then left with a atrophied right shoulder. But, in reality, many muscles throughout the body had atrophied because of her overall inactivity.

A combination of trigger point injections (TPI), stretch and spray (S&S), and physical therapy got her on her way.

At that time she could actively abduct the shoulder to 135 degrees and the neck problem was clearing.

One day she reached up to the third shelf of her cupboard (150 of forward flexion and 160 of abduction) to pick up a five-pound bag of baking flour. Over the next three days progressive and severe pain began to radiate down her right arm. This activated the second BARRIER.

Evaluation revealed that she had activated a latent trigger point in the infraspinatus muscle. This trigger point and the others that will be mentioned were all generated by her accident. The infraspinatus trigger point was relieved with appropriate therapy. That facilitated her housework.

Feeling encouraged, she booked a night of bowling with some of her friends. By the time she had finished her second line of bowling, she noticed a pulling sensation in her posterior right flank and some mild discomfort just above the waistline on the right side. The bowling, a routine activity for her, had activated the third BARRIER to her recovery. Upon retiring that evening she took two aspirins, and applied moist heat. At five a.m. the next morning she was awakened by sharp pains and muscle spasms in the same area. She had difficulty walking because of the pain. She saw her myofascial therapist who diagnosed trigger points in the right quadratus lumborum. This was quickly remedied by trigger point injections followed by stretch and spray to the effected muscle.

She was then feeling fine. She could do all of her activities of daily living and was getting along fine.

The ski season came up. She booked a weekend with a few friends. She was an intermediate skier, but stuck to the beginner runs the first day. After doing a number of easy runs, with a lot of right turns, she noticed the onset of cramping in the lateral right hip and radiation of pain down the outside of her right leg from the hip to the ankle. She began to limp, and needed to rest often. The pain and cramping was distressing and discouraging. The skiing, a routine activity for her, had activated the fourth BARRIER to her total recovery. Her friends took her to the nearest town where they found a physician familiar with MPS. He diagnosed a gluteus minimus trigger point. He injected the trigger points, stretch and spray the muscle, applied moist heat for 10 minutes, and sent her on her way.

Since that last BARRIER was removed, her recovery has been complete. She has returned to a fully active life style without any residual pain or restrictions.

REFERENCES

Baker, B. (1986). The muscle trigger: Evidence of overload injury. *Journal of Neurological & Orthopedic Medicine & Surgery, 7*: 31-43.

Barnes, B. (1976). *Hypothyroidism: The unsuspected illness.* New York: Thomas Crowell Company.

Dorland's Illustrated Medical Dictionary (1985) 26th ed. Philadelphia: WB. Saunders.

Farmer, T. (1985). *Neurological complications of vitamin and mineral disorders.* (p.1-8). In A. Baker & R. Joynt, (Eds.), *Clinical neurology,* Vol. 4, Chap. 60, Philadelphia: Harper & Rowe.

Fields, H. (1987). *Pain.* New York: McGraw Hill Book Company. (pp. 209-229).

Foley, K., & Portenoy, R. (1986). Chronic use of opioid analgesics in non-malignant pain: report of 38 cases. Pain. *Elsivier, 25*: 171-186.

Gilman, A., Goodman, L., & Gilman, A. (1980). (Eds.), *Goodman and Gilman's the pharmacological basis of therapeutics,* 6th. ed. New York: MacMillman Publishing Company, (494-583).

Houde, R. (1974). *The use and misuse of narcotics in the treatment of chronic pain.* (pp. 527-538). In J. Bonica (Ed.), Advances in neurology: An international symposium on pain. New York: Raven Press.

Jaffe, J., & Martin, W. (1985). In L. Goodman & A. Gilman (Eds.), *Goodman and Gilman's the pharmacological basis of therapeutics,* 7th. ed., New York: MacMillman Publishing Company. (p. 516).

Jeppsson, B., & Gimmon, Z. (1983). *Vitamins*. In J. Fischer (Ed.), *Surgical nutrition.* Boston: Little, Brown and Company. (pp. 241-282).

Lindblom, U. (1985). *Assessment of abnormal evoked pain in neurological pain patients and its relation to spontaneous pain: A descriptive and conceptual model with some analytical results* (p. 412). In H. Fields, R. Dubner, & F. Cervero, (Eds.), *Advances in pain research and therapy.* New York: Raven Press.

Mackley, R. (in press). *The role of trigger points and Myofascial Pain Syndrome in the management of head, neck, and face pain.* In M. Margoles (Ed.), *Conquering chronic pain.*

Margoles, M. (1983). The stress neuromyelopathic pain syndrome. *Journal of Neurological & Orthopedic Medicine and Surgery, 4*:317-322.

Margoles, M. (1983). *Pain charts: Spatial properties of pain.* (pp. 214-225). R. Melzack, (Ed.) *Pain measurement and assessment.* New York: Raven Press.

Margoles, M. (1984). *Opioid usage survey of the members of the American Pain Society,* unpublished data.

Margoles, M., & Margoles, M. (1984). The use of narcotic analgesics in the treatment of chronic orthopedic pain patients (COPP) - an informal and retrospective study of 95 patients. *Pain,* suppl. 2, S31.

Margoles, M. (1987). Cervical discs as perpetuating factors in chronic moderate to severe myofascial pain syndrome and SNPS. American Back Society newsletter, 2, 3-4.

Margoles, M. (1988). Colchicine usage in the treatment of patients with pain. *Journal of Neurological & Orthopedic Medicine & Surgery, 10*:913-18.

Margoles, M. (1988). Breaking colchicine tablets to make them more palatable. *Journal of Neurological & Orthopedic Medicine & Surgery, 9*:95.

Margoles, M. (1989). Vitamins by mouth and by injection in the treatment of patients with chronic pain. *Journal of Neurological & Orthopedic Medicine & Surgery, 10*:341-343.

Margoles, M. (1989). Comprehensive evaluation and treatment of the patient with Myofascial Pain Syndrome. *Journal of Neurological & Orthopedic Medicine & Surgery, 10*:344-346.

Margoles, M. (in press). *The stress neuromyeloencephalopathic pain syndrome (SNPS).* In M. Margoles (Ed.), *Conquering chronic pain.*

Margoles, M. (in press). The stress neuromyeloencephalopathic pain syndrome (SNPS): Update. *Journal of Neurological & Orthopedic Medicine & Surgery.*

Margoles, M. (in press). *Vitamin A toxicity in chronic pain patients.* In M. Margoles (Ed.), *Conquering chronic pain.*

Margoles, M. (in press). *Vitamin and mineral problems in patients with chronic pain.* In M. Margoles (Ed.), *Conquering chronic pain.*

Margoles, M. (in press). *Medication management in patients with chronic pain*. In M. Margoles (Ed.), *Conquering chronic pain.*

Margoles, M. (in press). *Sleep problems in patients with chronic pain*. In M. Margoles (Ed.), *Conquering chronic pain.*

Margoles, M. (in press). *Conquering chronic pain.*

Margoles, M. (in press). *Some important aspects of clinical and laboratory evaluation and treatment of patients with Myofascial Pain Syndrome.*

Margoles, M. (in press). *Advanced physical therapy techniques in the rehabilitation of patients with chronic pain*. In M. Margoles (Ed.), Conquering chronic pain.

Meyers, F., & Meyers, F. (1987). Management of chronic pain. *American Family Physician,* 35: 139-146.

Porter, J. & Jick, H. (1980). Addiction rare in patients treated with narcotics. *New England Journal of Medicine, 302,* 123.

Rask, M. (1980). Colchicine use in 500 patients with disk disease. *The Journal of Orthopaedic Surgery, 1*:1-19.

Rask, M. (1985). Colchicine use in 3,000 patients with diskal (and other) spinal disorders. *Journal of Neurological and Orthopedic Medicine & Surgery, 6*:1-8.

Simons, D. *Personal communication.*

Simons, D. (1984). *Myofascial Pain Syndromes and their treatment* (pp. 312-320). In J. Basmajian and R.L. Kirby, *Medical Rehabilitation*. Baltimore: Williams and Wilkins.

Smith, D. (1981, 1989). *Personal communication.*

Stimmel, B. (1985). Pain analgesia and addiction: An approach to the pharmacologic management of pain. *The Clinical Journal of Pain, 1*:14-22.

Tennent, F., & Ulemen, G. (1983). Narcotic maintenance for chronic pain, medical and legal guidelines. *Postgraduate Medicine, 73*:81-94.

Texidor, M., & Margoles, M. (in press). *The evaluation of vitamin/electrolyte for the management of chronic low back pain of myofascial origin.*

Travell, J., & Simons, D. (1983). *Myofascial pain and dysfunction: The trigger point manual*. Baltimore: Williams and Wilkins.

Travell, J. (1976). *Myofascial trigger points: Clinical view.* (p. 921). In J. Bonica and D. Albe-Fessard (Eds.), *Advances in pain research and therapy,* Vol. 1. New York: Raven Press.

Travell, J. *Personal communication.*

Travell, J. & Simons, D. (in press). *Myofascial pain and dysfunction: The trigger point manual,* Vol. 2. Baltimore: Williams and Wilkins.

Travell, J. & Simons, D. (1983). *Myofascial pain and dysfunction: The trigger point manual.* (p.61).Baltimore: Williams and Wilkins.

Chapter 16

NURSING AND PAIN MANAGEMENT

Kathleen Bellinger, R.N., Ed.D.
Mary Romelfanger, R.N., M.S.N.
Chris L. Algren, R.N., M.S.N., Ed.D.
Pamela C. Hagan, M.S.N., R.N., C.S.

Throughout time, nurses have been involved in the management of pain and suffering. Dr. Bellinger et al. describe the multifaceted role of the management of pain. The chapter emphasizes the systematic problem solving paradigm known as the nursing process. This chapter reviews the process of nurse decision-making as it is performed with patients and families. Special attention should be directed to the separate sections on pain management in infants, children, and in pain management of the elderly.

The reader will benefit from the many discussions of treatment options with an emphasis blending both behavioral and somatic concepts. The chapter concludes with a consideration of future trends such as research, professional practice, and regulations concerning practice.

Chapter 16

NURSING AND PAIN MANAGEMENT

Kathleen Bellinger, R.N., M.S., Ed.D.
Mary Romelfanger, R.N., M.S.N.
Chris L. Algren, R.N., M.S.N., Ed.D.
Pamela C. Hagan, M.S.N., R.N., C.S.

At every point in history where there is a record of nursing, the nurse has dealt with pain as a problem. Nurses diagnose and treat human responses based on professional standards and legal statutes. Pain crosses age, setting, cultural, geographic, economic, and educational boundaries. Pain management is a goal of many health care disciplines and a specialty within many professions including nursing. Historically, nurses have been recognized for their "caring" role.

The National Institutes of Health published a consensus statement in 1979 that stressed the "caring" role in pain management, not only the "curing" role. In the decade since the first statement, great strides have been made in the assessment and understanding of the multiple dimensions of pain and advances have been made in pharmacological and non-pharmacological methods to treat pain. The number of multidisciplinary pain centers has grown rapidly. The use of a multidisciplinary team of health professionals to treat pain has gained wide acceptance and has come to be known as "the integrated approach to the management of pain."

The current National Institutes of Health consensus statement expresses concern that the education of many professionals including nurses, physicians, dentists, and physical therapists does not put sufficient emphasis on contemporary pain assessment and management methods. There is a great need for communication and collaborative approaches among professionals (NIH, 1986).

This textbook is such a collaboration. Pain is an integrated response, therefore, pain management with contributions from each appropriate health discipline is best. Even when a sole practitioner is treating an individual, knowledge from the other disciplines is necessary.

The purpose of this chapter is to provide an overview of nursing and pain management practice. Since nurses use the systematic problem solving method-nursing process, nursing process is used as a framework for the chapter. Complete pain manuals specific to nursing practice are available. *Pain Clinical Manual For Nursing Practice* (McCaffrey & Bebe, 1989) is an excellent example.

This chapter fits together with others in this comprehensive textbook on pain management. Table I shows how the other chapters relate to the phases of the nursing process. The chapter, "Assessment and Diagnostic Techniques," for example, contains useful information for nursing ASSESSMENT and DIAGNOSIS. "The Role of Neural Blockade in the Management of Common Pain Syndromes" can aid the nurse to plan interdependent practice with a physician specialist and chapters such as "Post-Injury: The Return to Work Challenge" can assist the nurse with PLANNING, especially for referrals. Understanding the content in other chapters, "The Nonpharmacological Management of Chronic Pain via the Interdisciplinary Approach," and "Pharmacotherapeutic Management of Selected Pain Phenomenon" for example, are vital for IMPLEMENTATION of nursing practice. The EVALUATION phase of the process is enhanced through other chapters such as "Understanding and Treating Low Back Pain." Nurses, like all other pain management practitioners, benefit from reading each chapter, but the chapters have varying degrees of relevance based on the reader's particular discipline. The information in the chapters may be applied differently by those from various disciplines.

In this chapter, first the nursing process and then its use with pain management are explained. Because nursing management of pain occurs in a variety of settings both acute and chronic, with persons at each point in the life cycle and with persons who have differing medical diagnoses, content about acute intrapartum-postpartum pain management, post-surgical pain management, chronic, benign, and cancer pain management is included. Sections about special concerns of pain management in children and the elderly are also found in the chapter. Since "patient" is used by pain management practitioners from many disciplines and since "patient" is used in a majority of settings where nurses practice in the world, "patient" rather than "client" is used in this chapter. The rights and responsibilities associated with the use of "client" are intended. The complete nursing process is utilized by nurses with every patient but each of the specific sections emphasizes one or two phases of the process. An example of how research results can influence nursing practice standards and legal scope of practice follows. Nursing theory and models of advanced nursing practice are beyond the scope of this chapter.

Table I. Phases of Nursing Process and Chapter Relatedness by Number and Title

Assessment/Nursing Diagnosis

3. The Classification of Pain
5. Assessment and Diagnostic Techniques
11. Headaches: Muscle Contractions, Migraine, and Cluster
12. Orofacial Pain and Temporomandibular Disorders: Differential Diagnosis
14. Reflex Sympathetic Dystrophy
15. Myofascial Pain Syndrome
17. Lower Extremity Neuropathic Pain

Planning

10. The Role of Neural Blockade in the Management of Common Pain Syndromes
19. Orthopaedic Practice and the Use of Electronic Thermography
20. Manual Medicine: An Osteopathic Approach
22. Physical Therapy and Pain Management
23. Electromedicine: The Other Side of Physiology
24. Post-Injury: The Return to Work Challenge

Implementation

7. The Nonpharmacological Management of Chronic Pain Via the Interdisciplinary Approach
8. Pharmacotherapeutic Management of Selected Pain Phenomena

Evaluation

1. The Magnitude of the Pain Problem
2. The History of Pain Management
4. Multidisciplinary Pain Clinics
6. The Psychiatrist's Role in Pain Management
9. Understanding and Treating Low Back Pain
13. Hospice, Cancer Pain Management, and Symptom Control

NURSING PROCESS

In the United States during the 1960s students of nursing were taught a systematic method to provide nursing care. This method is called the nursing process. The phases in the process were assessment, planning, implementation, and evaluation. In the 1970s nurses recognized that just as physicians diagnose and treat medical problems, nurses diagnose and treat. Therefore, nursing diagnosis was added to the nursing process as an outcome of the assessment phase or as a separate phase between assessment and implementation. Nurse decision-making is performed step-by-step through the process but new information can result in a rapid return to a prior phase as shown (Fig. 1).

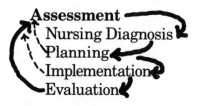

Assessment
  Nursing Diagnosis
  Planning
  Implementation
  Evaluation

Fig. 1. Nursing Process

Because nurses diagnose and treat human responses, nurses needed a classification system for nursing diagnoses. The North American Nursing Diagnosis Association (NANDA) accepted the task and has produced a list of nursing diagnoses based on clinical practice and nursing research. The NANDA list of accepted diagnoses currently contains 88 nursing diagnoses.

A nursing diagnosis can be an actual, potential, or possible diagnosis and consists of two or three parts. An actual nursing diagnosis contains a diagnostic label, the contributing factors and the signs and symptoms. Potential and possible nursing diagnoses consist of the potential nursing diagnosis and the related risk factors.

For those who want a reference that describes the concept of nursing diagnosis and the specific instructions for clinical use either of two sources may be useful (Carpenito, 1989b; Gordon, 1989). A quick reference to the 88 current diagnostic categories approved by NANDA plus 12 other diagnostic categories is recommended by Carpenito (1989a) and used by many nurses.

Pain and chronic pain are nursing diagnoses approved by NANDA. These diagnoses fit within the cognitive-perceptual functional health pattern. Table II contains other NANDA-approved nursing diagnoses by functional health patterns that are commonly concurrent diagnoses for patients with pain (acute) or chronic pain. Alteration in comfort is a nursing diagnosis recommended by Carpenito (1989a & 1989b) and Pain, self-care deficit is a nursing diagnosis proposed by Gordon (1989). Each of these diagnoses are used in this chapter for patients with pain-related nursing management problems.

NURSING MANAGEMENT OF CHRONIC BENIGN PAIN

Assessment & Planning

Pain is whatever an individual says it is, occurring whenever the individual says it does (McCaffery, 1968). Pain is subjective and personal. The practitioner can only observe signs and obtain information about symptoms. The pain belongs to the patient, not to the practitioner. The person with pain is the best judge of the existence, duration, and severity of the pain and of the success of pain management treatments.

The patient as expert judge rather than the professional practitioner can be difficult for the practitioner to accept. Until recently, pain has been viewed as a symptom, not as the diagnosis. Pain was considered by practitioners and patients as something that the practitioner should be able to cure or at least control. Many times the etiology of chronic pain is not determined or not determined quickly or easily after evaluating data obtained by history, examination, and sophisticated tests. The practitioners, as well as the patient, become frustrated. Many health care providers, including nurses, had little in their education about pain, particularly chronic pain, and pain relief. The information the nurse does have may be outdated as well as inadequate and pain relief may not be valued as a priority in the setting where the nurse practices.

The North American Nursing Diagnosis Association accepts chronic pain as a nursing diagnosis and the nurse is an integral player on the chronic pain management team whether the patient is being treated in a hospital, in an inpatient or outpatient program, or in the community by the patient's primary provider. Nurses are among the professionals with a long history of treating responses to pain. Nurses who work in community settings are likely to regularly help patients and families manage chronic pain. To do this, the nurse and others interested in pain management need to know the meaning pain has for the patient. No chemical or neurophysiological tests exist that can accurately measure pain. Since the question of whether the patient has "real pain" cannot be answered by the practitioner, the nurse, like the others on the pain management team, accept reports of pain from the patient. As a sound place to begin, the nurse must determine what the patient thinks is needed to deal with chronic pain. Results of one qualitative investigation with 25 patients in chronic pain indicate that people in pain want to talk with others in pain and to have an easy to reach source for information about coping with chronic pain for themselves and for their families. Nurses, particularly those who are discharge planners or who work in the community, require current information on resources available to people in pain. Support groups established to assist individuals in pain or professionals who want a referral source for patients are needed. One such group in the United States that has chapters throughout the country is the National Chronic Pain Outreach Association. Nurses and physicians often serve as advisers or as coordinators for local chapters. If the pain management practitioners who advise or belong to the chapter are certified in pain management by the American Academy of Pain Management, they bring valuable knowledge and expertise that might not be available to many members of the group (Geevarghese & Bellinger, 1990).

Table II. NANDA Nursing Diagnosis Commonly Associated with (Acute) Pain and Chronic Pain

Health-Perception Health-Management Pattern	• Altered Health Maintenance • Noncompliance (Specify) • Potential for Injury
Nutritional-Metabolic Pattern	• Altered Nutrition: Potential for More than Body Requirements • Altered Nutrition: More than Body Requirements • Altered Nutrition: Less than Body Requirements
Elimination Pattern	• Constipation • Altered Urinary Elimination Pattern
Activity-Exercise Pattern	• Activity Intolerance • Fatigue • Impaired Physical Mobility • Diversional Activity Deficit • Altered Growth and Development
Sleep-Rest Pattern	• Sleep-Pattern Disturbance
Cognitive-Perceptual Pattern	• Sensory-Perceptual Alteration: Input Excess • Impaired Thought Processes
Self-Perception Self-Concept Pattern	• Fear (Specify Focus) • Anxiety • Hopelessness • Powerlessness (Severe, Moderate, Low) • Self-Esteem Disturbance • Body Image Disturbance • Personal Identity Disturbance
Role-Relationship Pattern	• Distrubance in Role Performance • Social Isolation/Social Rejection • Impaired Social Interation • Altered Family Processes
Sexuality-Reproductive Pattern	• Sexual Dysfunction • Altered Sexual Patterns
Coping-Stress-Tolerance Pattern	• Ineffective Coping (Individual) • Ineffective Family Coping

Adapted from Gordon, 1989, pp. iii-viii.

Regardless of setting, the nurse performs as patient advocate, health teacher, and counselor, as well as provider and coordinator of care. The nurse makes referrals to practitioners from other disciplines and accepts appropriate referrals. On the chronic pain management team, the nurse is a collaborator.

NURSING MANAGEMENT OF PAIN IN THE ELDERLY

Assessment and Nursing Diagnosis

For purposes of the discussion which follows, the term "elderly" refers to those persons 65 years of age or older. However, it is important to note that many of the physiologic changes associated with the aging process have an onset as early as the fourth decade. Therefore, although this discussion focuses on an age-related cohort, individual variation is a hallmark of any investigation of the sequelae of human aging.

The axiom "aging is not for sissies" may have found its origin in the many factors of aging that support the nursing diagnosis—alteration in comfort. Carpenito (1989b) states unequivocally that pain is omnipresent in the elderly. This is a particularly startling revelation in view of Wolanin's observation that pain is primary—until it is relieved, no person functions adequately (Wolanin, 1976). This discussion explores these concepts in more detail and addresses other factors which combine to make the elderly a population uniquely vulnerable to pain.

The myriad physiologic and pathophysiologic changes of human aging resulting in either acute or chronic pain may manifest themselves in a variety of ways in the elderly. Some of these manifestations are obvious and accompanied by typical signs and symptoms of a specific problem while some are subtle, atypical, or even paradoxical (Caird et al., 1987). While the mechanisms of pain have been well-described (Thompson, 1984), variation in pain perception in the elderly remains an area of contradictory subjective opinion and objective data (Carso, 1971; Matteson, 1988; Caird et al., 1987). However, it is generally accepted that pain threshold increases with age (Jacox, 1977; Carpenito, 1989b; McConnell, 1988; Charlton & Buckley, 1984).

In addition to an increased pain threshold, other factors are known to alter pain perception in the elderly. These include peripheral and central nervous system impairments, drug therapies, cognitive impairments, co-existing pathologies, individual psychophysiological or cultural, experiences, and adaptation (McConnell, 1988; Carpenito, 1989b; Caird et al., 1987; McCue, 1987).

Whether a result of increased pain threshold or other factors, certain conditions are reported to be less painful in older adults than in younger persons. Conditions frequently presenting with significant pain in younger persons but with only mild discomfort in the elderly include peptic ulceration, appendicitis, pneumonia, and mesenteric infarction. In the elderly these events may be heralded only by vague signs such as restlessness or confusion.

Another factor confusing the symptom pattern in the elderly is the tendency for pain to be referred to other sites in the body. Chest pain may be referred from abdominal or esophageal pathologies (Charlton & Buckley, 1984; Dymock, 1985), while abdominal pain may arise from musculoskeletal or spinal problems or abdominal wall entrapment syndromes. Back pain may be the presenting symptom of a host of pathologies including disc degeneration, arthritis, osteoarthritis, metastatic disease, and Paget's disease. These conditions may present as lower limb pain (Charlton & Buckley, 1984). Spondylosis of the cervical vertebrae may present as pain, muscular spasticity, or paresthesia in one upper limb (Pathy, 1985; Grahame, 1985).

Perhaps the most frequently cited clinical manifestation of paradoxical pain perception in the elderly is cardiac pain. Although elderly persons experiencing angina pectoris report the same need to cease exertion and similar dyspnea and pain radiation patterns as younger persons, they also report much less severe pain. It is postulated that the modified severity of pain results from either the presence of afferent degeneration of the heart or the occurrence of disease in the smaller coronary vessels which produces less pain than disease in the larger vessels (Carid et al., 1987).

Besides modified chest pain, it is not unusual for the elderly patient with clinically severe ischemic heart disease to present totally absent of pain. One study found 31 percent of the elderly patients who experienced myocardial infarction reported no pain while 40 percent reported clinically atypical symptoms (Caird et al., 1987; Charlton & Buckley, 1984). This phenomenon may be the result of the presence of multiple pathologies which severely limit activity, such as arthritis, Parkinsonism, blindness, or hemiplegia. The presence of other pathologies may also present the patient with other symptoms so noxious that chest pain is not noticed (Caird et al., 1987). Clearly, determining the origin of pain in the elderly presents a challenge to the health care practitioner and patient alike.

Pain is a subjective phenomenon. Although practitioners observe the elderly for behavioral manifestations of pain such as facial grimacing, positional guarding, etc., such observations, or even the perceptions of the experienced practitioner, are not reliable assessments of whether pain is present, and if so, how severe that pain may be. As is the case with non-elderly patients presenting with pain, the elderly patient's report of pain must be as accepted as the most reliable clinical description. This requires that the patient with pain be trusted (Wright & Gal, 1987). It has been reported that the inability of an elderly patient to walk on a broken thigh was ascribed to hysteria (Pitt, 1982).

While this is an extreme example of failure to trust, attributing pain to psychogenic origin may occur in those circumstances where no clear cut etiology for the pain is found. In reality, it is not always possible to discover an etiology for the discomfort experienced by patients. This reality can lead to frustration or guilt for the clinical practitioner, which in turn can lead to avoidance of the patient or minimization of the patient's pain by the practitioner—neither of which benefits either party (McConnell, 1988). Compounding the difficulty of establishing trust and gathering accurate data from the patient is the fact that older persons tend to be more reluctant to report pain than younger persons (Matteson, 1988; Charlton & Buckley, 1984; McConnell, 1988). Additionally, due to increased pain tolerance and adaptation, the elderly individual also does not tend to demonstrate expected objective signs of pain as readily as a younger person (Carpenito, 1989b). While this adaptive behavior by the elderly patient may be necessary for continued survival, particularly in the presence of chronic pain, it may lead to inaccurate assessment by the practitioner, ineffective pain management, and to reduced comfort and mobility and increasing dependence and isolation, anger and frustration, and in some cases, confusion by the patient (Pitt, 1982).

Although instruments have been developed to quantify and qualify pain experienced by the elderly and non-elderly (Wright & Gal, 1987; Kane & Kane, 1984), this remains an area of need for additional nursing research. Results of scientific investigation about the phenomenon of pain experienced by the elderly may assist the elderly to achieve the best possible quality of life. In summary, some of the factors which singly and in combination explain why the elderly population is at high risk for the nursing diagnosis alteration in comfort are presented in Table III.

NURSING MANAGEMENT OF PAIN IN INFANTS AND CHILDREN

Implementation

Although relieving pain is a primary goal of nurses, pain management in children has often been ignored and has received limited attention in the literature. Eland and Anderson (1977) documented the undertreatment of children in pain. The lingering myth that children do not experience pain has seemingly justified the lack of pain management in children by physicians and nurses. Despite increasing interest and research in this area, the 1986 Consensus Development Conference on the Integrated Approach to Pain Management noted that even when pain is reported by the child and assessed by the nurse, pain management may be inadequate (Stevens, 1989).

Although evaluating pain in infants and children is a critical component of pediatric nursing care, the nurse must be able to recognize pain and understand that children respond to pain with reactions that depend

Table III. Risk Factors Associated with Nursing Diagnosis—Alterations of Comfort in the Elderly

- Pain threshold increases with age
- Physiologic/patholphysiologic changes may alter perception of pain
- Pain in elderly may be reffered from site of origin
- Physiololologic changes of aging give rise to chronic pain
- Multiple pathologies may result in the paradoxical absence of pain
- Severe pain, chronic discomfort in the elderly may manifest as confusion
- Cultural/psychological expectations may diminish reporting of pain
- Concern for over-medication may result in insufficient pain management modalities
- Societal acceptance of pain in the elderly leads to avoidance or minimalization of pain
- Depression is present and most frequently associated with chronic pain
- Constellation of symptoms in chronic pain states includes behavior commonly associated with maladaptation to the aging process including: sleep disturbances, appetite disturbances, decreased libido, irritability, withdrawal of interests, weakening of relationships, and increased preoccupation with ill health
- Underreporting of symptoms
- Communication difficulties that increase history taking difficulties

on their age and cognitive processes. Because of the problems with the measurement of pain in children, assessment requires a multifaceted approach.

Research results indicate that children do experience pain and they respond behaviorally and physiologically. The pain behaviors, however, may be more subtle than those expressed by adults. Observation of these responses provides a basis for nursing assessment.

Behavioral changes such as irritability, loss of appetite, unusual quietness, disturbed sleep patterns, and changes in facial expression may indicate pain in children who are unable to report pain verbally. Children may also exhibit protective behaviors such as splinting or positioning. Parents are often the first to detect these subtle behaviors, and their input should be sought.

Physiologic responses such as flushed skin, increased temperature, pulse and blood pressure, restlessness, and dilated pupils may be associated with pain. These signs of automatic nervous system arousal are short-lived. The body adapts and a state of homeostasis follows. These physiological responses are only helpful, therefore, when they are combined with other assessment data.

Pediatric nurses have been very reluctant to rely on their own assessments of pain in children. When combined with lingering myths about children not experiencing pain and fears about addiction and respiratory depression, this reluctance can result in undermedication and unnecessary discomfort for children.

Medications used to manage pain in children include non-narcotic analgesics such as acetaminophen and aspirin. Narcotic agents such as meperidine hydrochloride and morphine may also be given. The ideal drug is easy to administer, has a rapid onset, and produces the desired degree of analgesia. Physiological parameters and ventilation should be minimally altered. Oral or rectal analgesics may be less traumatizing than those given by intramuscular injection. According to Eland (1988), narcotic sprays, skin patches, and popcicles are being developed.

Recently, anesthesiologists and surgeons have been administering regional nerve blocks intraoperatively to decrease pain in the immediate post-operative period. Use of ilioinguinal and iliohypogastric nerve blocks during inguinal hernia repairs and penile blocks for circumcisions permit a prolonged period of comfort without the administration of narcotics. The most commonly used agent, bupivacaine, has a duration of approximately six hours.

Epidural anesthesia has recently been adapted for use in pediatric patients having surgery below the umbilicus. Morphine or fentanyl is usually administered either by a single injection or repeatedly through a catheter placed in the epidural space via the caudal approach. The duration of analgesia is 12 to 24 hours. The nurse should observe for common side effects which include urinary retention, pruritis, and nausea.

In the United States, patient-controlled analgesia (PCA) is being used on a limited basis in the management of pain in adolescents. By using an infusion pump, patients can administer a small bolus of medication by simply pressing a button. The patient, however, cannot repeat a dose before a specified period of time. This permits individual titration and a relatively constant analgesic effect. This technique requires specific explanations to both the adolescent and parents.

By understanding children's responses to pain, pediatric nurses can choose appropriate pain relief measures which are individualized for the child. Because anxiety intensifies the sensation of pain, reducing fear and anxiety can alter the child's perception of pain. Explanations which increase the understanding of both the child and parents can help reduce fear and anxiety. Other measures, such as the presence of parents, family members, and security objects, help achieve the goal of providing emotional support for the child or fostering it within the child's existing support system.

Many of the noninvasive techniques for children are similar to those used with adult patients. Children, however, will eagerly participate in fantasy, "games," and new ideas. Distraction is a powerful pain relief measure. Therapeutic play, for example, distracts the child from fears, from a focus on self, and from pain. The nurse must remember, however, that the perception of pain is only altered during the distracting activity. When the activity ends, the pain may return.

Relaxation and imagery can be used as an approach to relieve pain in children who are capable of some degree of abstract thinking. Guided imagery requires patients to use their imaginations to create pleasant images such as swimming at the beach. Rocking infants and children, singing or talking in a soothing voice, or soothing music can produce relaxation.

Cutaneous stimulation may also be used as a noninvasive pain relief measure. Activities such as holding, stroking, or rubbing an injection site or the side opposite the part of the body that hurts often produces muscle relaxation, comfort, and sedation.

Other noninvasive measures such as hypnosis, humor, and coping skills training may help children who are experiencing chronic pain. These measures, however, have not been tested extensively in children.

A combination of the use of interaction between the child and parents, noninvasive techniques, and medication facilitates the development of an individualized plan for pain relief in children. Pain management can be facilitated by the nurse keeping a record that includes vital signs, time of pain relief measures, the measures used, and the child's response. The child's response to pain can then be evaluated more accurately.

NURSING MANAGEMENT OF ACUTE PAIN

Implementation

With a pregnant patient, the physician and nurse or nurse-midwife take histories, perform physical examinations, and obtain and assess laboratory data. Acute pain is a nursing diagnosis that is anticipated for the intrapartum and early postpartum periods, particularly with women for whom a cesarean section is probable. An alternate to the NANDA diagnosis, acute pain is suggested by Gordon (1989) pain, self-management deficit.

Health teaching and health counseling is done to promote a healthy outcome and to prevent unnecessary pain. Information about labor and delivery, anesthesia and analgesia for labor, vaginal delivery or cesarean section, noninvasive measures to prevent pain, and comfort measures for postpartum are part of the anticipatory guidance provided by the practitioner or obtained through classes taken elsewhere. Prepared childbirth classes, Lamaze for example, are given by qualified nurses. Nurses also teach classes for pregnant parents through local hospitals.

While there are many options to reduce pain during labor and delivery, epidural anesthesia is increasingly common, as is epidural or spinal anesthesia for cesarean sections. The nurse in labor and delivery counsels the patient about choices and supports the patient while the anesthesiologist or nurse anesthetist administers the regional anesthetic. Monitoring maternal pain relief, blood pressure, contraction pattern and fetal heart rate, repositioning the patient for comfort and safety, maintaining fluid and electrolyte balance, and providing information and support are performed by the nurse during labor, especially for those patients who have epidurals. An intermittent bolus of local anesthetics through the indwelling epidural catheter or a continuous drip epidural through the catheter using an epidural syringe pump or PCA pump can prevent acute pain without interfering with the patient's ability to push. The epidural anesthesia in effect for labor can be continued for a cesarean section. Spinal or epidural anesthesia with local anesthetics and narcotics are popular and safe for planned cesarean sections (Ackerman, Colclough, et al., 1989; Ackerman, Denison et al., 1990).

Single dose narcotics given via the epidural or spinal route after a cesarean section or after a vaginal delivery with a third or fourth degree laceration may result in less acute pain for the patient, earlier ambulation, and progression to oral analgesics sooner. Length of stay in the hospital may be shortened (Ackerman, Juneja, et al., 1989a; Ackerman, Juneja, et al., 1989b; Carmichael, Rolbin, & Hew, 1982). Standing order sets and clear communication among patient, nurse, and physician facilitates nursing activity to monitor and treat the possible side effects of intraspinal opioids. Respiratory depression is not common in this patient population and can be treated with intravenous naloxone. The more frequent occurrences of pruritis or nausea and vomiting can be treated with drugs such as hydroxyzine (Ackerman, Bellinger, et al., in press). Carpenito (1989a) includes pruritis, as well as nausea and vomiting as separate pain-related nursing diagnoses.

Acute pain is an expected nursing diagnosis after any surgery, not only a cesarean section. Historically, patients were admitted to a hospital at least one day before surgery. Today, many surgeries are performed in outpatient surgery (OP) or the patient is admitted within hours of the surgery and does not go to a room on a nursing unit until after discharge from the post anesthesia care unit (PACU), a post-operative admission (PO).

To improve surgical and anesthetic safety, reduce patient anxiety and fear of the unknown and prevent pain, a pre-admission testing visit is sometimes scheduled for the patient with an OP surgery or PACU nurse a few days before the surgery. Baseline data are obtained by the nurse to compare with intraoperative and post-operative vital signs. The nurse provides information, answers patient questions, and gives preoperative instructions to be followed by the patient prior to admission the day of surgery or after surgery. Individualized post-operative pain management techniques can be planned with the patient and family and communicated to the other members of the team. If the same nurse cares for the patient the day of surgery, patient anxiety is further reduced.

On post-surgical units, nurses perform non-invasive pain management treatments, such as cutaneous stimulation. Reinforcement of relaxation techniques and guided imagery may be used to support pharmacologic therapy. Nurse and patient scheduling, administration, and evaluation of the effectiveness of the analgesics selected by the nurse from those ordered by the physician is facilitated with the use of a medication flow sheet.

Parenteral analgesic therapy via a PCA pump and intraspinal opioids via a catheter inserted prior to surgery are preferred by many patients, nurses, and physicians. Medications can be given via the intraspinal route by the nurse on a prn basis or the catheter can be connected to a pump for continuous and/or patient-controlled dosing (Adams, 1985; Pageau, Mroz, et al, 1985).

The nursing care plan for pain management must be consistent with medical and other therapies planned for the patient. Nurses spend more time with the patient than any other practitioner therefore the nurse's roles as collaborator, coordinator, and evaluator influence acute pain management outcomes.

NURSING MANAGEMENT OF CHRONIC PAIN

Planning and Evaluation

The perception that pain is a high incidence phenomenon of cancer prevails in both professionals and those who have or will experience cancer. Unfortunately, accurate data are not available to determine the incidence or prevalence of cancer pain. Bonica (1984) combined data from multiple studies and estimated that millions of cancer patients worldwide experience pain of a moderate to severe level. It is suggested that 40 percent to 65 percent of patients in the intermediate stages of the disease have chronic pain while 55 percent to 95 percent of terminal cancer patients have pain. For those patients who do experience pain, over 50 percent indicate it is of a moderate or severe level. Cancer pain is multifaceted and is generally classified as pain from: direct tumor involvement; cancer therapy, or accompanying problems such as constipation; and sources other than cancer and/or cancer treatment (Foley, 1985).

Because cancer most often occurs at ages when other maladies develop which also cause pain, for example arthritis and chronic back problems, the practitioner must attempt to identify the source of each pain and intervene specifically. Cancer-related pain may be difficult to define by the individual experiencing it as well as the nurse who intervenes, therefore a thorough and accurate nursing assessment is paramount to the diagnosis and management of cancer pain.

The Standards of Oncology Nursing Practice emphasize the systematic and continuous collection of data to plan appropriate interventions with the patient (ANA:ONS, 1987). Cancer patients may underreport pain, if they think pain indicates their disease is not responding to treatment. Some patients simply do not want to complain even if analgesics are available for the pain and think it is an accompanying fate of the disease (Cleeland, 1984). Other variables such as financial concerns, anxiety, and limited family support may add to the perceived pain experienced because of the disease. Absence of standardized assessment tools make it difficult for nurses to consistently and effectively assess the extent of pain, evaluate the efficacy of the intervention, and to accurately communicate this information. Lack of knowledge about cancer pain etiology, as well as some attitudes toward pain and its management that may be held by nurses, can be barriers to adequate assessment. The Oncology Nursing Society recognized the need for a consistent approach to cancer pain management and addressed barriers to effective cancer pain management in its Position Paper on Cancer Pain (ONS, in press).

Cancer site and stage of disease factor into the incidence and prevalence of pain. As the disease progresses, patients with metastatic disease are more likely to experience pain, particularly those with bone involvement from primary infiltration or metastasis. Interference with organ function or structure or nerve invasion intensify pain. Terminal patients report significant increases in pain. It is evident that the management of cancer pain may need to be multimodal secondary to the many dimensions of its etiology. However, the treatment of acute and chronic cancer pain continues to remain primarily within the realm of pharmacologic management.

Analgesics are extremely effective in most patients when used correctly. The World Health Organization (WHO) recommends a three step "analgesic ladder" which emphasizes the use of standard drugs classified as non-opioids, weak opioids, and strong opioids (WHO, 1986). Sequential use of the drugs is advocated with the addition of a weak opioid in combination with the non-opioid or a strong opioid should the relief not be obtained. Adjuvant drugs are added if required for specific indications and they are often needed in patients with pain secondary to nerve injury. Non-opioid drugs such as the nonsteroidal anti-inflammatory drugs interfere with peripheral receptors by inhibiting prostaglandin release, thus reducing pain from resulting inflammation. Opioid drugs, narcotics, bind to receptors which interfere with the transmission of painful stimuli. Because of the difference in action, combination of the two types of drugs results in efficacious pain management. Adjuvant drugs are used to treat specific types of pain and to alleviate other symptoms which may occur in cancer patients. Anticonvulsants, antidepressants, and corticosteriods are used to reduce anxiety and depression which often exacerbate cancer pain and interfere with other activities of the patient.

Other interventions may be useful, particularly for pain that is not responsive to analgesics. Nerve blocks, transcutaneous nerve stimulation, and neuroablative techniques may benefit cancer patients.

Nurses in acute and chronic pain settings can add a unique perspective to the assessment and care of each cancer patient. Changes in a patient's comfort which occur each 24 hours can be observed, reported, and interventions evaluated more closely because of the increased contact made with the patient. Combining nursing therapies with behavioral therapies and pharmacotherapies offers a broader approach to pain management which is more effective than a single therapy. Nursing therapies which assist patients to meet multiple needs during a cancer pain experience are summarized in Table IV.

Table IV. Nursing Therapies for Cancer Pain

- Mobility/Positioning
- Environmental Manipulation
- Medication Administration
- Promotion of Sleep/Rest
- Maintenance of Hope
- Maintenance of Nutrition
- Stabilization of Mood
- Promotion of Self/ Control/Independence
- Supportive Suggestions for a Satisfying Sexual Expression

- Anticipatory Instruction to Prevent Pain
- Assessment/Communication/ Providing Information/ Documentation
- Thermal Techniques
- Touch
- Relaxation
- Distracting
- Staying
- Maintenance of Elimination
- Spiritual Support

Adapted from GRECC, 1986, pp. 14-18.

The Standards of Oncology Nursing Practice support nurse design of individualized physical and psychosocial interventions which are intended to achieve stated outcomes and are prioritized according to the patient's needs. The nurse also collaborates and communicates with appropriate members of the multidisciplinary team in designing the plan of care (ANA:ONS, 1987).

It is imperative that information as complete as possible be available to all practitioners involved in the alleviation of cancer pain or discomfort. Outcome criteria for the patient in relation to comfort state the patient will: (1) communicate alterations in comfort level; (2) identify measures to modify psychosocial, environmental, and physical factors that increase comfort and promote the continuance of valued activities and relationships; (3) describe the source of discomfort, the treatment, and the expected outcome of the proposed intervention; and (4) describe appropriate interventions for potential or predicable problems such as pain.

To do so requires a comprehensive approach to pain control for the cancer patient. Accountability and responsibility of the professionals involved with the care is demanded and advocated. The challenge is for the nurse to identify, assess, treat, evaluate at specific intervals, make alterations if necessary, and further evaluate. It is the professional and ethical responsibility of caregivers to assist the patient and family to identify and manage factors which promote comfort.

NURSING RESEARCH, PROFESSIONAL PRACTICE, AND LAW

Laws that regulate practice tend to lag behind practice innovation. Nurses are required to understand the legal statutes and professional standards that determine scope of nursing practice, including pain management practice. Often, clinical problems faced daily by the practitioner in the field result in small practice variations and clinical research that may lead to practice changes which affect broader areas of practice.

In one U.S. state for example, the Board of Nursing examined the Nursing Practice Act (KRS 314) and issued a scope of practice advisory opinion that it was not within registered nurse practice to remove epidural catheters. The literature search showed no research published on the safety of catheter removal by registered nurses (R.N.s) vs. certified registered nurse anesthetists (C.R.N.A.s) vs. anesthesiologists. The Board of Nursing needed empirical evidence and testimony from nurses and other experts before the opinion could be revised. The American Association of Nurse Anesthetists (AANA) and several other boards of nursing were also interested in the issue of administration of medications per intraspinal routes.

Results of an investigation conducted by Bellinger (1987) showed that 100 percent of the subjects who had epidural anesthesia (N = 1975) had the epidural catheters removed intact. The data that showed registered nurses safely removed the epidural catheters with one sample of subjects were examined by the AANA. The AANA Standard was revised to allow registered nurses to remove epidural catheters providing the nurse has the appropriate education and experience and an appropriate anesthesia policy exists in the work setting.

Findings from this research, other findings in the literature, and laws in other states were reviewed by the Board. Testimony, including testimony from a nurse certified as a Diplomate by the American Academy of Pain Management about nursing practice in that one state and practice throughout the United States was also considered before the Board of Nursing altered the practice advisory opinion to be consistent with the AANA Standard. Other related pain management nursing practice questions were posed, and after examination of the evidence the statement was revised again. Registered nurses who have the appropriate education and experience may administer the intraspinal analgesics ordered for patients in acute and chronic pain and local anesthetic drugs ordered for patients in chronic pain providing there is an agency policy to support the practice. These changes in legal practice improve comprehensive, cost-effective care and affirm advancement in nursing practice. A simple, descriptive quantitative study that was prompted by a pain management clinical problem in the hospital setting can be linked directly to pain management practice in the community where medication is administered to patients in the home by home health nurses.

END NOTE

The United States Congress created The Agency for Health Care Policy and Research (AHCPR) in December 1989 as the federal government's focal point for health services research. The AHCPR replaces the National Center for Health Care Technology Accessment. The agency's mission is to enhance the quality of patient care services by generating knowledge that can be used to meet society's health care needs. The AHCPR is responsible for developing and updating guidelines that will be used to manage clinical conditions. The clinical guidelines are being formulated as part of AHCPR's Medical Treatment Effectiveness Program (MEDTEP) which also includes database development, effectiveness and outcome research, and dissemination of research findings and guidelines. MEDTEP was developed to improve the effectiveness and appropriateness of the health care services and procedures. Pain-related guidelines are among the first set of seven guidelines currently in development. A nursing advisory panel was convened to provide the nursing profession's perspective on the role of nurses in the MEDTEP initiative, particularly related to guideline design. Nurse clinicians, educators, researchers, administrators, and professional nursing organization representatives comprise the panel (USPHS, 1990a; USPHS, 1990b).

Nurses are ubiquitous, just as pain and the need for pain management are ubiquitous. Nurses have more continuing contact with patients in pain than any other practitioners. Nurse practice and research are vital and integral components of pain management practice and nurses are key participants who are helping to determine how the health care system in the United States and throughout the world deals with pain management.

REFERENCES

Ackerman, W. E., Bellinger, K., Juneja, M. M., & Herold, J. (in press). Extradural opioid utilization in the parturient. *Louisville Medicine.*

Ackerman, W. E., Cololough, G. W., Guiler, J., Guiler, D., Aken, J., & Juneja, M. M. (1989). Epidural fentanyl for management of pain caused by uterine manipulation for elective cesarean section. *Anesthesiology Review* 16(1), 41-45.

Ackerman, W. E., Dension, D. D., Juneja, M. M., Herold, J., Sweeney, N. J., & Nicholson, C. J. (1990). Alkalinization of for chloroprocaine for epidural anesthesia: Effects of pCO2 on constant pH. *Regional Anesthesia,* (3), 89-93.

Ackerman, W. E., Juneja, M. M., Cololough, G. W., Guiler, J. M., & Guiler, D. (1989a). A comparison of epidural fentanyl, butorphanol for the management of post-cesarean section pain. *Anesthesiology Review,* 16(3), 37-40.

Ackerman, W. E., Juneja, M. M., Kaczorowski, D. M., & Cololough, G. W. (1989b). A comparison of the incidence of pruritis following epidural opioid administration in the parturient. *Canadian Journal of Anaesthesiology,* 36(4), 388-391.

Adams, S. (1985). Intensive care nursing: Epidural anesthesia. *Nursing Mirror,* 160(10), 38-41.

American Nurses Association: Oncology Nursing Society. (1987). *Standards of oncology nursing practice.* Kansas City, MO: ANA.

Bellinger, K. (1987, July). *Removal of epidural catheters by R.N.s: Safety and scope of practice.* Sigma Theta Tau International Research Congress, Edinburgh, Scotland.

Bonica, J. J. (1984). Treatment of cancer pain: Current status and future needs. *Pain,* 2:196.

Caird, F. I., Dall, J. C., & Williams, B. O. (1987). The cardiovascular system. In J.C.Brocklehurst (Ed.), *Textbook of geriatric medicine and gerontology* (3rd ed.). (pp. 230-267). Edinburgh: Churchill Livingstone.

Carmichael, F. J., Rolbin, S. H. & Hew, E. M. (1982). Epidural morphine for analgesia after cesarean section. *Canadian Anaesthesia Society Journal,* 29(4): 359-363.

Carpenito, L. J. (1989a). *Handbook of nursing diagnosis.* Philadelphia: J. B. Lippincott Company.

Carpenito, L. J. (1989b). *Nursing diagnosis application to clinical practice* (3rd ed.). Philadelphia: J. B. Lippincott Company.

Charlton, J. E., & Buckley, F. P. (1984). Management of chronic pain. In J.G. Evans & F.I. Caird (Eds.), *Advanced geriatric medicine* (Vol. 4., pp. 17-32). Bath: Pittman Press.

Cleeland, C. S. (1984). The impact of pain on the patient with cancer. *Cancer,* 54(11):2635-2641.

Corso, J. F. (1971). Sensory processes and age effects in normal adults. *Journal of Gerontology* 26:90-105.

Dymock, I. W. (1985). The gastrointestinal system--the upper gastrointestinal tract. In J.C. Brocklehurst (Ed.), *Textbook of geriatric medicine and gerontology* (3rd ed.). (pp. 508-519). Edinburgh: Churchill Livingstone.

Eland, J. (1988). Pharmacologic management of acute and chronic pain. *Issues in Comprehensive Pediatric Nursing,* 11:93-111.

Eland, J., & Anderson, J. (1977). The experience of pain in children. In A. Jacox (Ed.), *Pain: A sourcebook for nurses and other health professionals.* Boston: Little, Brown & Company.

Foley, K. M. (1985). The treatment of cancer pain. *New England Journal of Medicine,* 313:84-95.

Geevarghese, K. P., & Bellinger, K. (1990). On pain, *Louisville Medicine,* 37(11):71-74.

Geriatric Research, Education and Clinical Center (GRECC) & Durham Veterans Administration Medical Center. (1986, March). *Cancer pain.* (3rd ed.), Durham, NC: Cancer Pain Study Committee.

Gordon, M. (1989). *Manual of nursing diagnosis 1988-1989.* Saint Louis: C.V. Mosby Company.

Grahame, R. (1985). The musculoskeletal system - disease of the joints. In J.C. Brocklehurst (Ed.), *Textbook of geriatric medicine and gerontology* (3rd ed.). (pp. 795-819).

Jacox, A. (1977). Sociocultural and psychological aspects of pain. In A. Jacox (Ed.), *Pain: A sourcebook for nurses and other health professionals.* Boston: Little, Brown & Company.

Kane, R., & Kane, R. (1984). *Assessing the elderly.* Lexington MA: Lexington Books.

Matteson, M. A. (1988). Age-related changes in the special senses. In M.A. Matteson & E.S. McConnell (Eds.), *Gerontological nursing concepts and practice* (pp. 311-329). Philadelphia: W.B. Saunders.

McCaffery, M. (1968). Nursing practice theories related to cognition, body pain, and man-environment interaction. Los Angeles: University of California, Students' Store.

McCaffery, M., & Beebe, A. (1989). *Pain: Clinical manual for nursing practice.* Saint Louis: C.V. Mosby Company.

McConnell, E. S. (1988). Nursing diagnoses related to physiological alterations. In M.A. Matteson & E. S. McConnell (Eds.), *Gerontological nursing concepts and practice.* (pp. 331-428). Philadelphia: W.B. Saunders.

McCue, J. D. (1987). Medical screening of the relatively asymptomatic elderly patient. In C. S. Rogers & J. D. McCue (Eds.), *Managing chronic disease.* (pp. 391-399). Oradell: Medical Economics Books.

National Institutes of Health. (1986). *The integrated approach to the management of pain: Consensus development conference statement Vol. 6.,* No. 3. Washington, D.C.: Author.

Oncology Nursing Society. (in press). Position paper on cancer pain. Pittsburgh, PA: Author.

Pageau, M. G., Mroz, W. T., & Coombs, D. W. (1985). New analgesic therapy. *Nursing* 85(4):46-49.

Pathy, M. J. (1985). The central nervous system--clinical presentation and management of neurological disorders in old age. In J.C. Brocklehurst (Ed.), *Textbook of geriatric medicine and gerontology* (3rd ed.). (pp. 795-819). Edinburgh: Churchill Linvingstone.

Pitt, B. (1982). *Psychogeriatrics: An introduction to the psychiatry of old age.* (2nd ed.). (pp. 2-14; 31-38). Edinburgh: Churchill Livingstone.

Stevens, B. (1989). Nursing management of pain in children. In R. Foster, M. Hunsberger, & J. Anderson (Eds.), *Family-centered nursing care of children* (p. 877.). Philadelphia: W.B. Saunders.

Thompson, J. W. (1984). Pain: Mechanisms and principles of management. In J. G. Evans, & F. I. Caird (Eds.), *Advanced geriatric medicine* (Vol. 4., pp. 3-16). Bath: Pittman Press.

U. S. Department of Health and Human Services--Public Health Service. (1990b, February). AHCPR program note-Nursing advisory panel for guideline development: Summary (OM90-0063). Washington, D. C.: U. S. Government Printing Office.

U. S. Department of Health and Human Services--Public Health Service. (1990a, March). AHCPR program note-Medical treatment effectiveness research (OM90-0059). Washington, D. C. Government Printing Office.

Wolanin, M. O. (1976). Nursing assessment. In I.M. Burnside (Ed.), *Nursing and the aged* (pp. 398-420). New York: McGraw Hill Book Company.

Wright, A. B., & Gal, P. (1987). Assessment and treatment of pain. In C. S. Rogers & J.D. McCue (Eds.), *Managing chronic disease* (pp. 28-34). Oradell: Medical Economics Books.

World Health Organization. (1986). Cancer pain relief. Geneva Switzerland: Author.

Chapter 17

LOWER EXTREMITY NEUROPATHIC PAIN

Earl L. Cherniak, D.P.M.; D. Sc. (Hon)

Doctor Cherniak reviews many of the classic neuropathies faced by clinicians when treating lower extremity peripheral neuropathic diseases. The discussion of these syndromes includes commentary on sensory, motor, reflex, and vasomotor symptoms. These problems often lead to patients presenting with anesthesia, numbness and an unsteady gait.

A table and illustrations help the reader differentiate neuropathic pain from trauma, vascular insufficiency, metabolic disease, as well as several other important etiological factors. The reader benefits also from a review of methods of clinical examination and suggestions for treatment.

Chapter 17

LOWER EXTREMITY NEUROPATHIC PAIN

Earl L. Cherniak, D.P.M.; D. Sc. (HON)

Neuropathic pain is part of the symptom complex known as peripheral neuropathy. Sensory loss, muscle weakness, atrophy, and decreased tendon reflexes are more common than pain in neuropathic disease. The general term neuropathy pertains to disturbances and pathologic changes in the peripheral nervous system. This system includes the cranial nerves, the spinal nerves with their roots and rami, the peripheral nerves, and the peripheral components of the autonomic nervous system. Etiologic factors of peripheral nerve disease can number in the hundreds.

The diseases of the peripheral nervous system create a syndrome of sensory, motor, reflex, and vasomotor symptoms (Bradley & Walton, 1974). In dealing with sensory abnormalities, there are positive and negative phenomena of sensation. The negative phenomena are found where there is a significant loss of large myelinated nerve function. The patient complaints include anesthesia, numbness, edematous sensations, and unsteady gait. These patients develop painless skin lesions, ulcerations, and burns. They have neuropathic joints directly caused by the lack of pain and temperature sensations. The protective reflexes are diminished or absent.

The positive phenomenon found in peripheral neuropathic disease is pain. Direct pressure or injury of a nerve will cause a stimulation of the afferent, pain-conducting fibers.

The "pins and needles" sensation, paraesthesia, is caused by a spontaneous discharge of the large myelinated fibers. The "burning feet" sensation found in diabetes, thiamine deficiency, uremia, alcoholism, malabsorption, and carcinoma, is difficult to understand. Other sensations described include the following: contact dyasthesiae, hyperaglesia, and hyperpathia. In contact dyasthesiae, skin contact produces an uncomfortable pricking sensation. In hyperaglesia, the patient has an abnormally low threshold of pain. Hyperpathia is observed when the pain threshold is raised and tolerated but once exceeded, the pain is severe.

The sensation of "restless legs" is found in some neuropathies. The legs are uncomfortable, painful, and have a burning sensation. It is found in mild neuropathies.

Table I. Lower Extremity Neuropathic Pain

Trauma
 Nerve Entrapments
 Causalgia
 Phantom Limb Syndrome
 Reflect Sympathetic Dystrophy

Vascular Insufficiency
 Ischemic Neuropathy

Metabolic Diseases
 Diabetes Mellitus
 Fabry's Disease
 Uremic Neuropathy
 Hepatic Neuropathy
 Thyroid Disease

Hereditary Neuropathies
 Amyloid Neuropathy
 Hereditary Sensory Neuropathy
 Friedrich's Ataxia
 Hereditary Motor Sensory
  Neuropathy

Motor Neuron Disease
 Amyotrophic Lateral Sclerosis

Neuropathies Associated with Paraproteinemias
 Multiple Myeloma
 Macroglobulinemia
 Cryoglobulinemia

Neuropathies caused by Nutritional Deficiencies
 Neuropathic Beriberi
 Pellagra
 Strachan's Syndrome
 Alcoholic Neuropathy
 Burning Feet Syndrome

Neuropathy Associated with Connective Tissue
 Rheumatoid Neuropathy

Neuropathies caused by Toxins
 Arsenic Neuropathy
 Lead Neuropathy
 Mercury Neuropathy

Neuropathies caused by Carcinoma
 Carcinomatous Neuropathy

PERIPHERAL NERVE ENTRAPMENTS

Entrapment neuropathies refer to those lesions caused directly by entrapment in the fibro-osseous tunnels or damage caused by stretching, angulation and friction (Dawson, Hallet & Millender, 1983). As we examine the entrapment neuropathies we will discover one or more of these etiologic factors present. Aguayo feels that the peripheral nerves are especially vulnerable to injury due to their long and superficial courses. Usually, compression neuropathies affect only single nerves that are anatomically susceptible to compression and trauma.

INTERDIGITAL NERVE ENTRAPMENT

Interdigital neuropathies are also known as neuroma, Morton's toe, and Morton's neuroma (Burns & Stewart, 1982). It usually is found in the third metatarsal interspace but has been described in others (Silverman, 1987). It was the earliest entrapment neuropathy described. The interdigital nerves are prolongations of the medial and lateral plantar nerves. As the nerve passes dorsally, it changes its course over and against the deep transverse ligament, that structure that binds the metatarsal heads together. It is felt that the pressure of the ligament against the nerve causes the development of the neuroma. A recent study by Bossley and Cairne suggests the involvement of an intermetatarsal bursa in the formation of the lesion (Addante, Peicott, Wong, & Brooks, 1986). It is the inflammatory process of the bursa that causes the secondary fibrosis associated with the neuroma. It is appropriate to mention at this point that the lesion heretofore known as a neuroma is not a tumor but a benign fibrosis of the nerve comprised of perineural, epineural, and endoneural fibrosis with loss of myelinated nerve fibres.

Pain is evident over the fourth metatarsal head that radiates to the end of the fourth toe. Of course, this will vary depending on the intermetatarsal site of the lesion. I have had patients complain of an ingrown toe nail when, in actuality, their pain was caused by a neuroma. At times pain will extend proximally into the lower leg. The pain can be excruciating. Carlton (1952) had mentioned in his lectures that Morton had a classic description of the person suffering from this entrapment circa 1876. The woman with high button shoes would immediately sit on the curb, quickly remove her shoe and massage her forefoot for relief.

The treatment of interdigital neuroma is conservative management at first: wide shoes, metatarsal padding, physical therapy, and anti-inflammatory drugs, locally and systemically. Steroid/anesthetic injections often alleviate the symptoms for prolonged periods of time. If these measures fail, surgical excision of the lesion is necessary (Gaynor et al., 1989).

PLANTAR NERVE ENTRAPMENT

The medial and lateral plantar nerves are formed by the division of the posterior tibial nerve. The posterior tibial nerve is covered by the laciniate ligament, the flexor retinaculum, in the passageway known as the tarsal tunnel, the area between the medial malleolus and tendo-achilles. The entity described as tarsal tunnel syndrome is in actuality the posterior tarsal syndrome. It involves the posterior portion of the posterior tibial nerve that affects the sensation to the sole of the foot (Dowling & Skaggs, 1982). The entity known as anterior tarsal syndrome is caused by the entrapment of the distal portion of the deep peroneal nerve. This was first described by Kopell (Kopell & Thompson, 1963). The anterior

From Kopell, H.P. and Thompson, W.A.L.: *Peripheral Entrapment Neuropathies.*
Baltimore, Williams and Wilkins Company, 1963.

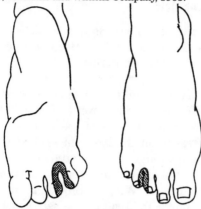

Fig. 1. Sensory distribution of an interdigital nerve.

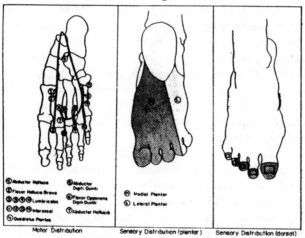

Fig. 2. Plantar nerves—motor and sensory distribution.

tarsal tunnel syndrome causes pain to the dorsum of the foot (Goodman
& Kehr, 1983). Tarsal tunnel syndrome and posterior tarsal syndrome
cause pain and tingling sensation in the sole of the foot and toes that is
followed by a burning sensation and accompanying ankle pain. Some
patients complain of these symptoms at rest while others experience
them after ambulation and standing. Tinel's sign, light compression at
the area of entrapment, can simulate the tarsal tunnel syndrome pain.
The area compressed is inferior and anterior to the medial malleolus.

Treatment consists of physical therapy, immobilization of the foot and
ankle with strapping, anti-inflammatory drugs, local and systemic, and
orthotics. If these measures fail, surgical intervention is necessary to
release the nerve beneath the laciniate ligament and retinaculum.

DEEP PERONEAL NERVE ENTRAPMENT

If the trunk of the deep peroneal is entrapped before the division of the medial branch, the patient experiences pain in the great toe. If there is an entrapment of the lateral branch, the patient experiences mid-foot pain in the tarsal area. The entrapment of the deep peroneal nerve is usually on the dorsum of the foot in the area of the base of the first metatarsal bone.

The etiologic factors are trauma, direct pressure from a tight ill-fitting shoe or cast, violent plantar flexion, and inversion of the foot.

Treatment regime consists of immobilization and anti-inflammatory drugs. If these fail, surgical intervention is required.

SUPERFICIAL PERONEAL NERVE ENTRAPMENT

This nerve is a division of the common peroneal nerve at the fibular neck. As the nerve descends it separates into two branches that pierce the deep fascia. The entrapment occurs at the opening in the deep fascia.

The patient complains of a burning pain in the antero-lateral aspect of the lower leg and dorsum of the foot.

Etiologic factors are ill-fitting footwear, boots, and direct trauma.

Treatment program includes efforts to reduce the tension on the peroneal nerve and the lateral musculature of the leg. This can be accomplished by eversion strapping, shoe wedging, and orthotics. Anti-inflammatory drugs are prescribed. As a last resort, surgical intervention is needed.

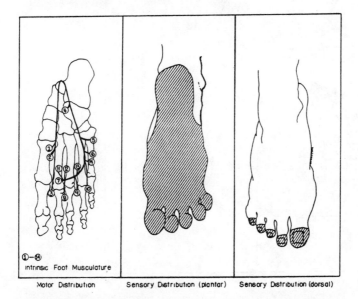

Motor Distribution | Sensory Distribution (plantar) | Sensory Distribution (dorsal)

Fig. 3. Posterior tibial nerve at ankle—motor and sensory distribution.

From Kopell, H.P. and Thompson, W.A.L.: *Peripheral Entrapment Neuropathies.* Baltimore, Williams and Wilkins Company, 1963.

COMMON PERONEAL NERVE ENTRAPMENT

The common peroneal nerve is a bifurcation of the sciatic nerve. The common peroneal nerve passes down the lateral aspect of the thigh and pierces the deep fascia at the fibula neck. Its sensory distribution is to the dorsum of the foot and the antero-lateral aspect of the lower leg.

Etiologic factors causing this entrapment are direct injury, tight and constricting footwear, e.g., boots, fracture of the fibula neck, constant compression of the area as found in bed-ridden patients, muscle injury, lesions occupying the popliteal fossa, and violent muscle contractions. Tinel's sign at the site of entrapment will simulate a radiating pain to the affected area.

Treatment requires stabilization of the foot in an everted position to avoid stress on the peroneal muscles. This can be affected by strapping of the foot and leg, shoe wedges, and orthotics. Systemic and local anti-inflammatory drugs can be utilized. If these measures are ineffective, operative neurolysis is required.

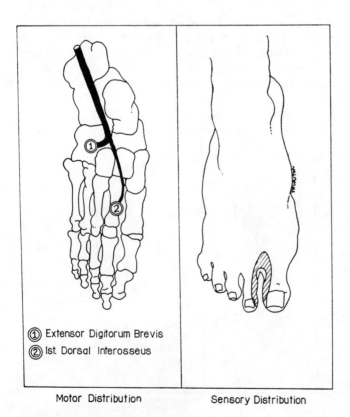

① Extensor Digitorum Brevis
② 1st. Dorsal Interosseus

Motor Distribution   Sensory Distribution

Fig. 4. Termination deep peroneal nerve—foot—motor and sensory distribution.

From Kopell, H.P. and Thompson, W.A.L.: *Peripheral Entrapment Neuropathies.* Baltimore, Williams and Wilkins Company, 1963.

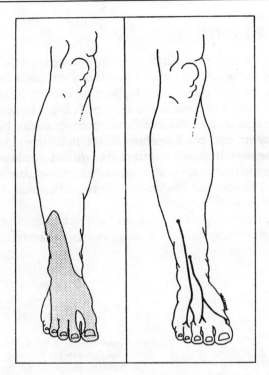

Fig. 5. Termination of superficial peroneal nerve—sensory distribution and fascial emergence.

From Kopell, H.P. and Thompson, W.A.L.: *Peripheral Entrapment Neuropathies.* Baltimore, Williams and Wilkins Company, 1963.

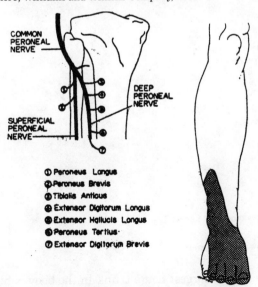

Fig. 6. Common peroneal nerve—motor and sensory distribution.

SAPHENOUS NERVE ENTRAPMENT

The saphenous nerve is one of the three sensory branches of the femoral nerve. The nerve has a long course and penetrates the fascia above the medial aspect of the knee. According to Dawson, Hallett & Millender (1983), the entrapment may occur as the nerve exits from Hunter's canal.

Pain is experienced in the medial calf and can be simulated by Tinel's sign at the area of entrapment. The etiologic factors for this entrapment are injuries of the medial knee structures, e.g., medial meniscus, cartilage and ligamentous structures, and operative trauma from vascular and knee surgery. Koppel and Thompson note the entrapment in adults over 40 with thigh obesity and genu varum.

Treatment regime consists of rest, physio-therapy, and anti-inflammatory drugs. If these conservative methods are not successful, surgical intervention is necessary.

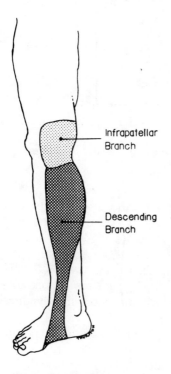

From Kopell, H.P. and Thompson, W.A.L.: *Peripheral Entrapment Neuropathies.* Baltimore, Williams and Wilkins Company, 1963.

Infrapatellar Branch

Descending Branch

Fig. 7. Distribution of the saphenous nerve.

SCIATIC NERVE ENTRAPMENT

The sciatic nerve being the largest nerve trunk in the body is highly vulnerable to entrapment. It originates from the lumbo-sacral plexus, lumbar 4 to sacral 3. The entrapment occurs as the sciatic nerve crosses the sciatic notch, leaving the pelvis.

The patient has marked pain with hip motion. It is often mistaken for a herniated disc.

The etiologic factors include direct injury to the area. The injury could be invasive, e.g., shrapnel or from a low gluteal intramuscular injection. It may be caused by a fall, low back derangement, or prolonged regional pressure.

Treatment consists of support to the area and anti-inflammatory medication, both local and systemic. Operative neurolysis is necessary if conservative measures fail.

OBTURATOR NERVE ENTRAPMENT

The entrapment of the obturator nerve occurs as it passes through the obturator canal. The nerve originates in the lumbar plexus, roots of lumbar 2, 3 and 4. It divides into anterior and posterior branches at the obturator canal.

The patient complains of pain radiating from the groin distally involving the medial aspect of the thigh.

The etiologic factors are compression from a fractured pelvis, obturator hernia, inflammatory processes, forceps delivery or fetal head pressure during labor, and complications from genito-urinary surgery.

The treatment regime consists of rest and anti-inflammatory medication. Surgical intervention is necessary if these methods fail.

LATERAL FEMORAL CUTANEOUS NERVE ENTRAPMENT

This nerve is formed from the branches of the lumbar 2 and 3 nerves. The entrapment occurs as the nerve passes at the lateral end of the inguinal ligament. It is the opening formed by the attachment of the inguinal ligament of the anterior superior iliac spine. The entrapment is also known as meralgia paresthetica. The patient has a burning pain at the antero-lateral aspect of the thigh. This sensation is exacerbated with the wearing of clothes and stockings. Etiologic factors include direct trauma to the area, fracture of the anterior ilium, short limb syndrome, and pelvic tilt.

Treatment program consists of conservatively changing the postural position, support, and anti-inflammatory medication. Surgical intervention is necessary if the conservative measures are not successful.

ILIO INGUINAL NERVE ENTRAPMENT

The nerve entrapment is located medial to the antero-iliac spine of the pelvis. It causes a burning pain in the lower abdomen that radiates distally to the medial aspect of the thigh. The pain also radiates into the scrotum and labia majora.

From Kopell, H.P. and Thompson, W.A.L.: *Peripheral Entrapment Neuropathies.*
Baltimore, Williams and Wilkins Company, 1963.

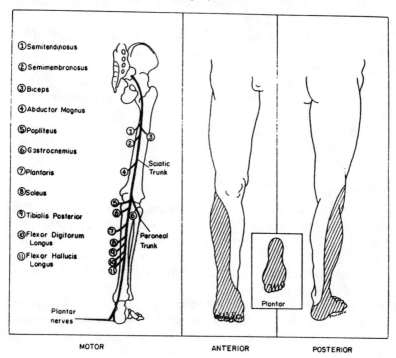

Fig. 8. Sciatic nerve—motor and sensory distribution.

The etiologic factors include direct trauma and a low incision for a hernia repair or appendectomy. Koppel and Thompson (1963) state that changes in the shape of the femoral head could cause problems that affect hip rotation and induce this entrapment. Other theories mentioned include compensatory tightening of the abdominal muscles, limited hip extension, and downward pelvic angulation.

Treatment regime includes support, anti-inflammatory drugs, and neurolysis.

CAUSALGIA

Causalgia is a term first introduced by Weir Mitchell in 1872 during the time of the American Civil War. Soldiers experienced severe burning pain in the area of an injured nerve and beyond. The pain was exacerbated by external and psychologic stimuli. Investigators classify causalgia as major or true causalgia and minor causalgia depending on the severity of pain. Major causalgia is found most commonly in war injuries, e.g., shrapnel wounds, while minor causalgia is more common in lesser domestic wounds (Seddon, 1972).

From Kopell, H.P. and Thompson, W.A.L.: *Peripheral Entrapment Neuropathies.*
Baltimore, Williams and Wilkins Company, 1963.

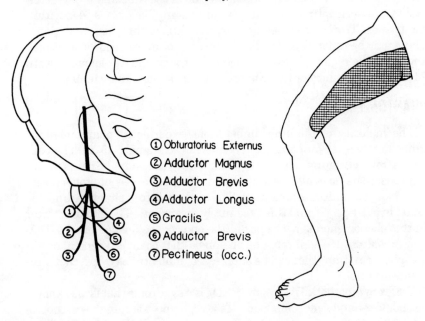

① Obturatorius Externus
② Adductor Magnus
③ Adductor Brevis
④ Adductor Longus
⑤ Gracilis
⑥ Adductor Brevis
⑦ Pectineus (occ.)

Fig. 9. Obturator nerve—motor and sensory distribution.

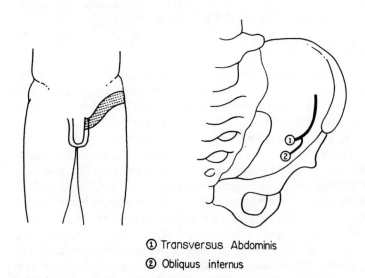

① Transversus Abdominis
② Obliquus internus

Fig. 10. Ilioinguinal nerve— motor and sensory distribution. In this diagram the placement of the lateral portion of the sensory zone is somewhat lower than in the usual case.
From Kopell, H.P. and Thompson, W.A.L.: *Peripheral Entrapment Neuropathies.*
Baltimore, Williams and Wilkins Company, 1963.

Major causalgia affects the distal portion of the limb and is characterized by an excruciating, constant, burning pain. The pain is deep within the tissues. Trophic changes appear; the skin is thin, red, and glossy. There may be reflex sweating and hyperkeratotic cutaneous lesions may appear in the region of nerve distribution. Causalgia can appear within 24 hours after injury or remain latent, up to 45 days, after injury.

PHANTOM LIMB

The majority of all limb amputations experience "phantom limb" immediately after amputation (Thomas & Cavanaugh, 1975). The pain varies from a tingling sensation to lancinating or cramplike pains. Burning sensations have also been recorded. Most of these symptoms disappear two years after amputation. The more painful "phantom limb" is found in older people and this type rarely disappears. The etiologic factor in this phenomenon is neuromas at the ends of the divided nerves (Bradley & Walton, 1974). It must be presumed that there is a central origin for "phantom limb" that can be suppressed, many times by psychotherapeutic agents.

Reflex Sympathetic Dystrophy (RSD), is a syndrome that is also known as shoulder-hand syndrome, Sudeck's atrophy, post-traumatic osteoporosis, traumatic vasospasm, and acute bone atrophy. RSD affects the limbs and causalgia is included in this syndrome. In these cases there exists trophic and vasomotor changes, hyperhidrosis with osteoporosis. There may or may not be predisposing factors with RSD, carcinoma, myocardial infarction, and bursitis (Berkow & Fletcher, 1987).

ISCHEMIC NEUROPATHY

It has long been recognized that vascular insufficiency and peripheral neuropathy have a definitive relationship. The neuropathy associated with large artery disease is classified as acute or chronic. Acute ischemia involves the obstruction of major arteries, aorta, and major limb arteries. This can be caused by an embolus, thrombus, laceration, or compression. The chronic ischemic disorders are caused by insidious vascular disease, severe atherosclerosis, and thromboangiitis obliterans. The resulting neuropathy is referred to as "ischemic neuritis" (Daube & Dyck, 1975).

Arterial occlusion caused by embolism and thrombosis includes pain in its classic symptomatology. The pain involved has been described as being an aching type of pain to a severe, sharp pain. The major arterial occlusions caused by trauma are commonly seen in war casualties. The younger patients usually develop good collateral circulation and neuropathic pain lasts for a short period of time. In older patients and more severe injuries, this is not the case. These patients develop persistent, burning pain after the acute painful onset.

Volkmann's ischemic contracture is a post-traumatic contracture of the muscles of the arm and hand caused by ischemic damage to the muscle. A similar condition has been described in the lower extremity that usually involves the flexor hallicus longus muscle. The condition involves the peroneal and tibial nerves. The pain caused by this condition is excruciating. A similar condition to this affects the anterior tibial muscle and is known as the anterior tibial syndrome. Vascular occlusion could be caused by pressure within the anterior compartment with resultant vascular occlusion or by an occlusion caused by an embolus or thrombus of the anterior tibial artery. It is thought that anterior tibial syndrome is a result of excessive walking or running.

Ischemic neuritis can also be caused by drug injection and the inadvertent injection into the artery causing a thrombosis of the vessel with a resultant ischemia of the nerve and neuritis. It is more common in the upper extremity. Tourniquet paralysis is frequently accompanied by nerve damage. The pneumatic tourniquet has eliminated many of the problems previously seen. The condition still exists because of poor tourniquet technique. The nerve damage and resultant ischemic neuritis are caused by nerve compression.

Other occlusive arterial neuropathies are found in barbiturate and carbon dioxide poisoning, frostbite, renal dialysis ultrainfiltration, decompression sickness, and coma.

The pain caused by ischemic neuritis in peripheral vascular disease varies from a diffuse, tingling, burning pain to sharp, lightning pains (Daube & Dyke, 1975). These neuropathies are not uncommon with others and there is no direct evidence linking arteriosclerosis obliterans to nerve fiber damage.

An ischemic neuritis is found in patients suffering with thromboangiitis obliterans, also known as Buerger's disease. The disease is characterized by a phlebitis and periarteritis that causes severe vascular changes, many times resulting in gangrene and amputation. Episodes of ischemic neuritis pain accompany this disease.

FABRY'S DISEASE

This inherited metabolic disorder is found in boys and young men. The major symptom is severe burning and intense pain sensations in the feet and lower legs. Ambulation is often impossible. Dermatologic manifestations, reddish purple dermatitis of the upper thigh, lower abdomen, subungual, oral mucosa, and conjunctiva angiectases, may appear. Patients with this disease develop hypertension, cerebral vascular disease, renal dysfunction, and cardiomegaly. The life span is 40 to 50 years (Brady & King, 1975).

DIABETIC NEUROPATHY

Generally speaking, diabetic neuropathy is rarely found in juvenile diabetics and its incidence increases with age (Brenner, 1987). Brenner states that after 25 years of diabetes, 50 per cent of the patients displayed some evidence of neuropathy and an average of 19 per cent of the remaining patients developed it each year (Scarlet & Blais, 1989). Neuropathic pain can be lancinating, burning, aching, dull, crushing, or cramp-like. Patients in my practice with severe neuropathic pain will avoid any contact with their feet. The pain is relieved with ambulation (Bradley & Walton, 1974). Patients complain that they are walking on red-hot coals while others feel that they are walking on balls of cotton. There is a correlation between diabetic neuropathy and control of the disease: neuropathy improves with control (Thomas & Eliasson, 1975). Distal symmetrical sensory polyneuropathy is the most common neuropathy found in diabetes mellitus. It is caused by a dysfunction of the small fibers.

UREMIC NEUROPATHY

The extent and reporting of cases of renal neuropathy has increased since the early 1960s with the advent of hemodialysis and renal transplantation for the treatment of chronic renal failure. The incidence is greater in males and there is a correlation with the length and severity of the renal disease. Clinicians are investigating an increase in neuropathy with hemodialysis. A majority of the patients complain of muscle cramps and restless legs syndrome. The early symptoms described are distal dyesthesias and painful, raw, and tingling sensations in the toes. Overall burning sensations in the soles of the feet are not uncommon (Asbury, 1975).

HEPATIC NEUROPATHY

In itself, the neuropathy that is associated with liver disease may be a symptom of disorders that involve both the liver and nerve tissue. Examples of this include infectious mononucleosis, celiac disease, periarteritis nodosa, and acute arsenic poisoning. Neuropathic pain is rarely present and then only in cases of biliary cirrhosis (Asbury, 1975).

NEUROPATHY ASSOCIATED WITH THYROID DISEASE

Neuropathic extremity pain is present in patients suffering with hypothyroidism. This symptom disappears with thyroid hormonal therapy. Patients with hypothyroidism, myxedema, and thyrotoxicosis suffer with painful muscle cramps. It is less frequent in hyperthyroidism and is almost always eliminated with the treatment of the endocrine disease. Neuropathic pain has also been observed in patients with acromegaly. It is felt that bone and cartilage proliferation causes the compression of the nerves. There is evidence of this in the upper extremity development of carpal tunnel syndrome. A direct relationship exists between the severity of neuropathic pain and the size of the pituitary tumor; with the reduction of the tumor the pain decreases. Some investigators have found a defect in the metabolism of the peripheral nerves (Bastron, 1975).

AMYLOID NEUROPATHY

Amyloidosis is the extra-cellular deposition of the fibrous protein amyloid in one or more sites of the body (Cohen & Benson, 1975). Invasion of the substance causes severe pathophysiologic changes in the organ systems affected. The classification of amyloid neuropathies falls under two major headings: nonhereditary amyloidosis and hereditary amyloidosis. The clinical course of the disease depends on the organ system(s) involved. Infiltration into the renal system is the most serious and has the highest mortality rate. Involvement of the lower extremities is seen in hereditary amyloid neuropathies, Portuguese, Japanese, Swedish, Greek, and American types. Patients display both sensory and motor problems in the legs. Early symptoms are paresthesias, numbness, burning sensations, and lancinating pain into the lower limbs. In Portugal, the disease at first was called "mal dos pesinhos" (foot disease). Further investigation disclosed the other manifestations of the disease. Amyloid involvement of the other body systems causes interference with a gastrointestinal mobility, impotence, cardiac ischemia, kidney dysfunction, and optic involvement.

HEREDITARY SENSORY NEUROPATHY (HSN)

This disorder is inherited and affects the peripheral sensory neurons. The classic symptom is plantar ulceration of the foot. These lesions drain with a purulent exudate and can be present for years. Although these lesions may be painless, the accompanying infections, cellulitis, lymphangitis, and osteomyelitis are not. Lancinating pains in the leg and foot are common with this disease. Other characteristics of the disease are peroneal muscle atrophy and pes cavus type feet. In some cases, there is distinct sensory loss. With proper management, those afflicted with HSN can live normal life spans. HSN II is seen in young children and has the same symptomatology as HSN. The children develop stress fractures and there is involvement of the distal ends of the toes, and ulcerations. The distal phalanges appear broad, short, and deformed. It is felt that the onset of the disease is at birth (Dyck & Ohta, 1975).

FRIEDREICH'S ATAXIA

This disease was first described in 1863. At approximately the time of puberty, there is a weakness in the lower extremities, unsteady gait, and imbalance. As the patient gets older, there is upper limb involvement with speech difficulties. Patients describe stabbing and cutting pains in the legs and the characteristics of "restless legs." The patient's life span is 30 to 40 years.

HEREDITARY MOTOR AND SENSORY NEUROPATHY

Dyck (1975) classifies these inherited, progressive, symmetrical, and non-focal group of disorders as HMSN, hereditary motor and sensory neuropathy. A number of diseases are in this category: progressive muscle atrophy, peroneal form of progressive muscular atrophy, progressive neural muscular atrophy, and hypertrophic neuropathy, Roussy and Levy Syndrome, spastic paraplegia with peroneal muscular atrophy, hereditary sensory neuropathy, spinocerebellar degeneration, etc. For the most part, these diseases exhibit sensory symptoms. Some patients with the peroneal form of progressive muscle atrophy have severe lancinating pains. The same holds true in patients with Charcot-Marie-Tooth type of hypertrophic neuropathy, termed HMSN Type I by Dyck and Lambert. They suffer with lancinating pains and burning, pricking sensations. This disease is characterized by atrophy of the foot and leg muscles. Patients develop pes cavus and hammer toes with painful tylomata and corns on the plantar aspect of the metatarsal-phalangeal articulations and at the dorsum of the toes.

AMYOTROPHIC LATERAL SCLEROSIS

ALS is a motor neuron disease of unknown etiology (Mulder, 1975). Mulder prefers to use the term "motor neuron disease" rather than "amyotrophic lateral sclerosis." There is a progressive wasting degeneration of the musculature and degeneration of the corticospinal tracts and anterior horn cells. The symptoms of the disease usually occur first in the lower extremities. There is a cramping of the musculature that may precede the atrophic weakness of the muscle (Berkow & Fletcher, 1987). This disease is found in males over the age of 40 and it is usually terminal in two to five years after the onset. There is a five year survival rate in 20 per cent of the patients.

MULTIPLE MYELOMA

Symmetrical neuropathic pain occurs early in cases of this malignant disease. It is sometimes evident in the upper extremity. There is a proliferation of plasma cells that invade and replace bone marrow and other tissue. Patients develop anemia, renal failure, infection, and compression of the spinal cord and roots. Death usually ensues in 18 months from time of diagnosis (McLeod & Walsh, 1975).

MACROGLOBULINEMIA

This condition is characterized by an increase of macroglobulin in the blood. It is found in the elderly and characterized by weight loss, fatigue, mucosal bleeding, and anemia. There is a generalized wasting away of the musculature. Patients experience paraesthesias, pain, and muscle cramping.

CRYOGLOBULINEMIA

The symptoms of this disorder are similar to those of Raynaud's phenomenon: sensitivity to cold, color changes, bleeding, malaise, arthralgia, and in severe cases, gangrene. The upper extremities are more commonly affected. Neuropathic pain in the lower extremity is usually asymmetrical paresthesias, tingling toes, and muscle pain. As in Raynaud's, the disorder is more severe in cold weather. The etiologic factor is the presence in the serum of the protein, cryoglobulin.

NEUROPATHIC BERIBERI

For the most part, beriberi is characterized by a sensory loss. There are, however, instances where pain is prominent and intense. The neuropathy is caused by dietary deficiency of Vitamin B-1 and thiamine. It is characterized by a paralysis of the feet and hands. The disease affects both the heart and peripheral nerves. Depending on the presence of edema, it is classified as "wet" or "dry" beriberi (Victor, 1975).

PELLAGRA

The etiology of this disease is a severe niacin deficiency. Pellagra has cutaneous, gastro-intestinal, central nervous system, mucosal, and neuropathic manifestations. There is early pain and tenderness in the feet and calves of the legs. A characteristic "glove and stocking" loss of vibratory and superficial sensation is present.

STRACHAN'S SYNDROME; SYNDROME OF AMBLYOPIA, PAINFUL NEUROPATHY AND OROGENITAL DERMATITIS

This nutritional disorder was first described by Dr. H. Strachan in Jamaica in the late 1800s. Patients complain of severe burning in the palms and soles. Other symptoms include dimness of vision, atrophy of the hand and foot musculature, gastro-intestinal problems, and progressive sensory loss. During World War II the syndrome was identified in

Japanese prisoner of war camps. Although it has not been proven, many investigators feel that a riboflavin deficiency causes Strachan's Syndrome.

ALCOHOLIC NEUROPATHY

The etiologic factors in this neuropathy are the abuse of alcohol and dietary deficiency. Neuropathic pain has been described as being a dull, constant ache or intermittent, sharp, lancinating pain in the feet and/or legs. The more common complaint is that of severe burning in the feet. Other clinical characteristics that may be present are anemia, motor and sensory loss, excessive perspiration of the soles, dryness and pigmentation of the skin, rhinophyma, and muscle atrophy.

BURNING FEET SYNDROME

This condition was commonly described by incarcerated American, British, and Canadian soldiers in Japanese prisoner of war camps during the Second World War. The symptoms include an early, chronic pain over the metatarsal-phalangeal articulations that later extends as lancinating, sharp pains into the legs. These pains are more severe at night. It is felt that the syndrome is caused by a vitamin deficiency but the specific vitamin(s) have not been identified. It is thought to be caused by a Vitamin B deficiency (Victor, 1975).

RHEUMATOID NEUROPATHY

There is a high frequency of neuropathic involvement of the lower extremities in patients with long-standing rheumatoid arthritis. It is difficult to distinguish the neuropathic pain from the joint pain usually experienced by the rheumatoid arthritic. Rheumatoid neuropathy is usually mild and symmetrical with symptoms of tingling and numbness. Less commonly found is mononeuritis multiplex that causes severe and sudden pain radiating into the course of the involved peripheral nerve. Conn and Dyck (1975) list the following clinical features of rheumatoid arthritis associated with neuropathy: long standing rheumatoid arthritis, rheumatoid nodules, skin vasculitis, change in clinical status, rapid decrease in corticosteroids, high titer of rheumatoid factor, and diminished serum complement.

ARSENIC NEUROPATHY

For the most part, mild neuropathies associated with arsenic ingestion and/or exposure are painless. The patient may have paresthesia or anesthesia and muscle weakness. Severe neuropathy symptoms include intense pain or painful paresthesias of the feet. Other symptoms include a brownish discoloration of the skin, hyperkeratoses of the soles of the feet, edema of the feet, and brittle nails with a distinguishable transverse white striae and Mee's lines. The acute stage of arsenical intoxication involves gastro-intestinal, renal, and respiratory symptoms (Goldstein, McCall, & Dyck, 1975).

LEAD NEUROPATHY

Sensory symptoms are rarely found in lead intoxication. Lower extremity symptoms are more common in children than adults. The patient may have painful joints and muscles rather than nerve tenderness. Weakness and footdrop is common with this problem.

MERCURY NEUROPATHY

This problem is rare. Patients will complain of edematous, aching joints, weakness of the extremities, paresthesias, and sensory disturbances in the legs and feet.

CARCINOMATOUS NEUROPATHY

The incidence of peripheral neuropathy in cancer patients is thought to be more common than previously stated. According to McLeod (1975), the dominant symptoms are numbness and paresthesias of the extremities and sensory ataxia. Burning and aching pains may also be present.

SUMMARY

There are virtually hundreds of causes of peripheral nerve disease including trauma, metabolic diseases, vascular insufficiency, hereditary diseases, motor neuron diseases, nutritional deficiencies, and toxins. A symptom complex associated with peripheral nerve disease is peripheral neuropathy. Most of the sensory abnormalities are negative phenomena usually characterized by a loss of sensation. The positive phenomena are pain that varies from "pins and needles" and burning sensations to sharp and severe pain. Clinical evaluation with appropriate tests are essential to determine the treatment regime for the pain associated with the peripheral nerve disease.

REFERENCES

Addante, J., Peicott, P., Wong, K., & Brooks, D. (1986). Interdigital Neuromas. *JAPA, Vol. 76,* No. 9. (pp. 493-495).

Altman, M., & Hinkes, M. (1982). Heel Neuroma. *JAPA, Vol. 72,* No. 3. (pp. 517-519).

Asbury, A. (1975). *Hepatic neuropathy.* (pp. 993-997). In *Peripheral neuropathy.* Philadelphia: W.B. Saunders Company.

Asbury, A. (1975). *Uremic neuropathy.* (pp. 982-985). *In Peripheral neuropathy.* Philadelphia: W.B. Saunders Company.

Bannister, R. (1973). *Brian's clinical neurology.* London: Oxford University Press.

Bastron, J. (1975). *Neuropathy in diseases of the thyroid.* (pp. 999-1009). In *Peripheral neuropathy.* Philadelphia: W.B. Saunders Company.

Beito, S., Krych, S., & Harkless, L. (1989). Recalcitrant heel pain. *JAPA. Vol. 79,* No. 7. (pp. 336-339).

Berkow, R., & Fletcher, A. (1987). *Merck manual.* Merck, Sharp and Dohme.

Bradley, W., & Walton, J. (1974). *Disorders of peripheral nerves.* Oxford: Blackwell Scientific Publications.

Brady, R., & King, F. (1975). *Fabry's disease.* (pp. 914-915). In *Peripheral neuropathy.* Philadelphia: W.B. Saunders Company.

Brewer, M. (1987). *Management of the diabetic foot.* Baltimore: Williams and Wilkins.

Burns, A., & Stewart, W. (1982). Morton's neuroma. *JAPA, Vol. 72,* No. 3. (pp. 135-141).

Carlton, F. (1952). *Lectures.* Temple University, School of Podiatry.

Cohen, A., & Benson, M. (1975). *Amyloid neuropathy.* (pp. 1067-1091). In *Peripheral neuropathy.* Philadelphia: W.B. Saunders Company.

Conn, D., & Dyck, P. (1975). *Angiopathic neuropathy in connective tissue diseases.* (pp. 1149-1165). In Peripheral neuropathy. Philadelphia: W.B. Saunders Company.

Daube, J., & Dyck, P. (1985). *Neuropathy due to peripheral vascular diseases.* (pp. 714-729). In *Peripheral neuropathy.* Philadelphia: W.B. Saunders Company.

Dawson, D., Hallett, M., & Millender, L. (1983). *Entrapment neuropathies.* Boston: Little, Brown and Company.

Dowling, G., & Skaggs, R. (1982). Neurilemoma (Schwannoma) as a Cause of Tarsal Tunnel Syndrome. *JAPA, Vol. 72,* No. 1. (pp. 45-48).

Dyck, P. (1975). *Inherited neuronal degeneration and atrophy affecting peripheral motor, Sensory and automic neurons.* (pp. 825-867). In *Peripheral neuropathy.* Philadelphia: W.B. Saunders Company.

Dyck, P., & Ohta, M. (1975). *Neuronal atrophy and degeneration predominantly affecting peripheral sensory neuron.* (pp. 791-824). In *Peripheral neuropathy.* Philadelphia: W. B. Saunders Company.

Dyck, P., Thomas, P., Lambert, E., & Bunge, R. (1975). *Peripheral neuropathy.* Philadelphia: W.B. Saunders Company.

Gaynor, R., Hake, D., Spinner, S., & Tomczal, R. (1989). Comparative analysis of conservative versus surgical treatment of morton's neuroma. *JAPA. Vol. 79,* No. 1. (pp. 27-30).

Goldstein, N., McCall, J., & Dyck, P. (1975). *Metal neuropathy.* (pp. 1227-1262). In *Peripheral neuropathy.* Philadelphia: W.B. Saunders Company.

Goodman, C., & Kehr, L. (1983). Bilateral tarsal tunnel syndrome. *JAPA. Vol. 73*, No. 5. (pp. 256-259).

Goodman, C., & Kehr, L. (1988). Bilateral tarsal tunnel syndrome. *JAPA. Vol. 78,* No. 6. (pp. 292-294).

Haymaker, W., & Woodhall, B. (1953). *Peripheral nerve injuries.* Philadelphia: W.B. Saunders Company.

Kopell, H., & Thompson, W. (1963). *Peripheral entrapment neuropathies.* (pp. 14-76). Baltimore: Williams and Wilkins.

Lee, B., & Crowhurst, J. (1987). *Entrapment neuropathy of the first metatarsophalangeal joint. Vol. 77,* No. 12. (pp. 657-659).

Mathers, L. (1985). *The peripheral nervous system.* Menlo Park: Addison-Wesley Publishing Company.

McGlamry, E. (1974). *Reconstructive surgery of the foot and leg.* New York: Intercontinental Medical Book Corp.

McLeod, J. (1975). *Carcinomatous neuropathy.* (pp. 1301-1313). In *Peripheral neuropathy.* Philadelphia: W.B. Saunders Company.

McLeod, J., & Walsh, J. (1975). *Neuropathies associated with paraproteinemias and dysproteinemias.* (pp. 1012-1029). In *Peripheral neuropathy.* Philadelphia: W. B. Saunders Company.

Miller, H., Abadesco, L., & Heaney, J. (1983). Morton's neuroma symptoms from a rheumatoid nodule. *JAPA. Vol. 73,* No. 6. (pp. 311-312).

Mulder, D. (1975). *Motor neuron disease.* (pp. 759-770). In *Peripheral neuropathy.* Philadelphia: W.B. Saunders Company.

Pace, J., & Spinoa, F. (1989). Benign schwannoma of the foot. *JAPA. Vol. 79,* No. 6. (pp. 293-294).

Rakow, R. (1979). *Podiatric management of the diabetic foot.* Mount Kisko: Futura Publishing Company.

Roth, R., & Harford, G. (1980). Peripheral nerve and dermatomal sensory innervation of the lower extremities. *JAPA. Vol. 70,* No. 5. (pp. 215-223).

Scarlet, J., & Blais, M. (1989). Statistics on the diabetic foot. *JAPA. Vol. 79,* No. 6. (pp. 306-307).

Seddon, H. (1972). *Surgical disorders of the peripheral nerves.* Edinburgh: Churchill Livingstone.

Sidlow, C., Frankel, S., Chioros, P., & Hamilton, V. (1989). Electroacupuncture therapy for stump neuroma pain. *JAPA, Vol. 79,* No. 1. (pp. 31-33).

Silverman, I. (1987). Three neuromas of one foot. *JAPA, Vol. 77,* No. 7. (pp. 353-354).

Stewart, J. (1987). *Focal peripheral neuropathies.* New York: Elsevier.

Thomas, P., & Cavanaugh, J. (1975). *Neuropathy due to physical agents.* (p. 739). In *Peripheral neuropathy.* Philadelphia: W.B. Saunders Company.

Thomas, P., & Eliasson, S. (1975). *Diabetic neuropathy.* (pp. 956-981). In *Peripheral neuropathy;* Philadelphia: W.B. Saunders Company.

Tisa, V., & Pauli, C. (1980). Neurilemoma of a digit. *JAPA, Vol. 70,* No. 10. (pp. 524-526).

Victor, M. (1975). *Polyneuropathy due to nutritional deficiency and alcoholism.* (pp. 1030-1066). In *Peripheral neuropathy.* Philadelphia: W.B. Saunders Company.

Yale, I. (1974). *Podiatric medicine.* Baltimore: Williams and Wilkins Company.

Yater, W., & Oliver, W. (1954). *Fundamentals of internal medicine.* New York: Appleton, Century, Crofts Inc.

Chapter 18

THE TREATMENT OF PAIN IN THE GERIATRIC AGE GROUP

Joseph A. Kwentus, M. D.

Dr. Kwentus reports that although pain may be a normal part of the aging process, the complaints of pain are not necessarily more common within the normal elderly population. Successful pain management for older patients is dependent upon obtaining a clear understanding of any underlying pathology, knowledge of the aging process, and a cross-cultural awareness of both perception and patient report of pain. The clinician must be aware of social factors, potential of depression, and sensitive to treatment tailored to an elderly patient, i.e., careful pharmacologic monitoring.

Chapter 18

THE TREATMENT OF PAIN IN THE GERIATRIC AGE GROUP

Joseph A. Kwentus, M. D.

Despite evidence to the contrary, the fallacy persists that pain is one of the expected consequences of normal aging. Although older people are more prone to painful illnesses such as trigeminal neuralgia, peripheral neuropathy, arthritis, and a variety of degenerative diseases, there is no evidence that pain complaints are necessarily more common in normal elderly. As a result of the fallacy that older people utter pain complaints more frequently than others, significant medical and surgical pathology including life threatening illnesses such as appendicitis may be overlooked. The key to geriatric pain management is an understanding of the pathology of the underlying etiologic disease event coupled with an understanding of age-related changes in how pain presents and how the older patient perceives and tolerates it. Secondly, there are dramatic changes in the pharmacokinetics of all classes of analgesic medications in the elderly because of alterations in the aging liver and kidney. In addition, pharmacodynamics are also markedly altered and serum levels of a variety of drugs may be well tolerated in younger patients but will result in delirium in the elderly. The social context in which the pain situation is occurring must also be considered. Secondary gain from painful problems and chronic pain may be related to the unique social situation of the elderly and, for some, the expression of pain complaints may represent an attempt to deal with loneliness, or with a fear of physical deterioration or the closeness of death. Pain complaints in the elderly may be exacerbated by coexisting depression. Finally, special problems that the elderly patient may have with communication or confusion may further complicate the evaluation of painful syndromes.

PAIN PHYSIOLOGY IN THE ELDERLY

Although geriatric illness is typically multi-system and chronic, there are surprisingly few studies on the special manifestations of pain in the elderly. Studies of age and thermal pain threshold using the projection lamp technique, which exposes subjects to radiant heat, reveals that the pain threshold of elderly patients may actually be increased by 12-20% when compared to younger people. This experiment is not able to determine whether the differences are due to changes in the mechanisms of pain perception or in the thermal properties of the skin of elderly people because the skin of the elderly has increased thermal dispersion. Several studies using electrical stimulation of teeth suggest that differences in pain sensitivity between younger and older people are of small magnitude. Actually attitude, judgment, and other cognitive factors may be more important than physiologic changes and are difficult to differentiate. In general, older people show slow reaction time and seem unwilling to respond to painful stimuli. The fact that no age differences in density or morphology of nociceptor endings have been found supports the view the basic processes of nociception are influenced only minimally by age.

ANALGESIC MANAGEMENT IN THE ELDERLY

In order to understand the management of analgesics in the elderly it is necessary to consider each class of analgesic medication used in older people separately. Alteration of receptors, changes in plasma protein binding, and prolonged clearance render the elderly patient more sensitive to both the analgesic effect and the side effects of narcotics. The narcotics must therefore be used in smaller doses in elderly patients. The response of elderly patients to morphine, for example, is fourfold that of young adults. Narcotic side effects, such as respiratory depression, cough suppression, and clouding of mental functions are more likely in older patients and occur at lower doses. Careful attention to diet and a prophylactic bowel regimen are essential to avoid constipation. Constipation may be serious in elderly patients taking narcotics and may result in mental status changes.

Mental status should be closely monitored because changes may reflect opiate intoxication. Again using morphine as a prototype, clearance of the drug from plasma is only one-half that of younger patients; this may lead to substantial accumulation. In patients with renal disease, meperidine may accumulate and cause symptoms ranging from alteration of mood to serious neurologic impairment. Because of their excessively long half-life, drugs such as methadone easily accumulate in the elderly and are best reserved for chronic pain in the terminally ill. Partial agonist, such as pentazocine are limited in higher dosage ranges by psychomimetic properties and may precipitate narcotic withdrawal if introduced to a patient receiving chronic opiates.

Since morphine is the standard for analgesic studies, dosages of other narcotics can be determined on the basis of morphine equivalents. In patients with mild to moderate pain, oral drugs such as codeine or oxycodone are preferred. For severe pain, parenterally administered drugs are more effective. Narcotic analgesia should be carefully adjusted by gradually increasing the dose until the patient obtains maximum relief for at least four hours. The dose should be given before pain recurs to avoid anticipatory anxiety and behavioral reinforcement of drug use. The total dose of any narcotic can be reduced by the concomitant use of nonsteroidal anti-inflammatory drugs (NSAIDs), hydroxyzine, or less commonly, amitriptyline.

Non-narcotic analgesics, such as nonsteroidal anti-inflammatory-drugs may also present special problems in the elderly. The safety margin between therapeutic and toxic levels is narrower in the elderly. Elderly patients may have reduced albumin levels. NSAIDs are bound to albumin and thus equivalent doses may produce higher serum levels in the elderly. NSAIDs may also displace other drugs from protein-binding sites prducing unexpected and undesirable effects. NSAIDs may cause upper GI side effects and may precipitate GI bleeding. Bleeding time is increased and may alter anti-coagulant treatment. There is also salt and water retention which may interfere with antihypertensive therapy. All NSAIDs may have CNS effects to which the elderly may be more prone. Some, such as indomethacin, are more likely to cause depression and confusion.

Benzodiazepines are best avoided in the treatment of pain syndromes unless there is evidence of musculoskeletal pain with spasm. Benzodiazepines have increased half-life in the elderly and may produce sedation, drowsiness, and decreased cognitive performance. If longer half-life drugs are used these effects can persist for some time after drugs are withdrawn. Lorazepam and Oxazepam have shorter half-lives and are more easily metabolized in elderly people.

Antidepressants are often used as adjuncts for pain management in the elderly. Drugs such as amitriptyline have independent analgesic action which is useful in nondepressed patients. In the elderly, low doses should be used to avoid side effects. Serum levels may be monitored to prevent overdosing. Potentially serious adverse reactions which may be encountered include severe constipation, postural hypotension, urinary retention and anti-cholinergic delirium. Postural hypotension is particularly worrisome because of the possibility of a fall with subsequent broken hip.

Other drugs used in the management of pain in the elderly include phenothiazines, anticonvulsants, and corticosteroids. Phenothiazine are useful for denervation pain, and thalamic pain, and are often used concomitantly with antidepressants in the treatment of herpetic neuralgia.

Tardive dyskinesia is a special risk in the elderly patient. Anticonvulsants such as carbamazepine may be effective for trigeminal neuralgia or for denervation neuropathy. Nausea and sedation can limit compliance. Bone marrow depression and other adverse effects may limit use. Corticosteriods are used,as needed, for medical indications and should be avoided for symptomatic treatment because of the potential for osteoporosis, hypothalamic-pituitary suppression, decreased resistance to infection, and risk of diabetes mellitus.

PSYCHOSOCIAL CONSIDERATIONS OF PAIN IN THE ELDERLY

Stress, depression, decreased resources, limited cognitive resourcefulness, and physical illness may lead to an intensification of the discomfort and suffering associated with pain. Evidence that pain-related psychosomatic complaints are more frequent in the elderly further complicates the issue. The older pain patient is not only at risk for reduced psychologic adaptability and increased comorbidity, but is also at considerable risk for loss of family and friends as well as losses of social and economic resources. The expression of pain may be the focus for obtaining attention. Families and physicians can unwittingly encourage a "sick role" and, in these cases, family therapy can be beneficial.   The probability of pain-related behaviors is higher in the patient who is unable to establish a trusting and secure relationship. It is sometimes difficult to determine whether reports of pain in older people stem from nociceptive processes or the need for security. Complaints may be a form of attachment behavior, i.e., increased questioning, demanding and anger.   Some elderly patients who complain of chronic pain have long-standing personality disorders. As an older person turns inward and withdraws from external concerns, preoccupation with bodily functions may occur. Obsessive-compulsive, dependent and narcissistic traits may be accentuated. Although there may be an organic basis for the pain, the pain behaviors have proven so "useful" that they continue unabated, even after partial or complete resolution of the cause. Although pain complaints may serve to manipulate friends, relatives, and physicians pain should be considered a manifestation of personality disorder only if the personality disorder is well-established throughout life and only if other etiologies are ruled out.

Central processes are very important in the perpetuation of chronic pain syndromes. The naturally occurring amines, norepinephrine, dopamine, and serotonin are important both in the central modulation of pain perception and the etiology of affective disorders. Serotonergic neurons in the periaqueductal gray, nucleus raphe magnus, and nucleus reticularis mangnocellularis exert a negative feedback on pain. Since these biologic amines undergo oxidative deamination to inactive compounds bymonamine oxidase (MAO), and since MAO activity increases after age

45, the availability of neurotransmitter at postsynaptic sites that affect mood and pain perception is reduced in elderly people. The physiologic and pharmacologic interdependence of pain and depression are of great potential clinical importance. Studies have determined that 59% of patients requesting treatment for depression also have recurring benign pain, and conversely, 87% of patients in chronic pain clinics have depression. This interdependence may be enhanced in the elderly, in whom both pain-producing peripheral pathologies and depression are more frequent. Even when the patient denies depression, the hallmarks may be observed. If the depression is autonomous, there may be sleep disturbance, early morning awakening, psychomotor retardation or agitation, and anorexia or weight loss. Pain complaints may be the patient's way of explaining loss of interest, low energy, poor concentration and inappropriate guilt.   Perhaps the major clinical precaution to be maintained in the treatment of elderly pain patients is protection of the elderly patient from drug abuse. Persons over the age of 65 constitute about 12% of the population, but receive over 25% of all prescribed drugs. They are the largest regular users of sedatives and hypnotics. Drugs used in pain treatment must be considered as a possible cause of a reversible chronic brain syndrome. Drug-related problems in older patients include excessive self-medication. Because the older patient often receives treatment from several physicians for different disorders, the patient can become physically dependent to sedatives or narcotics without any one doctor's knowledge. Thus, it is necessary for all treating physicians to perform a systematic review of the "brown bag" of pills that many of the elderly can produce on request.

CONCLUSION

Clinical effectiveness in the treatment of the elderly pain patient is based on an individualized treatment plan based on a thorough knowledge of the patient's history. Important information comes from a thorough psychosocial history and from a good system review. Many personality traits are established in childhood and adolescence, and casual conversation about early life may be very revealing. Most older people relish the opportunity to discuss their past. Reviewing medical illnesses and surgical procedures that patient has experienced allows the physician to get a feeling for how the patient both responds to treatment and relates to helping professionals. A multimode approach is most likely to be helpful. It is interdisciplinary by definition. Consultation from anesthesiology, neurosurgery, rehabilitation, neurology, internal medicine, psychiatry, psychology, social services, and physical or occupational therapy may be required. Nonpharmacologic treatment, such as physical therapy, family therapy, biofeedback, stress management, transcutaneous neurostimulation, and appropriate exercise, is often superior to pain medication or nerve blocks. For some patients there may be a role for in-patient behavior modification in a pain treatment unit. Whenever drug therapy is used, the unique pharmacodynamic and pharmacokinetic characteristics of the elderly must be considered and the possibility of drug-drug interactions debated. Organic mental pathology should be investigated and treated and the possibility of co-existing autonomous depression should be investigated. Pain discomfort and suffering must never be equated with the processes of normal aging, but should be as vigorously treated in the older individual as in the young.

99990005